AF527162

New Frontiers in Plastic and Cosmetic Surgery

New Frontiers in Plastic and Cosmetic Surgery

Editors

Alberto Di Giuseppe MD
Institute of Plastic and Reconstructive Surgery
School of Medicine, University of Ancona
Ancona, Italy

Melvin A Shiffman MD JD
Chair, Section of Surgery
Newport Specialty Hospital
Tustin, California, USA

Foreword
José Guerrerosantos

JAYPEE *The Health Sciences Publisher*
New Delhi | London | Panama | Philadelphia

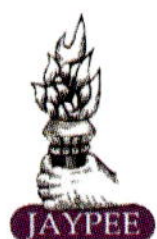

Jaypee Brothers Medical Publishers (P) Ltd

Headquarters
Jaypee Brothers Medical Publishers (P) Ltd.
4838/24, Ansari Road, Daryaganj
New Delhi 110 002, India
Phone: +91-11-43574357
Fax: +91-11-43574314
E-mail: jaypee@jaypeebrothers.com

Overseas Offices

J.P. Medical Ltd.
83, Victoria Street, London
SW1H 0HW (UK)
Phone: +44-20 3170 8910
Fax: +44(0)20 3008 6180
E-mail: info@jpmedpub.com

Jaypee-Highlights Medical Publishers Inc.
City of Knowledge, Bld. 237, Clayton
Panama City, Panama
Phone: +1 507-301-0496
Fax: +1 507-301-0499
E-mail: cservice@jphmedical.com

Jaypee Medical Inc.
The Bourse
111, South Independence Mall East
Suite 835
Philadelphia, PA 19106, USA
Phone: +1 267-519-9789
E-mail: jpmed.us@gmail.com

Jaypee Brothers Medical Publishers (P) Ltd.
17/1-B, Babar Road, Block-B, Shaymali
Mohammadpur, Dhaka-1207
Bangladesh
Mobile: +08801912003485
E-mail: jaypeedhaka@gmail.com

Jaypee Brothers Medical Publishers (P) Ltd.
Bhotahity, Kathmandu, Nepal
Phone: +977-9741283608
E-mail: kathmandu@jaypeebrothers.com

Website: www.jaypeebrothers.com
Website: www.jaypeedigital.com

Inquiries for bulk sales may be solicited at: jaypee@jaypeebrothers.com

New Frontiers in Plastic and Cosmetic Surgery

First Edition: **2015**

ISBN: 978-93-5152-776-3

Printed at: Ajanta Offset & Packagings Ltd., New Delhi

Dedicated to

Irving Rappaport MD DMD *who was my mentor and dear friend. He taught me so much over the years about plastic surgery technqiues, cosmetic surgery techniques, reconstruction techniques, and the future course of medicine and surgery. His death in January 2015 at the age of 90 was a loss to all who knew him including those he trained as residents, the whole Orange County Community and University of California, Irvine.*

Melvin A Shiffman

Contributors

Paolo Balercia MD
Maxillofacial Surgery Department
Ospedali Riuniti Umberto
I-Lancisi-Salesi
Ancona, Italy

Alexander Berghaus MD
Head, Department of
Oto-Rhino-Laryngology
Head and Neck Surgery
Grosshadern Campus
Ludwig-Maximilians-University
Munich, Germany

Giovanni Di Benedetto MD
Department of Plastic and Reconstructive
Surgery, Marche Polytechnic University
Medical School
Ancona, Italy

Manuela Bottoni MD
Department of Plastic and
Reconstructive Surgery
Marche Polytechnic University
Medical School
Ancona, Italy

Carlo Carusi MD
Division of Plastic and
Reconstructive Surgery
Campus Bio-Medico University of Rome
Rome, Italy

Anı Cinpolat MD
Adana Numune Training and
Research Hospital
Department of Plastic, Reconstructive
and Aesthetic Surgery
Adana, Turkey

George Commons MD
Private Practice
1515 El Camino Real, Suite C, Palo Alto
California, USA

O Koray Coskunfirat MD
Professor
Plastic and Reconstructive Surgery
Akdeniz University School of Medicine
Department of Plastic and
Reconstructive Surgery
Dumlupınar Bulvarı
Antalya, Turkey

Salvador Rodríguez-Camps Devís MD
Division Chief of Aesthetic and Plastic
Surgery, University Hospital
"Casa de Salud"
Valencia, Spain

Diane I Duncan MD
Private Practice
Plastic Surgery Associates of Fort Collins
Fort Collins, Colorado, USA

Matteo Gioacchini MD
Department of Plastic and
Reconstructive Surgery
Marche Polytechnic University
Medical School
Ancona, Italy

Riccardo Girotto MD
Maxillofacial Surgery Department
Ospedali Riuniti Umberto
I-Lancisi-Salesi
Ancona, Italy

Alberto Di Giuseppe MD
Institute of Plastic and Reconstructive
Surgery, School of Medicine
University of Ancona
Italy, Ancona

Luca Grassetti MD
Department of Plastic and
Reconstructive Surgery
Marche Polytechnic University
Medical School
Ancona, Italy

José Guerrerosantos MD
Professor of Plastic Surgery
University of Guadalajara
Guadalajara, México

Karens Harkaway MD
Private Practice
8001 Route 130 South
Delran, New Jersey, USA

Aurelia Isac MD
Senior Surgeon Plastic Surgery
University Hospital for Plastic
Surgery and Burns
Calea Grivitei 218
Bucharest, Romania

Cristina Isac MD
Assistant Professor of Plastic Surgery
University of Medicine and Pharmacy
"Carol Davila"
Bucharest, Romania

Florin Isac MD
Professor Plastic Surgery
Senior Surgeon, Plastic Surgery
University Hospital for
Plastic Surgery and Burns
Calea Grivitei 218, Bucharest, Romania

Brian Kinney MD
Private Practice
Plastic and Reconstructive Surgery
120 South Spalding Drive Suite 330,
Beverly Hills, California, USA

Doug McBurney MD
Private Practice
15589 East Dorado Place
Centennial, Colorado, USA

Marco Messi MD
Maxillofacial Surgery Department
Ospedali Riuniti Umberto
I-Lancisi-Salesi, Ancona, Italy

Miguel L Modolin MD
Assistant Professor
Division of Plastic Surgery
Hospital das Clínicas
São Paulo University
Faculty of Medicine
São Paulo, Brazil

R Stephen Mullholland MD
Private Practice
66 Avenue Road Suite 4 Upper Level
Toronto, Ontario, Canada

D Alex Munnoch MD
Honorary Clinical Professor
Australian School of Advanced Medicine
Macquarie University
Sydney, Australia
Consultant Plastic Surgeon and Chair
of the British Lymphology Society
Department of Plastic Surgery
Ninewells Hospital
Dundee, United Kingdom

Paolo Persichetti MD
Chief of the Division of Plastic and Reconstructive Surgery
Campus Bio-Medico University of Rome School of Medicine
Rome, Italy

Anna Petropoulos MD
Private Practice
The New England Facial and Cosmetic Surgery Center
Danvers, Massachusetts, USA

Dirk F Richter MD
Assistant Professor, Director
Dreifaltigkeits-Hospital Wesseling
Academic Teaching Hospital of the University of Bonn, Department of Plastic and Reconstructive Surgery
Wesseling, Germany

Alessandro Scalise MD
Department of Plastic and Reconstructive Surgery, Marche Polytechnic University Medical School
Ancona, Italy

Mark V Schaverien MD
Specialty Registrar in Plastic Surgery
Department of Plastic Surgery
Ninewells Hospital
Dundee, United Kingdom

Melvin A Shiffman MD JD
Chair, Section of Surgery
Newport Specialty Hospital
Tustin, California, USA

Pierfranco Simone MD
Division of Plastic and Reconstructive Surgery
Campus Bio-Medico University
Rome, Italy

Aris Sterodimas MD
Head, Plastic and Reconstructive Surgery Department, IASO General Hospital
Affiliated with the Athens Medical University, Athens, Greece
Director
Regenerative Plastic Surgery Institute
IASO General Hospital
Athens, Greece

Alexander Stoff MD
Assistant Professor, Dreifaltigkeits-Hospital Wesseling, Academic Teaching Hospital of the University of Bonn
Department of Plastic and Reconstructive Surgery
Wesseling Germany

Matteo Torresetti MD
Department of Plastic and Reconstructive Surgery
Marche Polytechnic University Medical School
Ancona, Italy

Fernando Velasco-Laguardia MD
Fellow, Dreifaltigkeits-Hospital Wesseling, Academic Teaching Hospital of the University of Bonn, Department of Plastic and Reconstructive Surgery
Wesseling, Germany

Dennis Wolf MD
Private Practice
98 Harley Street
London, United Kingdom

Foreword

For several years Dr Alberto Di Giuseppe and Dr Melvin A Shiffman, world-renowned plastic surgeons, have enthusiastically co-published books on reconstructive and plastic surgery. This recent publication on *New Frontiers in Plastic and Cosmetic Surgery* contains unique ideas developed by a select group of board-certified plastic surgeons in the field of surgical techniques for the treatment of body deformities.

The use of adipose tissue grafts and its stem cell components, though not a new surgical technique, offers new applications today. Also novel is the use of a cosmetic surgery procedure as a solution to an upper extremity chronic lymphedema problem, or Vaser liposuction techniques by performing minimally invasive maneuverings for neck and chin lift treatment.

Reconstruction of exenterated orbit with vascularized temporalis muscle flap, some new rhinoplasty techniques using deep temporal fascia, and secondary deformities correctable by otoplasty are reported. Several cosmetic breast surgery techniques are presented too. Also striking is the use of perforator flaps in several cases of reconstructive surgery.

Limb research also suggests strongly the use of combined reconstructive surgery techniques and correction of flaccidness in cases of brachioplasty after postbariatric surgical treatment.

We will all learn from the authors' teachings and, consequently, will conduct better deformity treatments affecting patients.

José Guerrerosantos MD
Professor of Plastic Surgery
University of Guadalajara
Guadalajara, México

Preface

Plastic Surgery, one of the youngest monospecialties in medicine, has historically been innovative to a drastic extent by introducing and adding the treatment of external appearance of mankind into medical sciences of healing patients of exclusively functional diseases. Science and progress cannot exist without innovative ideas and their creators, but all innovations are based on the experience and established knowledge of our predecessors. Many promising new findings will not survive forever or be rejected after a while or even innovated by the original authors or others. Many old techniques on the other hand have never been neglected. The coexistence of both: old and new is the secret of good science. This book targets new forms of therapy in cosmetic and plastic surgery that promotes support of the intrinsic, autologous, regenerative potential of human biological systems. Included are subjects involving stem cells, liposuction, head and neck surgery, and surgery of the breast, body, and extremities. All fields of surgical practice will benefit from the work of the international experts contributing chapters in the book.

Alberto Di Giuseppe MD

Acknowledgments

I would like to thank my wife, Pearl, and my dog, Bruno, for putting up with my constant time on the computer authoring and editing and lack of time with them.

I would also like to thank Shri Jitendar P Vij (Group Chairman), Ms Chetna Malhotra Vohra (Associate Director) and Ms Angima Shree (Development Editor) of M/S Jaypee Brothers Medical Publishers (P) Ltd., New Delhi, India.

Melvin A Shiffman

Contents

Section 1: Stem Cells

1. Tissue Engineering with Adipose-Derived Stem Cells (ADSCs) in Plastic and Reconstructive Surgery: Current and Future Applications **3**
Aris Sterodimas
- Technique *3*
- Discussion *9*

Section 2: Liposuction

2. Liposuction for Chronic Lymphedema of the Upper Limb **15**
Mark V Schaverien, D Alex Munnoch
- Background *15*
- Preoperative Assessment and Inclusion Criteria *15*
- Liposuction Technique *15*
- Postoperative Care *16*
- Patient Demographics *16*
- Limb Volume Outcomes *16*
- Psychological Outcomes *17*
- Discussion *19*

Section 3: Head and Neck

3. Vaser-Assisted Minimally Invasive Neck–Chin Lift **25**
Alberto Di Giuseppe, George Commons
- Guidelines for Vaser-Assisted Neck Contouring *25*
- Technique *25*
- Postoperative *27*
- Procedure *27*
- Clinical Cases *27*

4. Endoscopically Assisted Temporalis Muscle Transfer Harvesting for Orbit Reconstruction **38**
Riccardo Girotto, Marco Messi, Paolo Balercia
- Anatomical Basis *38*
- Surgical Technique *38*

5. Augmentation Rhinoplasty **44**
José Guerrerosantos
- Cartilage Grafts in Rhinoplasty *44*
- Clinical Cases *46*
- Multiple Ways to use Fascia Graft in Aesthetic Rhinoplasty *48*
- Rolled Fascia Graft *51*
- Clinical Cases *52*
- Cartilaginous Spreader Grafting *56*

- Fragmented Cartilage Graft Wrapped with Fascia in Primary Rhinoplasty *60*
- Fragmented Cartilage Wrapped with Fascia in Secondary Rhinoplasty *68*
- Case of Deformed Dorsum due to Application of Cartilage Graft in a Very Superficial Cavity *68*
- Clinical Case *69*
- Patients with Depressed Dorsum due to Excessive Resection in the Nose's Back in Primary Aesthetic Rhinoplasty *70*
- Clinical Cases *70*

6. Total Resection of the Alar Cartilages and Temporal Fascia Technique in Rhinoplasty **77**

Salvador Rodríguez-Camps Devís

- Technique *83*
- Results *92*
- Discussion *92*

7. Correction of Auricular Deformities after Failed Otoplasty **95**

Alexander Berghaus

- Analysis of Deformities after Otoplasty *95*
- Undercorrection *95*
- Overcorrection *96*
- Distorted Proportions *97*
- Formation of Edges *97*
- Deformities with Skin Defects *98*
- Deformities with Loss of Cartilage and Skin *100*

8. Focal Nerve Lesions with a Monopolar Radiofrequency Device for Cosmetic Enhancement **102**

Diane I Duncan, Doug McBurney, Brian Kinney

- The Device *102*
- Safety *102*
- History *103*
- History of Cosmetic Nerve Ablation *103*
- Anatomy *104*
- Potential Use for Brow Lifting *105*
- Technique: Treatment Protocols on Label *105*
- Case Studies *106*

Section 4: Breast

9. Stem Cell Fat Transfer for Mastoplasty using Vaser Ultrasound and Office Devised Stem Cell **113**

Alberto Di Giuseppe, Dennis Wolf

- Stem Cell Niche Therapy using Adipose Tissue *114*
- Patient Selection *116*
- Patient Assessment *116*
- Selection of Anesthesia *116*
- Incisions for Infiltration *120*
- Levels of Infiltration *120*
- Method of Infiltration *120*
- Volume Ranges *121*
- Donor Areas for Fat Harvesting *121*
- Technique *123*
- Breast Fat Augmentation *124*
- Limits of Technique *127*
- Complications *129*

10. "Scarless" Mastopexy: Using Heat-Mediated Tissue Tightening to Lift the Breast **136**

Diane I Duncan

- Evolution of Technique *136*
- Technique *136*
- Results *137*
- Asymmetry Treatment *139*
- The Modest Result *139*
- Discussion *140*
- Complications *142*

11. Inverted "T" Superior Pedicle Technique with Inferior-Based Dermal Adipose Flap for Reduction Mammaplasty **144**

Paolo Persichetti, Pierfranco Simone, Carlo Carusi

- Patient Selection *144*
- Surgical Procedure *145*
- Postoperative Care *148*
- Complications *148*

12. A Novel Approach in Male Breast Contouring after Massive Weight Loss: The Central Pedicled Breast Reduction Technique **152**

Alexander Stoff, Fernando Velasco-Laguardia, Dirk F Richter

- Preoperative Management *152*
- Preoperative Marking *152*
- Surgical Technique *154*
- Discussion *157*

Section 5: Body

13. Perforator Flaps for Pressure Sore Treatment **163**

Luca Grassetti, Matteo Torresetti, Matteo Gioacchini, Manuela Bottoni, Alessandro Scalise, Giovanni Di Benedetto

- Preoperative and Postoperative Management *164*
- Superior Gluteal Artery Perforator Flap *164*
- Inferior Gluteal Artery Perforator Flap *166*
- Posterior Thigh Perforator Flaps *170*
- First and Second Perforator of the Profunda Femoris Artery Perforator Flap *170*
- First Medial Perforator of the Profunda Femoris Artery Perforator Flap or Adductor Flap *172*
- Authors' Procedure Technique and Results *176*
- Results *179*
- Discussion *180*

14. Gluteal Perforator Flaps for Coverage of Pressure Sores **186**

O Koray Coskunfirat, Anı Cinpolat

- Gluteal Vascular Anatomy *187*
- Superior Gluteal Artery Perforator *187*
- Inferior Gluteal Artery Perforator *187*
- Preoperative Preparation *188*
- Surgical Technique *188*
- Postoperative Care *190*

15. Using Radiofrequency Energy for Heat-Mediated Tissue Tightening: Minimally Invasive and Noninvasive Modalities **191**

Diane I Duncan, Anna Petropoulos, Brian Kinney, Karen S Harkaway, R Stephen Mullholland

- RF Basics *191*
- Technique *194*

- Noninvasive RF Devices *199*
- Reaction Device by Viora *202*
- Reaction Device and RF Energy Applicators *203*
- Endymed RF Device *204*

Section 6: Extremities

16. Carpal Tunnel Syndrome **213**

Cristina Isac, Aurelia Isac, Florin Isac

- Definition and Anatomy *213*
- Symptoms *213*
- Examination *213*
- Types of Treatment *214*
- Surgical Treatment *214*
- Endoscopic Carpal Tunnel Release *216*
- Postoperative Care *216*
- Complications *216*
- Prognosis *218*

17. Improved Double Fusiform Resection Technique for Postbariatric Brachioplasty **219**

Miguel L Modolin

- Surgical Technique *219*
- Complications *222*

18. Body Dysmorphic Disorder **226**

Melvin A Shiffman

- Symptoms *226*
- Consequences of BDD *226*
- Associated Disorders *227*
- Etiology *227*
- Screening Tools for BDD *227*
- Treatment *228*
- Discussion *228*

Index *231*

Section 1

Stem Cells

Chapter Outline

- Tissue Engineering with Adipose-Derived Stem Cells (ADSCs) in Plastic and Reconstructive Surgery: Current and Future Applications

1 Tissue Engineering with Adipose-Derived Stem Cells (ADSCs) in Plastic and Reconstructive Surgery: Current and Future Applications

Aris Sterodimas

INTRODUCTION

Until very recently, most scientists and clinicians believed that damaged or diseased human tissue could only be replaced by donor transplants or with totally artificial parts. Tissue engineering (TE) promises a more advanced approach in which organs or tissues can be repaired, replaced, or regenerated for more targeted solutions. This approach also responds to clinical needs that cannot be met by organ donation alone.

Tissue engineering combines the principles of bioengineering, cell transplantation, and biomaterial engineering for the unique goal of generating bioartificial tissues and organs. Within just a few years, the possibility that the human body contains cells that can repair and regenerate damaged and diseased tissue has gone from an unlikely proposition to a virtual certainty.[1] Tissue engineering aims to provide an alternative better means of treatment for tissue and organ damage through combining both biological and artificial components in such a way that a long-lasting repair is produced. In plastic and reconstructive surgical applications, adipose tissue has become central to an increasing number of translational efforts in TE.[2] The growing interest in this area of research has resulted in the exploration of many novel research and clinical applications that utilize adipose-derived stem cell (ADSC) products obtained from this tissue source. Adipose-derived stem cells could also become the focus of an array of therapeutic solutions for many disease conditions, such as those affecting bone, cartilage, muscle, and neural expanding the possible indications and translational potential of tissue, cell-based, and regenerative medicine strategies.

After the introduction of liposuction, adipose tissue harvesting has become easier.[3] ADSCs, because of their pluripotentiality and unlimited capacity for self-renewal, have allowed significant advances for distinct reconstructive procedures in the recent years. It contains a large number of multipotent cells, which is an essential prerequisite for stem-cell-based therapies. It has been described that stem and progenitor cells in the uncultured stroma-vascular fraction (SVF) from adipose tissue usually amount to up to 3% of the whole cells, and this is 2,500-fold more than the content of stem cells in bone marrow.[4] ADSCs can easily be isolated by tissue digestion and centrifugation steps, followed by the outgrowth of the plastic adherent fraction from the SVF.[5] Stromal-enriched lipograft (SEL), the new technique of TE using ADSCs has revolutionized various aspects in reconstructive and aesthetic surgery. Implied in the definition of TE is the use of stem cells, biomolecules, and biomaterials. The SEL is based on the use of ADSCs combined with a biomaterial that is the adipose tissue that has been processed to be used as a natural scaffold and biomolecules, cytokines, and growth factors, which are secreted by the stem cells and the adipose tissue.[6]

TECHNIQUE

Marking of the areas to be liposuctioned are made while the patient is in standing position. Preoperative sedation in the surgical suite is administered. Anesthesia consists of an epidural block and intravenous sedation. The patient is placed in prone position. After the injection of normal saline wetting solution containing 1:500,000 of adrenaline by a small bore cannula and waiting 15 minutes, a 60-mL syringe attached to a 4-mm blunt cannula is inserted through small incisions in the abdominal area. Fat is aspirated by using the syringe method. The two thirds of the aspirated fat is used in order to isolate the SVF (Fig. 1.1). Digestion is done with 0.075% collagenase (Sigma, St Louis, MO, USA) in buffered saline and agitated for 30 minutes at 37°C in Celltibator (Medikan, Los Angeles, CA, USA). Separation of the SVF containing ADSCs is then done by

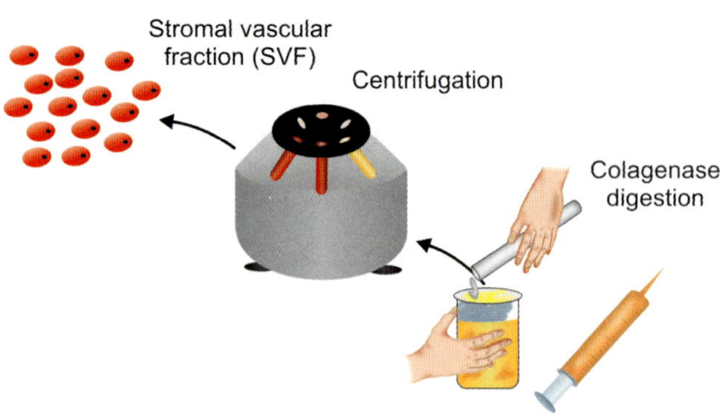

Fig. 1.1: SVF isolation from adipose tissue by collagenase digestion and centrifugation. (SVF: Stroma-vascular fraction).

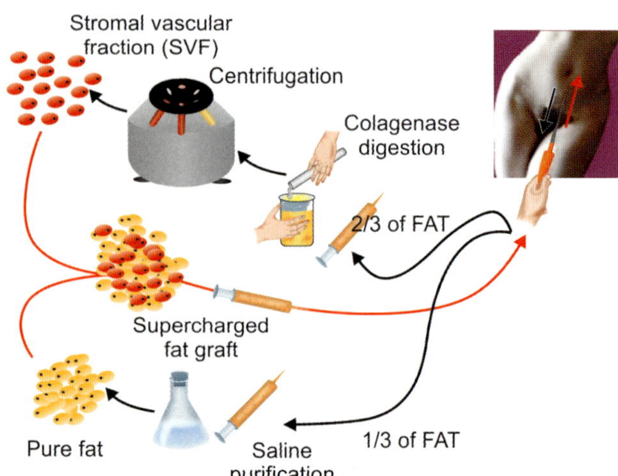

Fig. 1.2: Stromal-enriched lipograft technique.

using centrifugation at 1,200 × *g* for 5 minute.[7] The Lipokit Centrifuge (Medikan, Los Angeles, CA, USA) is used. The SVF is located in the pellet derived from the centrifuged fat at the bottom of the lipoaspirate. When human adipose stem-cell expansion is needed, the SVF is cultured in a very low human serum medium in order to allow rapid expansion of autologous ADSCs.[8] Biomaterials and biomolecules can then be used in order to guide the organization and differentiation of expanded ADSCs in the process of forming functional tissue.[9] Growth factors, differentiation factors, angiogenic factors, and gene-modulated factors are the main components of the biomolecules and need to be strategically integrated in to the future tissue engineered constructs.

In SEL, freshly isolated SVF is attached to the aspirated fat, with the fat tissue acting as a living bioscaffold before transplantation.[10] The remaining one third of the aspirated fat is treated in the following manner: with the syringe held vertically with the open end down, the fat and fluid are separated. Isotonic saline is added to the syringe, the fat and saline are separated and the exudate discarded. The procedure is repeated until the fat becomes yellow in color, free of blood, and other contaminants.[11-14] Mixing of the SVF-containing ADSCs and the purified fat is then done (Fig. 1.2). This whole procedure is done inside the operating theatre, by two tissue engineers, manually, and the time required is about 90 minutes. The adipose tissue graft enriched with SVF is woven into the targeted tissues (face, breast, and body), injecting only a tiny amount with each pass as in order to obtain the most reliable clinical outcome. Tissue planes are created by using specific cannulas in different trajectories, always from the deeper aspect to more superficial areas. The fat is injected as the cannula is withdrawn in order to avoid intravascular fat injection. Antibiotics, analgesics, and anti-inflammatory medications are prescribed during the following seven postoperative days.

Current Human Applications of ADSCs in Plastic and Reconstructive Surgery

Traditional facial rejuvenation techniques address the face by lifting the soft tissues in two dimensions. The element not routinely addressed, is reduction and atrophy of the facial soft tissues, particularly the subcutaneous fat layer.[15] This is the third dimension of facial aging. The SEL can achieve long-term volume replacement at the time of rhytidectomy and allows less aggressive surgical dissections in order to accomplish a more harmonious result (Figs. 1.3A to D). Successful applications of SEL in a series of patients for post-traumatic facial reconstruction have been published.[7] Parry-Romberg syndrome patient has been treated by SEL.[4]

In addition to the well-established procedure for breast enlargement with silicone implants, the augmentation by fat grafting has become established in recent years. The use of SEL for breast augmentation has gained attention due to further improvements in the fat preparation and processing (Figs. 1.4A to D). There are though concerns about possible role of ADSCs in promoting of tumor formation or recurrence mediated by mechanisms, such as angiogenesis, and tumor stromal cells. However,

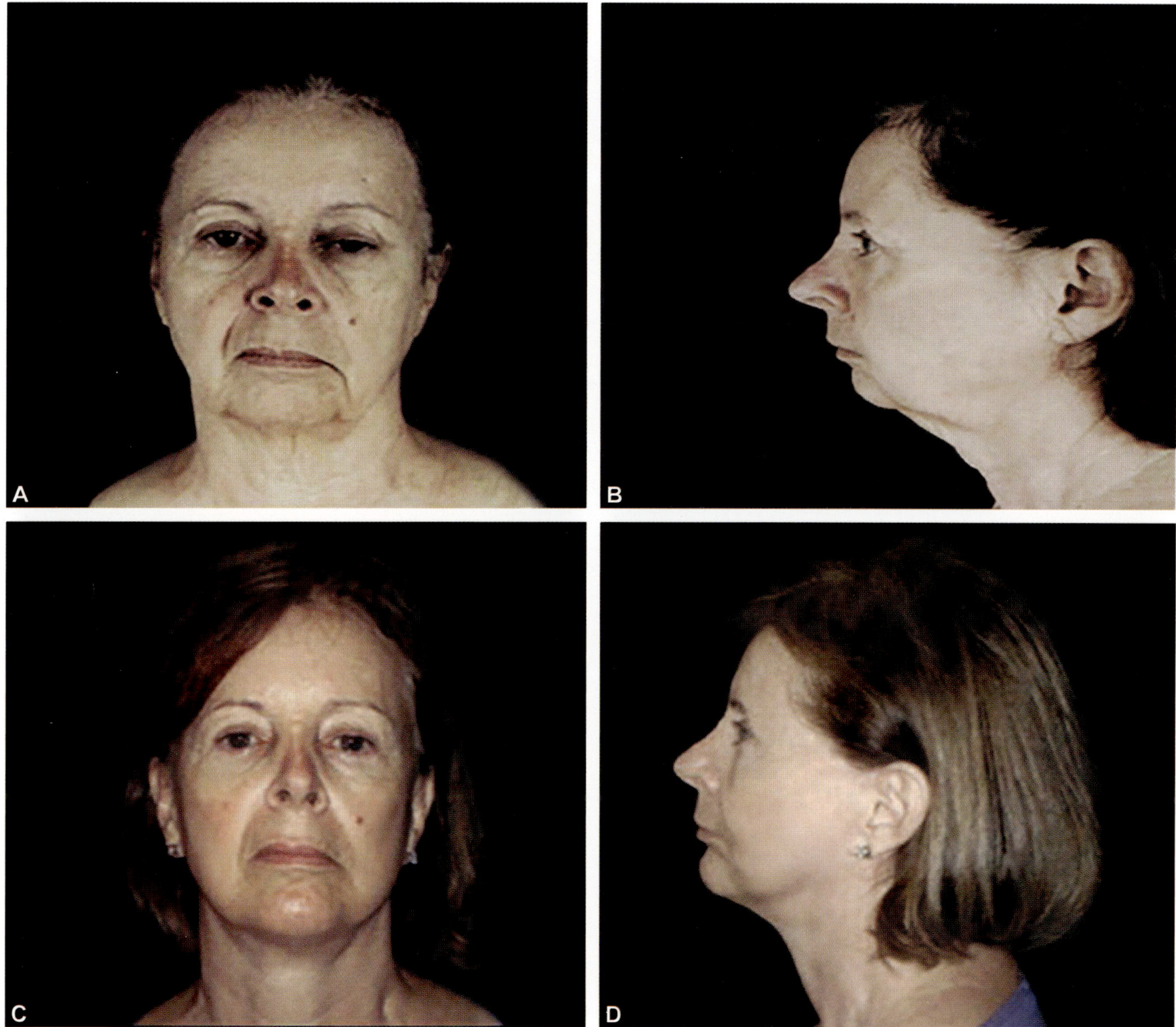

Figs. 1.3A to D: (A and B) Preoperative 72-year-old woman requesting facial rejuvenation. (C and D) Postoperative following facelifting assisted by stromal-enriched lipograft.

published clinical studies describing outcomes of fat grafting to the breast in >2,000 patients have not reported any increase in new or recurrent cancers.[16] Recently the concept of composite breast augmentation has been introduced where combining breast silicone implant insertion and simultaneous SEL has been done in 20 patients with aesthetically favorable results (Figs. 1.5A to D).

The combination of circumferential liposuction, SEL of buttocks, and/or lower limbs in a single surgical procedure has been performed successfully in the last 8 years, emphasizing the low rate of complications and the high overall patient satisfaction (Figs. 1.6A to D).

Despite advances in wound closure techniques and devices, there is still a critical need for new methods of enhancing the healing process to achieve optimal outcomes. Nonhealing and radiation exposed wounds remain a significant challenge for plastic surgeons. Recent studies suggest that ADSCs secret angiogenic cytokines in vitro and in vivo, including VEGF, HGF, and FGF2, which increase neovascularization and enhance wound healing

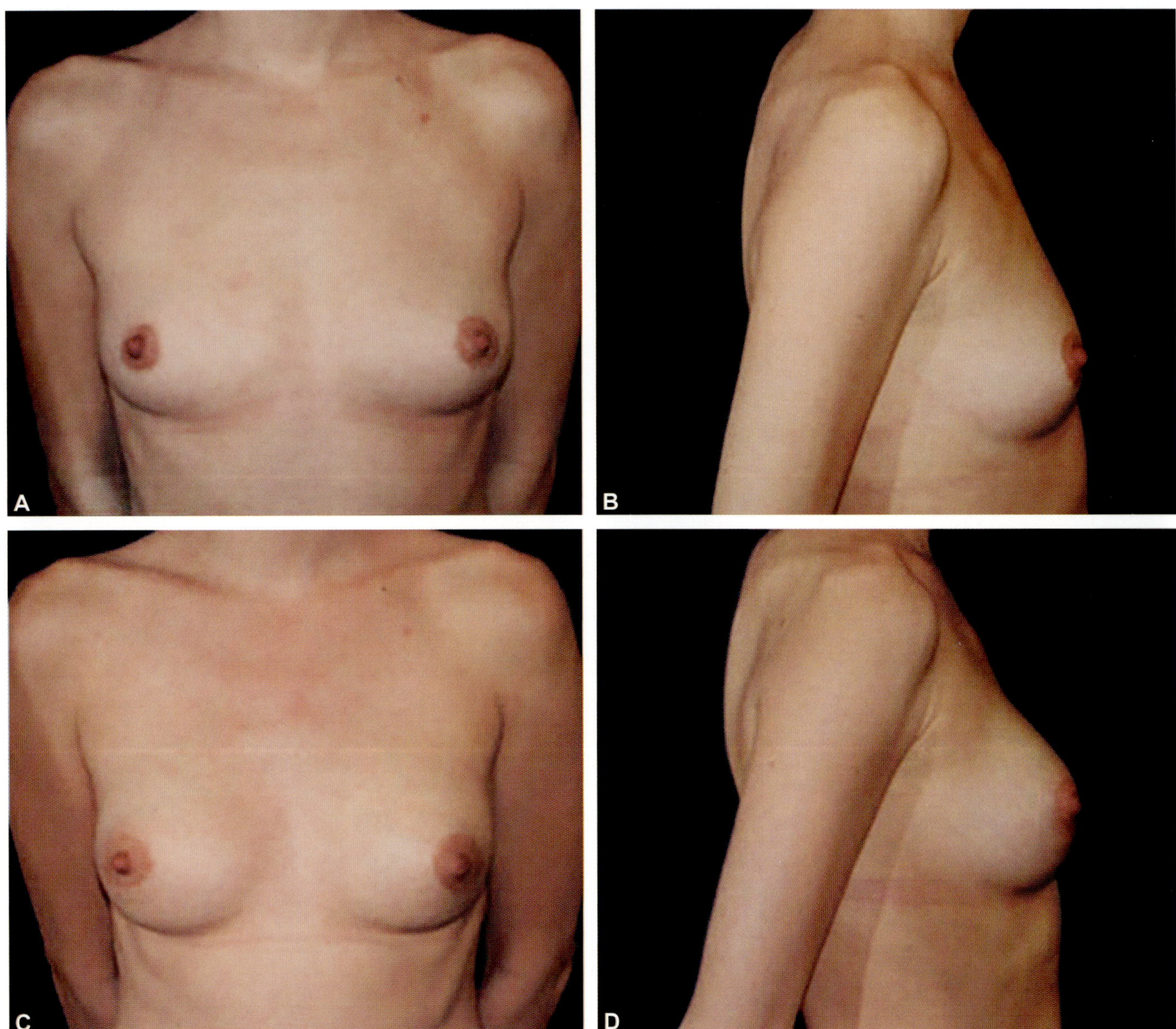

Figs. 1.4A to D: (A and B) Preoperative 22-year-old woman requesting breast augmentation. (C and D) Postoperative after breast augmentation by stromal-enriched lipograft.

in injured tissues.[17] Recently, autologous ADSCs, together with angiogenic and mitogenic factor of basic fibroblast growth factor and an artificial dermis, were applied over the excised irradiated skin defect and tested for patients who were uneventfully healed with minimal donor-site morbidity, which has lasted for >1.5 years.[18]

Reconstruction of large bony defects after tumor resection involves harvesting of autologous bone causing donor site morbidity and risk of infection. Recently clinical case where ectopic bone was produced using ADSCs in microvascular surgery for novel maxillary bone reconstruction has been reported.[19]

Future Human Applications of ADSCs in Plastic and Reconstructive Surgery

Facial volume enhancement for aesthetic and reconstructive purposes is probably going to be one of the near future applications of TE with ADSCs. Injectable microcarrier beads combined with ADSCs in order to form a minimally

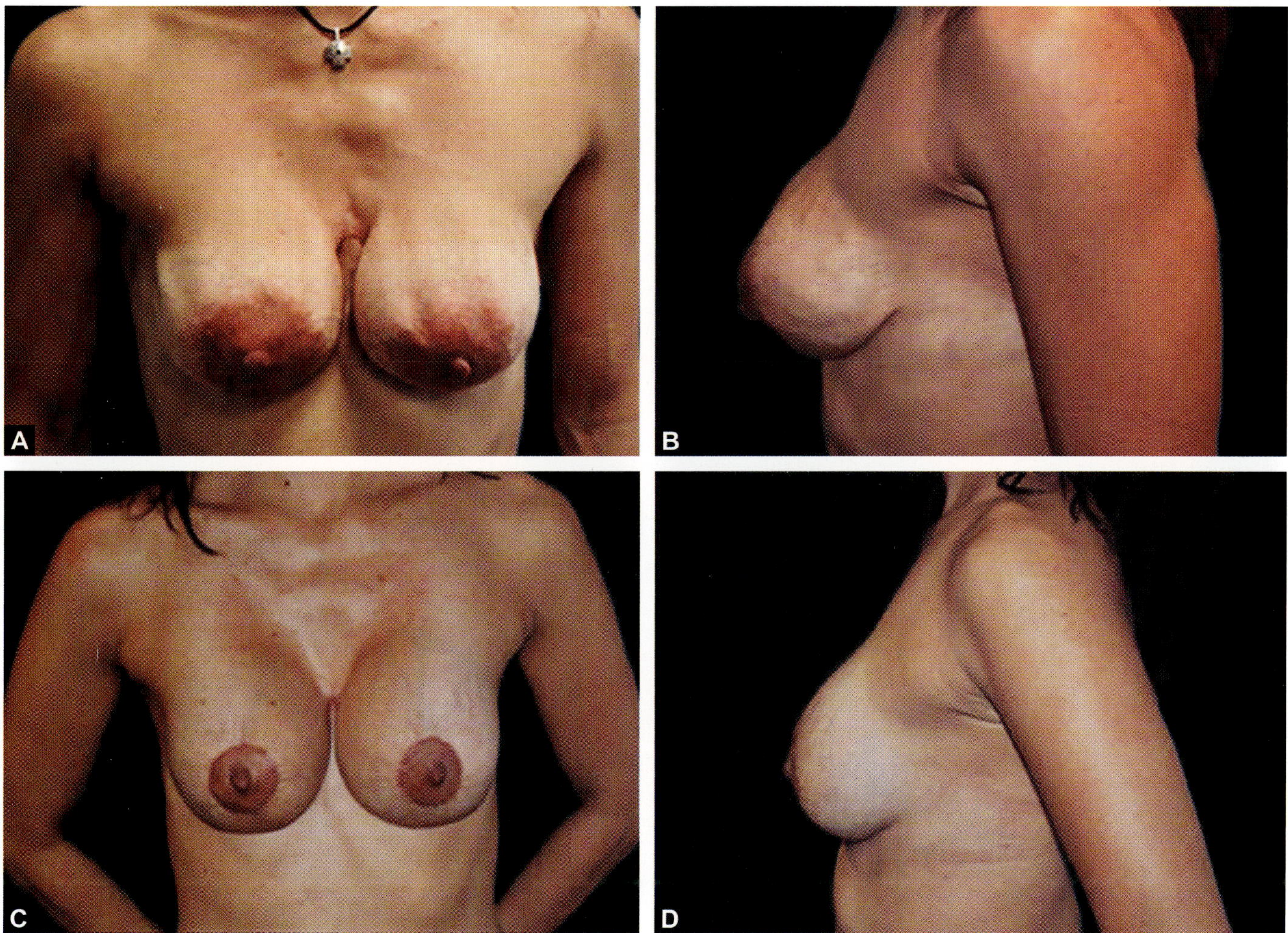

Figs. 1.5A to D: (A and B) Preoperative 29-year-old woman with pectus excavatum requesting breast augmentation revision and treatment of pectus. (C and D) Postoperative following composite breast augmentation combining silicone implant insertion and stromal-enriched lipograft.

invasive implant that will stimulate regeneration of host adipose cells and fill a soft-tissue void upon injection in vivo.[20] The system is comprised of cells seeded on hyaluronic acid biodegradable beads of an injectable size, resulting in a composite that may be injected into a patient through a syringe at the defect site. Stromal-enriched lipograft has been recently used as a nonsurgical alternative to the modeling of nasal shape and profile in secondary cases of rhinoplasty patients.[10]

Total auricular reconstruction represents one of the greatest challenges for the plastic and reconstructive surgery field. The ability to construct a fully satisfactory complete external ear has for centuries been an elusive goal. Tissue engineering using ADSCs could have the potential to provide ear-shaped cartilaginous constructs in the near future. Adipose-derived stem cells obtained by liposuction have been differentiated to chondrocytes, expanded in vitro and seeded onto biodegradable alginate and silk polymer ear-shaped scaffolds. Microporous three-dimensional (3D) scaffolds were fabricated by solvent casting technique using molds made through rapid prototyping from a normal ear CT image.[21] A recent published study has confirmed that the association of silk, alginate, and ADSCs is a reliable method to produce an engineered 3D auricular cartilage construct (Fig. 1.7).[22]

Breast augmentation or reconstruction based on ADSCs cultured on absorbable tailor-made breast scaffolds that are then implanted in vivo has been the target in the past years. Achieving simultaneous cellular proliferation and scaffold resorption can result in mature adipose

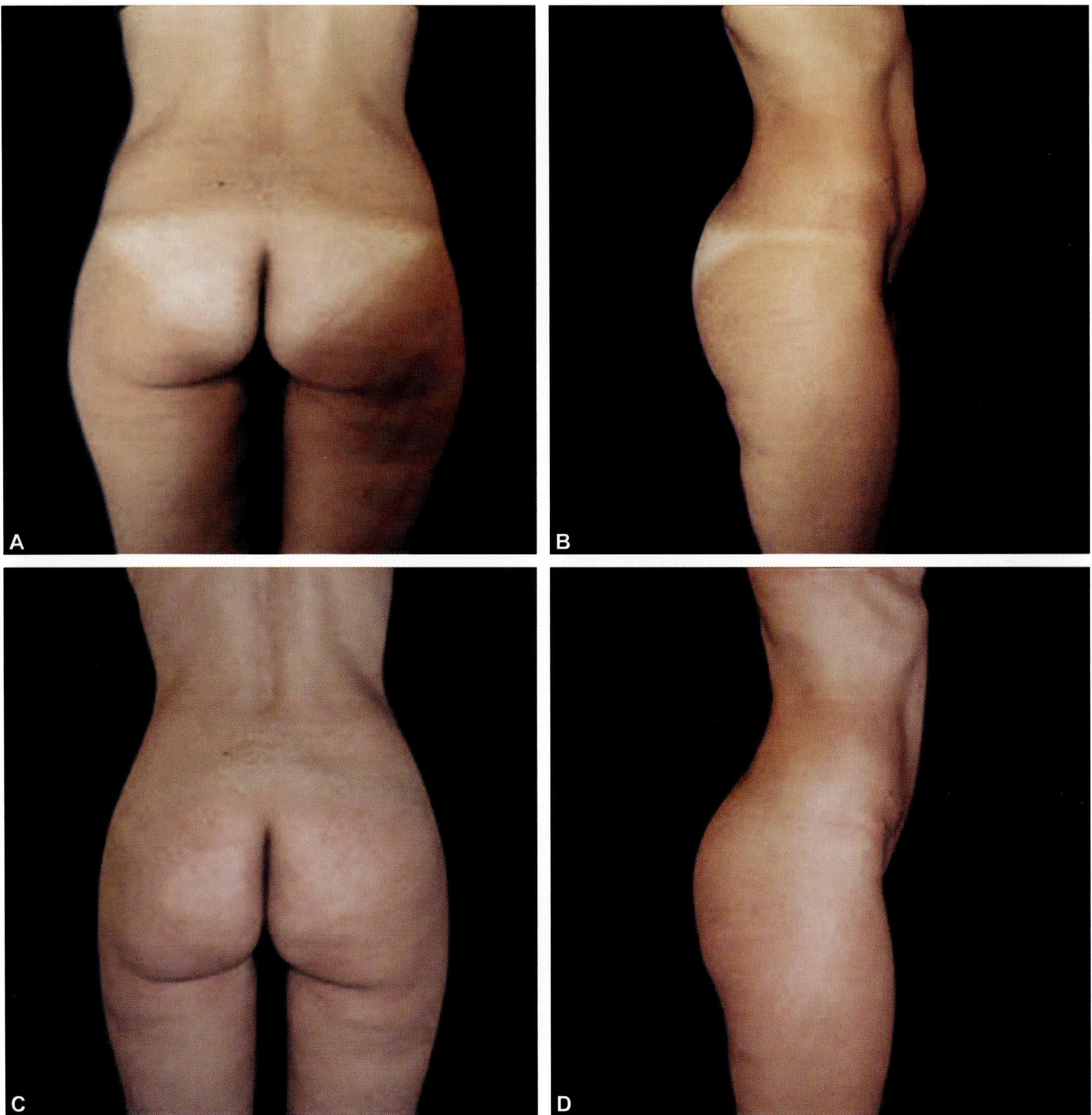

Figs. 1.6A to D: (A and B) Preoperative 31-year-old woman requesting body contouring. (C and D) Postoperative following body contouring by stromal-enriched lipograft.

tissue and possibly is superior to traditional fat grafting to the breast.[23] The future research is focusing on ADSCs-scaffold implantation into the patient in order to ideally restore the aesthetic function of the tissue by imparting a soft, smooth feel closely resembling that of natural breast (Fig. 1.8).

Use of a skin flap has been a common technique in reconstructive surgery for more than five decades. However, partial necrosis of its distal end is still a serious postoperative complication. Advances in the treatment of ischemia-reperfusion injury have created an opportunity for plastic surgeons to apply these treatments to flaps and

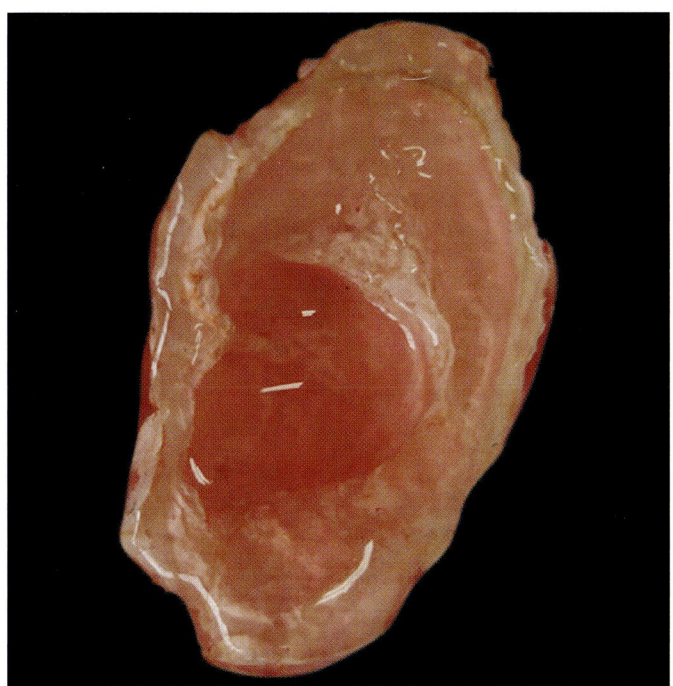

Fig. 1.7: Ear construct manufactured by auricular tissue engineering ready for implantation.

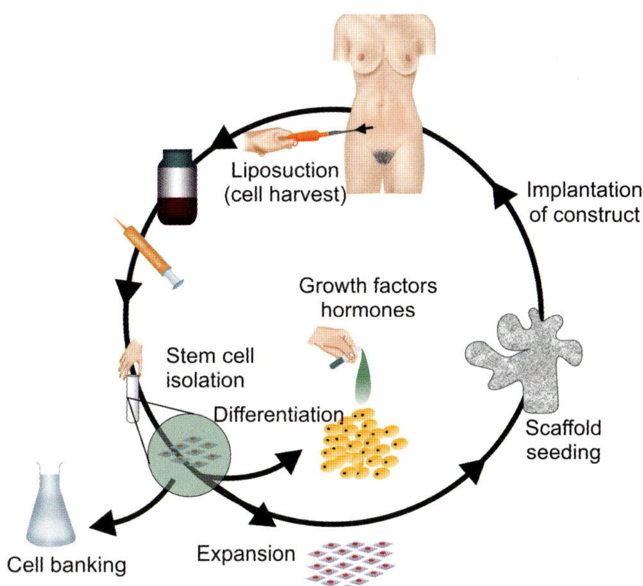

Fig. 1.8: Future breast tissue engineering based on stromal-enriched lipograft.

implanted tissues. A recent study reports that ADSCs treatment significantly enhances skin flap survival in the aftermath of ischemia to an extent that almost equals surgical results without ischemia. This effect is accompanied with a pronounced and significant angiogenic response and an improved blood perfusion to the flap.[24,25]

DISCUSSION

Tissue engineering using ADSC is a fairly young field of research that has shown huge potential so far. It is imperative to be humble enough to realize that TE combines several different fields of research, in themselves very complicated, as biology, medicine, chemistry, material science, and more.

The presence of ADSC cells in adipose tissue transplantation may contribute to neoangiogenesis in the acute phase by acting as endothelial progenitor cells or angiogenic-factor-releasing cells.[26] In vivo, ADSCs demonstrate the capacity to proliferate in response to a hypoxic insult remote from their resident niche, and this has been supported by in vitro studies showing increasing ADSCs proliferation with greater degrees of hypoxia. The number of functional ADSCs is likely to be important for tissue repair and remodeling and ADSCs differentiate into vascular endothelial cells that contribute to neoangiogenesis in the acute phase of transplantation. Adipose-derived stem cells also upregulate their proneovascular activity in response to hypoxia, and may harbor the capacity to home to ischemic tissue and function cooperatively with existing vasculature to promote angiogenesis.[4]

In 2011, the first study comparing the autologous fat grafting to SEL was published.[7] A group of 20 patients with congenital or acquired facial tissue defects were included in this study and randomly divided into two groups. Ten patients were treated with autologous fat transplantation, and the remaining 10 were treated with ADSC-enriched lipografts. Stromal-enriched lipografts produced superior results without the need for repeat treatment sessions, which were necessary with autologous fat transplantation. Even when large areas need reconstruction, like in head and neck cancers; it is possible to use the SEL technique as a TE method of reconstruction. The SEL technique also offer the possibility of prefabrication of flaps, reconstruction of auricular framework defects and fabrication of new skin for massive burns when SVF is used either alone or combined with other natural or synthetic biomaterials. In aesthetic plastic surgery, the SEL technique provides a safer alternative to allogenic implant use, resulting in the creation of a functional tissue that has a more natural look and carries fewer risks than currently available augmentation options.

One of the main obstacles in the progress of TE using ADSCs today is the vasculature system. Any biological structure of sizes larger than a couple of hundred microns in diameter needs a circulatory system for nutritional reasons. This is mirrored in the fact that the tissues that have found their ways to the clinical setting are all tissues and organs with the least complex blood circulation: fat, skin, cartilage, and bone. In order to succeed also with more complex organs and tissues, this problem needs to be resolved. Recent advances in nanotechnology may allow the development of nanostructured scaffolds with a cellular environment that maximally enhances not only cell expansion but also the neovascularization that is crucial for long-term maintenance of cell volume. Another obstacle is the limited materials that are currently available as carriers or scaffolds in the field of plastic and reconstructive surgery. Currently, fat tissue appears to be the best available natural biomaterial. Innovative synthetic materials, such as polypeptides or novel biodegradable polymers, need to be introduced. Advances in materials design may generate "smart" scaffolds that will control tissue topology and have surface modifications to stimulate cell attachment, differentiation, and growth.[27]

In 2009, the use of ADSCs to create induced pluripotent cells (iPS cells) was reported.[28] In their derivation of iPS cells from ADSCs, researchers cite the enormous clinical utility for an embryonic-like stem-cell population that can be easily derived and used without the ethical issues of an embryonic stem cell. Whether ADSC-derived iPS cells will be ultimately be used clinically will depend on a couple of important factors, namely, how easy is it to develop iPS lines and their safety.[29]

The apparent commercial and industrial interest on TE using ADSCs that has emerged lately should encourage the scientific community in adopting a disciplined strategy in pursuing this field and clinical trials can lead to optimization of it.[30] An interdisciplinary effort at and the government front will bring successful realization of this therapy in to the field of regenerative medicine.

CONCLUSION

There is a wealth of published clinical data showing safety, feasibility, and efficacy of the SEL technique. Adipose tissue stem-cell-based regenerative strategies hold tremendous promise, and this great potential must be balanced against stringent standards of scientific and clinical investigation, before developing "off-the-shelf" TE products. Further investigations should be encouraged toward bench side and bedside to resolve various issues.

REFERENCES

1. Sterodimas A, De Faria J, Correa WE, et al. Tissue engineering in plastic surgery: an up-to-date review of the current literature. Ann Plast Surg. 2009;62(1):97-103.
2. Sterodimas A, Pereira LH. Liposuction of the abdomen and trunk. In: Rubin JP, Jewell ML, Richter D, Uebel CO (Eds). Body Contouring and Liposuction. New York, NY: WB Saunders Elsevier; 2012. pp. 311-20.
3. Shiffman MA. Clinical applications of liposuction In: Illouz YG, Sterodimas A (Eds). Adipose Derived Stem Cells and Regenerative Medicine. Berlin: Springer-Verlag; 2011. pp. 31-44.
4. Sterodimas A, de Faria J, Nicaretta B, et al. Tissue engineering with adipose-derived stem cells (ADSCs): current and future applications. J Plast Reconstr Aesthet Surg. 2010;63(11):1886-92.
5. Sterodimas A, de Faria J, Nicaretta B, et al. Cell-assisted lipotransfer. Aesthet Surg J. 2010;30(1):78-81.
6. Sterodimas A. Adipose stem cell engineering. Clinical applications in plastic and reconstructive surgery. In: Illouz YG, Sterodimas A (Eds). Adipose Derived Stem Cells and Regenerative Medicine. Berlin: Springer-Verlag; 2011. pp. 165-80.
7. Sterodimas A, de Faria J, Nicaretta B, et al. Autologous fat transplantation versus adipose-derived stem cell-enriched lipografts: a study. Aesthet Surg J. 2011;31(6):682-93.
8. Parker AM, Shang H, Khurgel M, et al. Low serum and serum-free culture of multipotential human adipose stem cells. Cytotherapy. 2007;9(7):637-46.
9. Magarakis M, Shridharani SM. Fundamentals and Principles of biomolecules in adipose stem cell engineering. In: Illouz YG, Sterodimas A (Eds). Adipose Derived Stem Cells and Regenerative Medicine. Berlin: Springer-Verlag; 2011. pp. 103-9.
10. Sterodimas A. Stromal enriched lipograft for rhinoplasty refinement. Aesthet Surg J. 2013;33(4):612-14.
11. Pereira LH, Sterodimas A. Free fat transplantation for the aesthetic correction of mild pectus excavatum. Aesthetic Plast Surg. 2008;32(2):393-6.
12. Haroldo Pereira L, Sterodimas A. Aesthetic restoration of axillary contour deformity after lymph node dissection. J Plast Reconstr Aesthet Surg. 2008;61(2):231-2.
13. Pereira LH, Nicaretta B, Sterodimas A. Correction of liposuction sequelae by autologous fat transplantation. Aesthetic Plast Surg. 2011;35(6):1000-1008.
14. Nicareta B, Pereira LH, Sterodimas A, et al. Autologous gluteal lipograft. Aesthetic Plast Surg. 2011;35(2):216-24.
15. Citarella ER, Sterodimas A, Condé-Green A. Endoscopically assisted limited-incision rhytidectomy: a 10-year prospective study. J Plast Reconstr Aesthet Surg. 2010;63(11): 1842-8.
16. Fraser JK, Hedrick MH, Cohen SR. Oncologic risks of autologous fat grafting to the breast. Aesthet Surg J. 2011; 31(1):68-75.

17. Nie C, Yang D, Xu J, et al. Locally administered adipose-derived stem cells accelerate wound healing through differentiation and vasculogenesis. Cell Transplant. 2011;20(2): 205-16.
18. Akita S, Akino K, Hirano A, et al. Noncultured autologous adipose-derived stem cells therapy for chronic radiation injury. Stem Cells Int. 2010;2010:532704.
19. Mesimäki K, Lindroos B, Törnwall J, et al. Novel maxillary reconstruction with ectopic bone formation by GMP adipose stem cells. Int J Oral Maxillofac Surg. 2009;38(3):201-9.
20. Burg JLK, Cavin NM. Engineered scaffolds and matrices: tailored biomaterials for adipose stem cell engineering. In: Illouz YG, Sterodimas A (Eds). Adipose Derived Stem Cells and Regenerative Medicine. Berlin: Springer-Verlag; 2011. pp. 93-101.
21. Sterodimas A, de Faria J, Correa WE, et al. Tissue engineering and auricular reconstruction: a review. J Plast Reconstr Aesthet Surg. 2009;62(4):447-52.
22. Sterodimas A, de Faria J. Human auricular tissue engineering in an immunocompetent animal model. Aesthet Surg J. 2013;33(2):283-9.
23. Illouz YG, Sterodimas A. Autologous fat transplantation to the breast: a personal technique with 25 years of experience. Aesthetic Plast Surg. 2009;33(5):706-15.
24. Lu F, Mizuno H, Uysal CA, et al. Improved viability of random pattern skin flaps through the use of adipose-derived stem cells. Plast Reconstr Surg. 2008;121(1):50-58.
25. Reichenberger MA, Heimer S, Schaefer A, et al. Adipose derived stem cells protect skin flaps against ischemia-reperfusion injury. Stem Cell Rev. 2012;8(3):854-62.
26. Sterodimas A, Boriani F, Magarakis E, et al. Thirty-four years of liposuction: past, present and future. Eur Rev Med Pharmacol Sci. 2012;16(3):393-406.
27. Burnouf T, Goubran HA, Chen TM, et al. Blood-derived biomaterials and platelet growth factors in regenerative medicine. Blood Rev. 2013;27(2):77-89.
28. Lu F, Li J, Gao J, Ogawa R, et al. Improvement of the survival of human autologous fat transplantation by using VEGF-transfected adipose-derived stem cells. Plast Reconstr Surg. 2009;124(5):1437-46.
29. Goessler UR. Gene therapy used for adipose stem cell engineering. In: Illouz YG, Sterodimas A (Eds). Adipose Derived Stem Cells and Regenerative Medicine. Berlin: Springer-Verlag; 2011. pp. 111-19.
30. Sterodimas A, Illouz YG. Conclusions and future directions. In: Illouz YG, Sterodimas A (Eds). Adipose Derived Stem Cells and Regenerative Medicine. Berlin: Springer-Verlag; 2011. pp. 273-6.

Section 2

Liposuction

Chapter Outline

- Liposuction for Chronic Lymphedema of the Upper Limb

2 Liposuction for Chronic Lymphedema of the Upper Limb

Mark V Schaverien, D Alex Munnoch

BACKGROUND

Arm lymphedema is a well-recognized complication of axillary surgery for breast cancer, occurring in 9–41% of cases following axillary dissection,[1-5] and although the incidence is reduced following sentinel lymph node biopsy, it still occurs in 4–10% of cases.[4-7] The excess limb swelling can adversely affect the patient's daily activities and lead to measurable effects on quality of life.[8]

Patients diagnosed with lymphedema postoperatively are initially treated conservatively with complex decongestive therapy, which includes customized compression garments or bandaging that need to worn continuously, manual lymphatic drainage, and meticulous skin care, and moisturizing to reduce the risk of infections. Microsurgical techniques to improve the lymphatic drainage are becoming increasingly popular and have shown promising short-term results in the management of the edema. Techniques include lymphaticolymphatic or lymphaticovenous shunts,[9-17] and microvascular transplantation of lymphatic nodes either alone or with a free abdominal flap carrier.[18,19] Established chronic lymphedema, however, leads to secondary hypertrophy of the subcutaneous adipose tissue that will not respond to conservative measures or lymphatic bypass techniques.[20] Lipectomy was historically reserved for patients with chronic lymphedema to remove the hypertrophied subcutaneous fat. Debulking techniques, including the Charles, Homan, and Thompson procedures, were associated with unacceptable aesthetic appearance and scarring. Liposuction for the removal of the fat hypertrophy in chronic lymphedema was introduced by O'Brien and colleagues in 1989[21] and has been popularized by Brorson. Long-term data have demonstrated that the technique is effective at reducing limb volume with good cosmetic and functional outcomes, and with a low rate of complications, when used in conjunction with pressure garments.[22-25] The use of liposuction has also been shown not to further impair lymphatic function.[26,27]

Following training by Brorson, the Department of Plastic Surgery at Ninewells Hospital in Dundee set up a multidisciplinary surgical lymphedema service using liposuction over 7 years ago for the treatment of lymphedema of the upper and lower limbs. Here, we report the surgical technique and outcomes using liposuction for the treatment of chronic arm lymphedema following axillary surgery for breast cancer.

PREOPERATIVE ASSESSMENT AND INCLUSION CRITERIA

Patients must be compliant with wearing their pressure garments continuously and not have any pitting edema to be eligible for surgery. Those with active cancer, wounds, or infections are excluded. Preoperatively, the limbs are photographed and the excess volume calculated using conal measurements taken at 4-cm intervals, a method of limb volume estimation that has been shown to be a valid and reliable alternative to water displacement techniques.[28,29]

LIPOSUCTION TECHNIQUE

The liposuction technique and postoperative care are identical to that previously described by Brorson.[23] Liposuction is carried out under general anesthesia with intravenous steroid, given intraoperatively (8 mg dexamethasone) and antibiotic cover. Following arm exsanguination, an upper arm tourniquet is applied. Through multiple 3-mm stab incisions liposuction is performed without preinfiltration to the lower arm and distal part of the upper arm using a cannula designed by Brorson (Fig. 2.1). No liposuction is performed to the hand as effective compression is difficult to this area and recurrence usually occurs. Once the

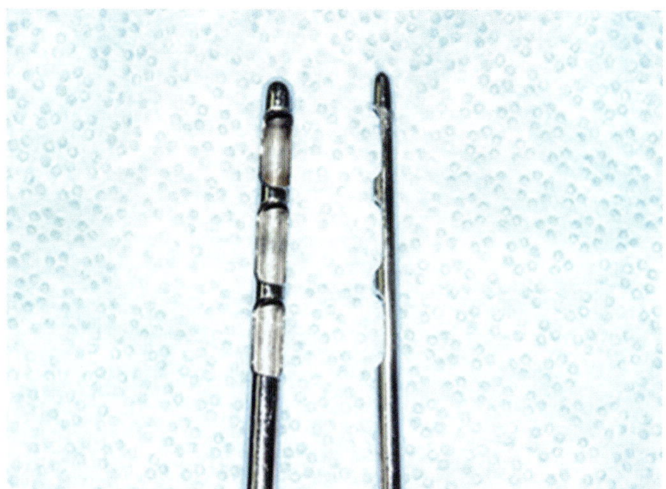

Fig. 2.1: Liposuction cannula designed by Bronson.

subcutaneous fat has been removed, a Jobst Elvarex Class 2 custom-made pressure garment is applied before releasing the tourniquet. Liposuction is then also carried out to the proximal part of the limb where required after infiltration with dilute local anesthetic and adrenaline (500 mL normal saline with 1 mg adrenaline and 20 mg 0.5% Chirocaine) in order to minimize blood loss. After completing the liposuction, the pressure garment is advanced to cover the whole limb. Incisions are left open to allow any fluid to egress and prevent hematoma formation.

The liposuction aspirate collected is allowed to separate within the collection container into supernatant fat and infranatant portions by gravitation sedimentation overnight, and then the volumes of each are measured to the nearest 10 mL.

POSTOPERATIVE CARE

The patient is given a 5-day course of antibiotics and analgesia as required and the limb is elevated. After 2 days, the garment is removed, the limb cleaned, and the pressure garments are renewed. At this stage, there is usually minimal bruising with the wounds healing well. A further dressing change is performed at day 4 when leakage from the small wounds has usually stopped and the patient is discharged home. Patients are then reviewed in the outpatient clinic at 2 weeks, 4 weeks, 3 months, 6 months, then 6 monthly to maximize pressure garment therapy. Patients need to wear the pressure garment continuously for 24 hours, then shower in the morning before applying a new garment. Compression garments need to be worn continuously for life, and should be supplied in a sufficient manner, based on individual patient requirements.

PATIENT DEMOGRAPHICS

Over the last 7 years, the authors have performed liposuction on 19 women with unilateral arm lymphedema, the dominant arm being affected in nine patients. Thirteen women had a mastectomy and four a wide local excision for breast cancer. Eighteen patients had an axillary dissection and 15 had postoperative radiotherapy, with the axilla irradiated in 12 patients, and 9 had adjuvant chemotherapy. One patient developed upper limb lymphedema following thyroidectomy.

The mean age at the time of liposuction was 59 years (range, 42–75). The lymphedema started at a mean of 2.6 years (range, 0–21) after surgery, and the mean duration between onset of lymphedema and liposuction was 7.8 years (range, 1–14). All 19 women had conservative treatment initially using compression garments, and in addition four had received pneumatic compression. No patients had previously undergone surgical procedures. Ten patients reported infective episodes preoperatively.

LIMB VOLUME OUTCOMES

The mean excess arm volume at admission was 1,350 mL (range, 620–2,428) and the ratio of the swollen arm to the unaffected arm was 1.48 (range, 1.2–1.8). The mean duration of surgery was approximately 2 hours (roughly 1 L of fat was aspirated per hour). At 2 weeks after surgery with continued application of compression garments, the mean volume reduction in our patient series is 1,144 mL. The mean percentage reduction compared with preoperative is 79%, corresponding to a mean ratio of operated to nonoperated arm of 1.11 (Table 2.1) (Figs. 2.2 and 2.3). There were no perioperative or postoperative complications.

At 1 year after surgery, the mean volume difference between operated and normal arms was 29 mL. This corresponds to a mean percentage difference of 101%, and a mean ratio of operated to nonoperated arm of 1.01, meaning that the volume in the operated and nonoperated limbs is virtually equivalent. At 2 years following surgery, there was a mean percentage difference of 109%, and a mean ratio of operated to nonoperated arm of 0.98. This reduction has been maintained for up to 7 years of follow-up with similar results to those of Brorson's Unit, and with excellent aesthetic results (Figs. 2.4 to 2.6). As can be seen in Figures 2.2 and 2.3, the volume reduction continues to improve with time as edema is treated by the compression garments and due to reversal of the compensatory muscle hypertrophy as the arm weight decreases. The importance of compliance with wearing the compression garments

Table 2.1: Mean volume and percentage reductions compared with preoperative measurements and normal arm with up to 7 years of follow-up

	2 weeks post-op (n = 19)	*4 weeks post-op (n = 19)*	*3 months post-op (n = 17)*	*6 months post-op (n = 15)*	*1 year post-op (n = 12)*	*2 years post-op (n = 11)*	*3 years post-op (n = 11)*	*4 years post-op (n = 11)*	*5 years post-op (n = 8)*	*6 years post-op (n = 5)*	*7 years post-op (n = 2)*
Arm volume difference (mL)	1144 (range, 487–2055)	1257 (range, 565–2057)	1244 (range, 523–2335)	1265 (range, 545–2246)	1381 (range, 489–1971)	1428 (range, 779–2263)	1499 (range, 705–2532)	1487 (range, 714–2357)	1474 (range, 937–2066)	1527 (range, 850–2245)	1227 (range, 917–1227)
Volume reduction normal arm (%)	79 (range, 40–118)	81 (range, 48–119)	87 (range, 54–125)	89 (range, 47–144)	101 (range, 69–148)	109 (range, 79–157)	118 (range, 74–164)	119 (range, 87–181)	126 (range, 76–174)	119 (range, 81–164)	129 (range, 74–183)
Ratio volume of operated to normal arm	1.11 (range, 0.92–1.36)	1.10 (range, 0.91–1.28)	1.07 (range, 0.92–1.25)	1.07 (range, 0.86–1.20)	1.01 (range, 0.85–1.13)	0.98 (range, 0.80–1.13)	0.94 (range, 0.75–1.10)	0.93 (range, 0.69–1.06)	0.91 (range, 0.70–1.15)	0.95 (range, 0.80–1.11)	0.95 (range, 0.76–1.14)

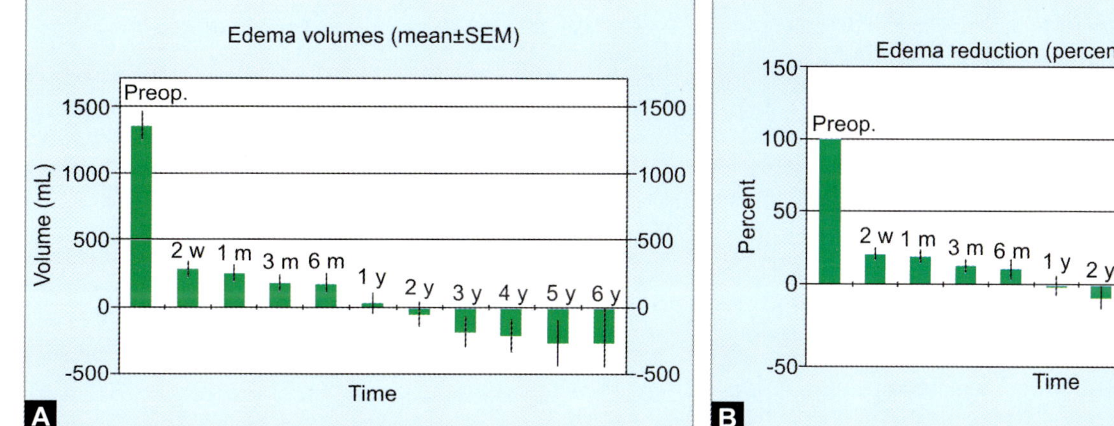

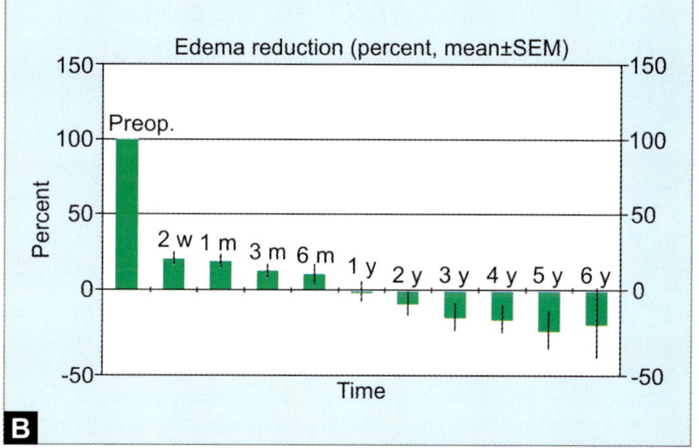

Figs. 2.2A and B: (A) Mean (standard error of mean) volume reduction with up to 7 years of follow-up. (B) Mean percentage edema reduction with up to 7 years of follow-up.

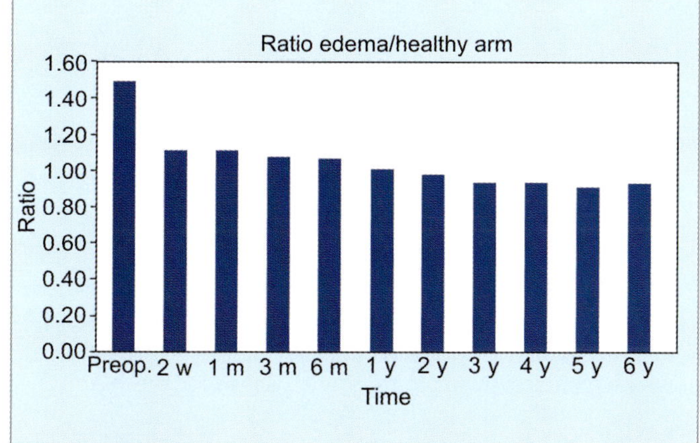

Fig. 2.3: Mean volume ratios of operated to normal arm with up to 7 years of follow-up.

continuously can be seen in Figure 2.7 comparing arm volumes in a compliant patient with a noncompliant patient.

The mean volume of aspirate removed below the tourniquet when it was inflated is 1,042 mL (range, 550–1900), and the mean proportion of fat in the aspirate is 88% (range, 58–100). The mean volume of aspirate removed without the tourniquet when tumescence was used is 736 mL (range 325–1,200) and fat comprised 68% (range, 40–83) percent of the aspirate. Thus, the total mean aspirate volume is 1,584 mL (range 600–2,600) (Fig. 2.8).

PSYCHOLOGICAL OUTCOMES

Eleven patients completed Hospital Anxiety and Depression Score questionnaires and a Visual Analogue Score

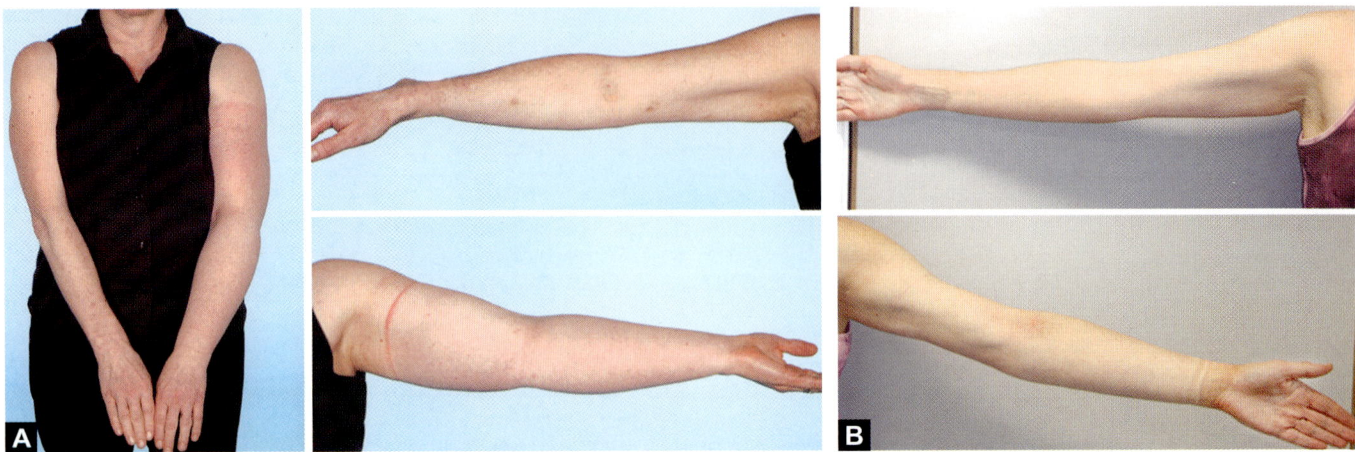

Figs. 2.4A and B: (A) Preoperative patient with left arm lymphedema following axillary surgery for breast cancer compared with the nonoperated right arm. (B) Two years postoperative following liposuction of left arm compared with the nonoperated right arm. The reduction in limb volume in the affected arm was 1,297 mL.

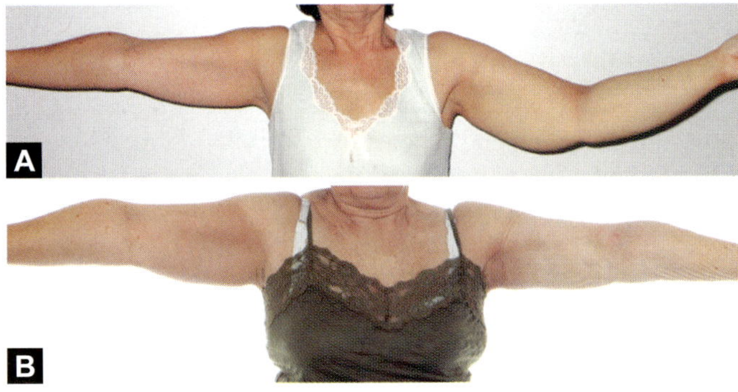

Figs. 2.5A and B: (A) Preoperative patient with left arm lymphedema following axillary surgery for breast cancer compared with the nonoperated right arm. (B) Three years postoperative following liposuction of the left arm compared with the nonoperated right arm. The reduction in limb volume in the affected arm was 1,297 mL.

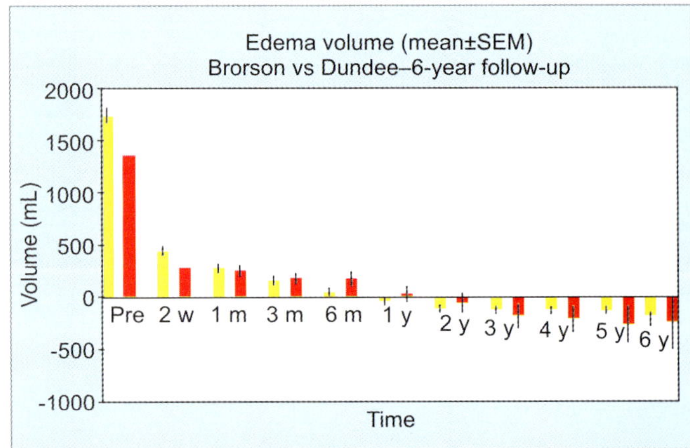

Fig. 2.6: Mean volume reduction for Dundee (red) compared with data available from Brorson (yellow) with 7 years of follow-up.

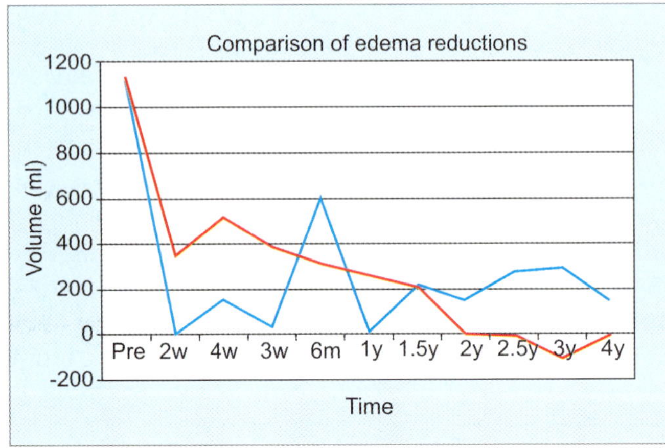

Fig. 2.7: Mean postoperative arm volume reduction of two patients demonstrating the importance of patient compliance with wearing pressure garments in long-term stable volume reduction (red line, compliant patient; blue line, noncompliant patient).

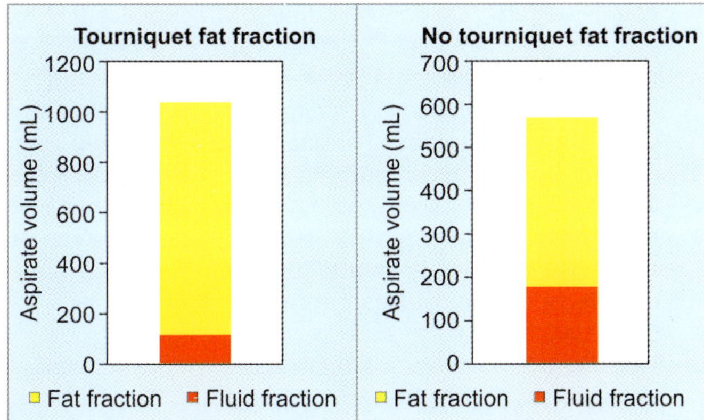

Fig. 2.8: Fat and fluid fractions from the aspirate above (with infiltration) and below (under tourniquet control) the tourniquet.

to assess psychological well-being preoperatively and at 3 months postoperatively. Anxiety scores reduced significantly from 9.09 to 4.60 (student's *t*-test; $p = 0.049$) as a result of surgery, and depression scores reduced from 5.73 to 1.70 (student's *t*-test; $p = 0.059$). The visual analog scores reflecting overall well-being had improved postoperatively from 64.60 to 81.20 (student's *t*-test; $p = 0.1$). Patients also expressed their delight at the improved function, reduced weight, and cosmetic appearance of their limbs. The most pleasing aspect from the patient's point of view is the ability to wear normal clothes (Figs. 2.4 and 2.5).

DISCUSSION

Liposuction has been shown to be an effective, reproducible, and long-lasting treatment for chronic upper limb lymphedema. From the authors' series at 2 weeks following surgery with continued application of compression garments, a mean volume reduction of 79% was achieved, equating to a 79% reduction when compared with the nonoperated arm. At 1 year the mean percentage volume reduction compared with the normal arm was 101%, meaning that the volume of both of the patients' arms was virtually equivalent, and this reduction was maintained up to 7 years after surgery (Table 2.1).

Lymphedema significantly impairs patient function and quality of life, and arm lymphedema is a well-recognized complication following axillary surgery for breast cancer. Although sentinel lymph node biopsy reduces this risk, it does not prevent it.[1-8] As well as axillary surgery, radiotherapy and chemotherapy increase the risk of development of lymphedema. Conservative methods including manual lymphatic drainage and compression bandaging are the mainstay of treatment to prevent the establishment of chronic lymphedema and subsequent subcutaneous fat hypertrophy.[20,30] Microsurgical procedures to improve the lymphatic drainage have demonstrated promising results in treating the tissue edema and have become increasingly popular recently, but cannot remove the fat once it is established.[9] Techniques including lymphaticolymphatic bypass surgery[10-12] and microvascular lymph node transfer, however, may cause donor site morbidity and may result in lymphedema in the donor limb.[18,19,31,32] Lymphaticovenular bypass surgery has shown good short-term results with low morbidity, but long-term efficacy has yet to be demonstrated.[13-17] The main disadvantage is the requirement for supramicrosurgical techniques for many of these approaches, requiring specialist skills, instruments, and operating microscopes,[16,17] and long-term results are needed as well as evidence of lymphatic function. Preliminary evidence also suggests that breast reconstruction alone may lead to the improvement of established lymphedema.[33-35]

Once nonpitting lymphedema becomes established it cannot be treated by compression treatment or microsurgical techniques and necessitates direct fat removal. Traditional excisional surgery leaves unacceptable scarring and liposuction has been shown to be efficacious where lipectomy is required. Liposuction has been shown through limb volume measurements, volume-rendered CT scans, and plethysmography to lead to complete reduction of the excess arm volume with long-lasting results.[20,22-25] The patient needs to continue to wear compression garments as liposuction alone will not reduce the future tendency to redevelop lymphedema and subsequent reaccumulation of subcutaneous fat. Patient compliance with wearing the customized pressure garments is critical for achievement of long-term stable edema reduction. Noncompliance leads to rebound increases in limb edema, whereas compliance leads to a consistent stable rate of volume reduction (Fig. 2.7). Provided that the liposuction is carried out axially with respect to the limb, the technique will not cause damage to the existing lymphatics within the limb.[26,27] A clinical study using lymphoscintigraphy demonstrated that liposuction was not associated with further impairment to an already impaired lymph transport in the lymphedematous upper extremity,[26] and a cadaveric study of the effect of liposuction techniques on the lymphatics of the lower extremity demonstrated that longitudinal liposuction with respect to the limb did not cause any major lesions of the epifascial lymph vessels.[27]

The authors' experience has found that liposuction for the treatment of arm lymphedema is effective and long-lasting, comparable with results previously demonstrated by Brorson. Liposuction combined with pressure garment therapy therefore is an effective treatment for chronic lymphedema with secondary fat accumulation. A dedicated team, careful patient selection and compliance with lifelong pressure therapy are essential to maintain the results of liposuction.

ACKNOWLEDGMENTS

The authors would like to thank SCN Susan Lundie and CN Marilyn Finnegan for their help in the lymphedema clinic.

REFERENCES

1. Kissin MW, Querci della Rovere G, Easton D, et al. Risk of lymphoedema following the treatment of breast cancer. Br J Surg. 1986;73(7):580-84.
2. Mazeron JJ, Otmezguine Y, Huart J, et al. Conservative treatment of breast cancer: results of management of axillary lymph node area in 3353 patients. Lancet. 1985;1 (8442):1387.
3. Fleissig A, Fallowfield LJ, Langridge CI, et al. Post-operative arm morbidity and quality of life: results of the ALMANAC randomised trial comparing sentinel node biopsy with standard axillary treatment in the management of patients with early breast cancer. Breast Cancer Res Treat. 2006;95 (3):279-93.
4. Langer I, Guller U, Berclaz G, et al. Morbidity of sentinel lymph node biopsy (SLN) alone versus SLN and completion axillary lymph node dissection after breast cancer surgery: a prospective Swiss multicenter study on 659 patients. Ann Surg. 2007;245(3):452-61.
5. Lucci A, McCall LM, Beitsch PD, et al. American College of Surgeons Oncology Group. Surgical complications associated with sentinel lymph node dissection (SLND) plus axillary lymph node dissection compared with SLND alone in the American College of Surgeons Oncology Group Trial Z0011. J Clin Oncol. 2007;25(24):3657-63.
6. Veronesi U, Paganelli G, Viale G, et al. A randomized comparison of sentinel-node biopsy with routine axillary dissection in breast cancer. N Engl J Med. 2003;349(6):546-53.
7. Wilke LG, McCall LM, Posther KE, et al. Surgical complications associated with sentinel lymph node biopsy: Results from a prospective international cooperative group trial. Ann Surg Oncol. 2006;13(4):491-500.
8. Brorson H, Ohlin K, Olsson G, et al. Quality of life following liposuction and conservative treatment of arm lymphoedema. Lymphology. 2006;39(1):8-25.
9. Suami H, Chang DW. Overview of surgical treatments for breast cancer-related lymphedema. Plast Reconstr Surg. 2010;126(6):1853-63.
10. Baumeister RG, Siuda S. Treatment of lymphedemas by microsurgical lymphatic grafting: what is proved? Plast Reconstr Surg. 1990;85(1):64-74.
11. Ho LC, Lai MF, Kennedy PJ. Micro-lymphatic bypass in the treatment of obstructive lymphoedema of the arm: case report of a new technique. Br J Plast Surg. 1983;36(3): 350-7.
12. Kleinhans E, Baumeister RG, Hahn D, et al. Evaluation of transport kinetics in lymphoscintigraphy: Follow-up study in patients with transplanted lymphatic vessels. Eur J Nucl Med. 1985;10(7-8):349-52.
13. Yamamoto Y, Sugihara T. Microsurgical lymphaticovenous implantation for the treatment of chronic lymphedema. Plast Reconstr Surg. 1998;101(1):157-61.
14. O'Brien BM, Sykes P, Threlfall GN, et al. Microlymphaticovenous anastomoses for obstructive lymphedema. Plast Reconstr Surg. 1977;60(2):197-211.
15. O'Brien BM, Mellow CG, Khazanchi RK, et al. Long-term results after microlymphaticovenous anastomoses for the treatment of obstructive lymphedema. Plast Reconstr Surg. 1990;85(4):562-72.
16. Koshima I, Inagawa K, Urushibara K, et al. Supermicrosurgical lymphaticovenular anastomosis for the treatment of lymphedema in the upper extremities. J Reconstr Microsurg. 2000;16(6):437-42.
17. Chang DW. Lymphaticovenular bypass for lymphedema management in breast cancer patients: a prospective study. Plast Reconstr Surg. 2010;126(3):752-8.
18. Becker C, Assouad J, Riquet M, et al. Postmastectomy lymphedema: long-term results following microsurgical lymph node transplantation. Ann Surg. 2006;243(3): 313-15.
19. Lin CH, Ali R, Chen SC, et al. Vascularized groin lymph node transfer using the wrist as a recipient site for management of postmastectomy upper extremity lymphedema. Plast Reconstr Surg. 2009;123(4):1265-75.
20. Brorson H, Ohlin K, Olsson G, et al. Adipose tissue dominates chronic arm lymphedema following breast cancer: an analysis using volume rendered CT images. Lymphat Res Biol. 2006;4(4):199-210.
21. O'Brien BM, Khazanchi RK, Kumar PA, et al. Liposuction in the treatment of lymphoedema: a preliminary report. Br J Plast Surg. 1989:42(5);530.
22. Brorson H. Liposuction in arm lymphedema treatment. Scand J Surg. 2003;92(4):287-95 Review.
23. Brorson H, Svensson H. Complete reduction of lymphoedema of the arm by liposuction after breast cancer. Scand J Plast Reconstr Surg Hand Surg. 1997;31(2);137-43.
24. Brorson H, Svensson H. Liposuction combined with controlled compression therapy reduces arm lymphoedema more effectively than controlled compression therapy alone. Plast Reconstr Surg. 1998;102(4);1058-67.
25. Damstra RJ, Voesten HG, Klinkert P, et al. Circumferential suction-assisted lipectomy for lymphoedema after surgery for breast cancer. Br J Surg. 2009;96(8):859-64.

26. Brorson H, Svensson H, Norrgren K, et al. Liposuction reduces arm lymphedema without significantly altering the already impaired lymph transport. Lymphology. 1998; 31(4):156-72.
27. Frick A, Hoffmann JN, Baumeister RG, et al. Liposuction technique and lymphatic lesions in lower legs: anatomic study to reduce risks. Plast Reconstr Surg. 1999;103(7): 1868-73.
28. Stanton A, Modi S, Mellor R, et al. Diagnosing cancer related lymphoedema in the arm. J Lymphoedema. 2006; 1(1):12-15.
29. Sander AP, Hajer NM, Hemenway K, et al. Upper-extremity volume measurements in women with lymphedema: a comparison of measurements obtained via water displacement with geometrically determined volume. Phys Ther. 2002;82(12):1202-12.
30. Brorson H, Ohlin K, Olsson G, et al. Breast cancer-related chronic arm lymphedema is associated with excess adipose and muscle tissue. Lymphat Res Biol. 2009;7(1):3-10.
31. Viitanen TP, Mäki MT, Seppänen MP, et al. Donor-site lymphatic function after microvascular lymph node transfer. Plast Reconstr Surg. 2012;130(6):1246-53.
32. Vignes S, Blanchard M, Yannoutsos A, et al. Complications of autologous lymph-node transplantation for limb lymphoedema. Eur J Vasc Endovasc Surg. 2013;45(5): 516-20.
33. Crosby MA, Card A, Liu J, et al. Immediate breast reconstruction and lymphedema incidence. Plast Reconstr Surg. 2012;129(5):789e-95e.
34. Blanchard M, Arrault M, Vignes S. Positive impact of delayed breast reconstruction on breast-cancer treatment-related arm lymphoedema. J Plast Reconstr Aesthet Surg. 2012;65(8):1060-3.
35. Abbas Khan MA, Mohan A, Hardwicke J, et al. Objective improvement in upper limb lymphoedema following ipsilateral latissimus dorsi pedicled flap breast reconstruction—a case series and review of literature. J Plast Reconstr Aesthet Surg. 2011;64(5):680-4.

Section
3

Head and Neck

Chapter Outline

- Vaser-Assisted Minimally Invasive Neck–Chin Lift
- Endoscopically Assisted Temporalis Muscle Transfer Harvesting for Orbit Reconstruction
- Augmentation Rhinoplasty
- Total Resection of the Alar Cartilages and Temporal Fascia Technique in Rhinoplasty
- Correction of Auricular Deformities after Failed Otoplasty
- Focal Nerve Lesions with a Monopolar Radiofrequency Device for Cosmetic Enhancement

3 Vaser-Assisted Minimally Invasive Neck–Chin Lift

Alberto Di Giuseppe, George Commons

GUIDELINES FOR VASER-ASSISTED NECK CONTOURING

Vaser-assisted neck contouring should only be performed by surgeons experienced with the Vaser system for fatty tissue emulsification. At least 10 cases of standard Vaser-assisted lipoplasty are recommended before moving to application to the face and neck.

Indications include patients seeking contouring of the neck and jowl areas who have heavy neck and/or chins with moderate to good skin tone and where extra volume is expected to be excess fatty tissue (Figs. 3.1A to C).

Informed Consent should include use of photos for educational purposes. Preoperative markings and planning using strategic plan for volume removal (locations) with incisions that are under chin and in front of/behind ears (bilaterally). Possible bilaterally in the neck at the lowest anticipated level of treatment (Fig. 3.2).

TECHNIQUE

Usually the technique is performed under local tumescent anesthesia and IV sedation. The operation is an office procedure.

Infusion

Infusion for the face/neck that has more vascular and more innervations than the typical fat layers in the body. Use epinephrine at 1:500,000 and lidocaine at 0.3–0.5%. The

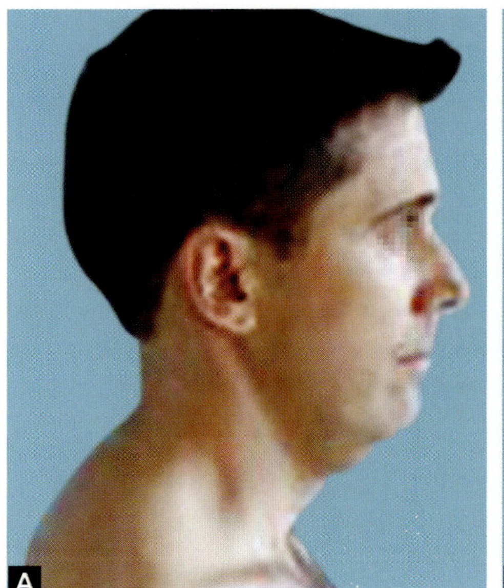

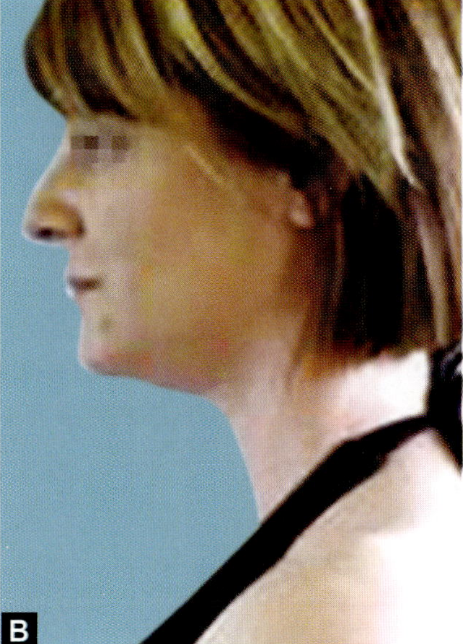

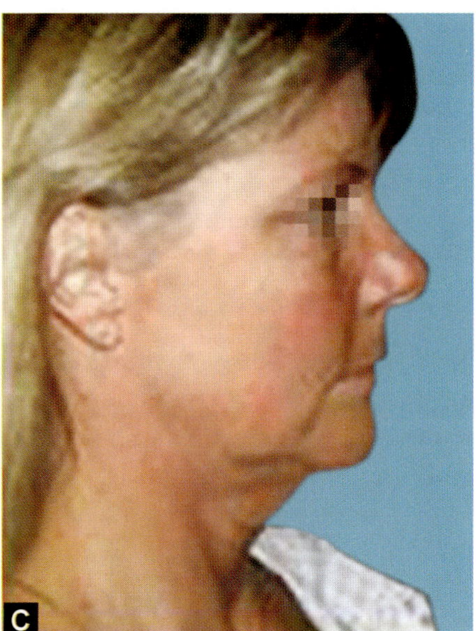

Figs. 3.1A to C: Indicated patients.

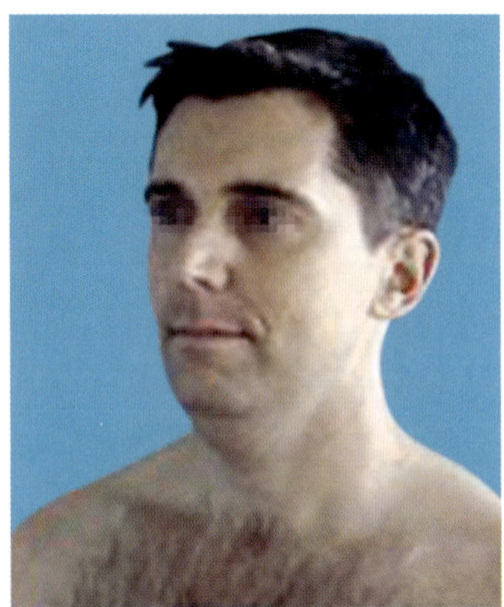

Fig. 3.2: Marking and incisions.

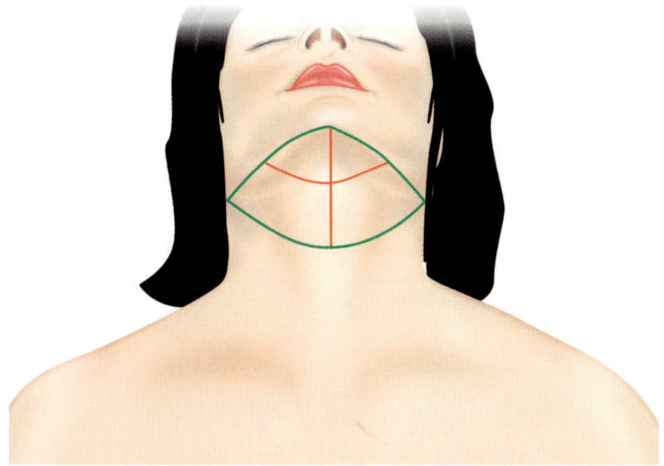

Fig. 3.3: Neck and chin is divided in four subunits. Each allows around 50 mL of tumescent, solution, or less.

neck and chin is divided into four subunits, each of which allows around 50 mL of tumescent infusion (Fig. 3.3). Wait 8–10 minutes (mandatory). Infuse with a small diameter blunt infusion cannula (2.0 mm or smaller, 14 gauge or smaller) and not a needle. Infuse uniformly and evenly into any and all locations where the Vaser or the suction cannula may be used. Typical expected infusion volume is 200–400 mL total (both sides and submental), depending on size of patient and areas to be treated. Infuse slowly at 100 mL/min.

Skin protection used in each incision. Use the black skin ports with the orange silicone discs. Suture the skin port disc into place (three anchor sutures) using 3-0 or 4-0 nylon. Make sure the knots are tight, as the silicone disc tends to cause the knots to unwind. These skin ports protect the incision edges and greatly reduce visible incision scarring. Stretch the incisions and tissues below the incision with a hemostat to ease insertion.

Vaser (Figs. 3.4 to 3.6)

Emulsification with 2.2 mm diameter (17 cm long) or 2.2 mm diameter (8 cm long) probes, 20–40% amplitude, Vaser mode. Begin with the short 2.2 probe if possible: 20% amplitude if face/neck is very soft, 30% amplitude for a moderate/average fat, and move to 40% amplitude if face is fibrous. Never exceed 40% with the 2.2 mm probes, they may break. Apply Vaser until targeted fat is emulsified, likely 2–3 minutes total per side depending on volumes, with an additional 2–3 minutes under the chin depending on how the Vaser was applied on the sides. Total Vaser time 6–10 minutes depending on patient and infused volumes. Try to achieve the targeted 6–10 minutes of Vaser time to minimize aspiration trauma.

Aspiration

Aspiration is with a 2.4 mm cannula with gentle port patterns. Avoid aggressive use of suction. Apply the suction only as long as it takes to remove the emulsified fluids and tissue. Expected aspiration volumes are 25–125 mL depending on infused volume, size of patient, and areas treated. Suction phase should be as short and atraumatic as possible. Remember: it is not what you take out but what you leave behind that is the key to smooth and even skin redraping and retraction. Two small stab incisions are sometimes placed in the lateral aspects of the neck at the lowest point of treatment and left open for drainage purposes. A small suction cannula with no vacuum applied is passed through the stab incisions to open channels into the treated areas.

Massage

Massage/press the treated areas to push any remaining free fluids out incisions.

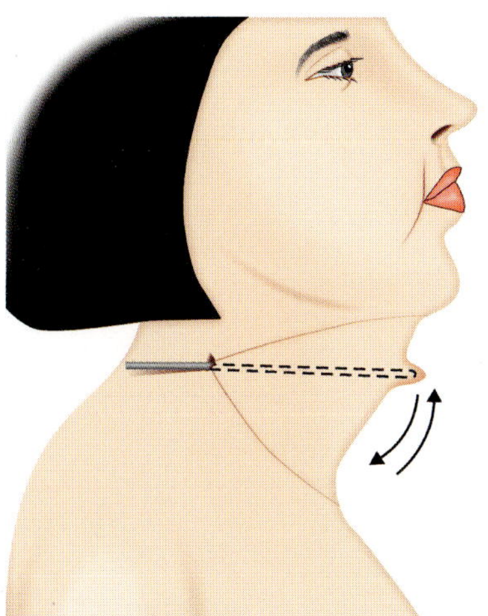

Fig. 3.4: Vaser 2.2 mm in action, set at 30% of power, through ear lobe incision.

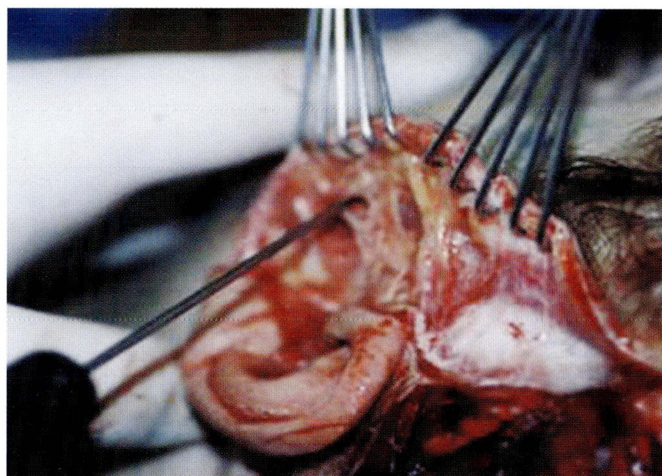

Fig. 3.5: Vaser undermining in a classic facelift.

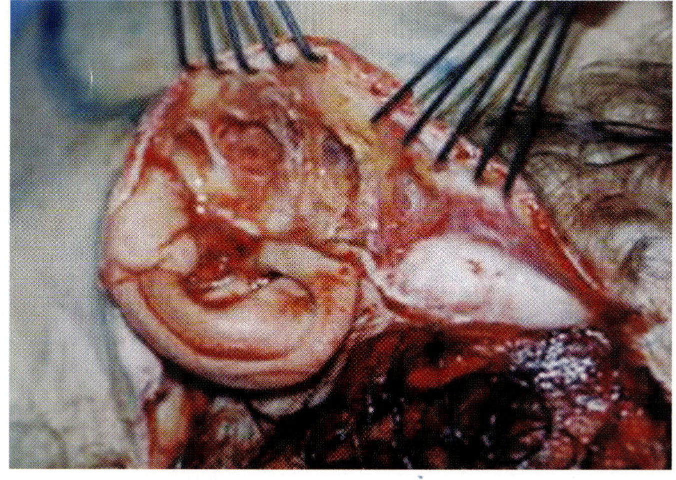

Fig. 3.6: Tunnels as appear after Vaser undermining.

POSTOPERATIVE

Postoperative taping/dressing/support: The key is gentle, even compression to help the skin redrape and settle into position and to prevent ripples or folds in the skin. Consider the following options: cotton pads with elastic wraps, cold compresses, silicone foam padding. Elastic face garments typically applied for 2–4 days, then overnight for 1–2 weeks, depending on preference. Keep head elevated at night.

Follow-up is 1 day, 1 week, 6 weeks, 6 months, as needed. External ultrasound and light massage may be beneficial. Protocol for external ultrasound: setting of 10 W for 5 minutes with small head, twice a week for minimum of 3 weeks.

PROCEDURE (FIGS. 3.7A TO Q)

Figure 3.8 is a 50-year-old patient, with heavy neck, heavy chin, lack of cheek definition, neck laxity, upper and lower blepharochalasis. Markings are shown and the procedure detailed in the photos.

CLINICAL CASES

See Figures (3.8 to 3.22).

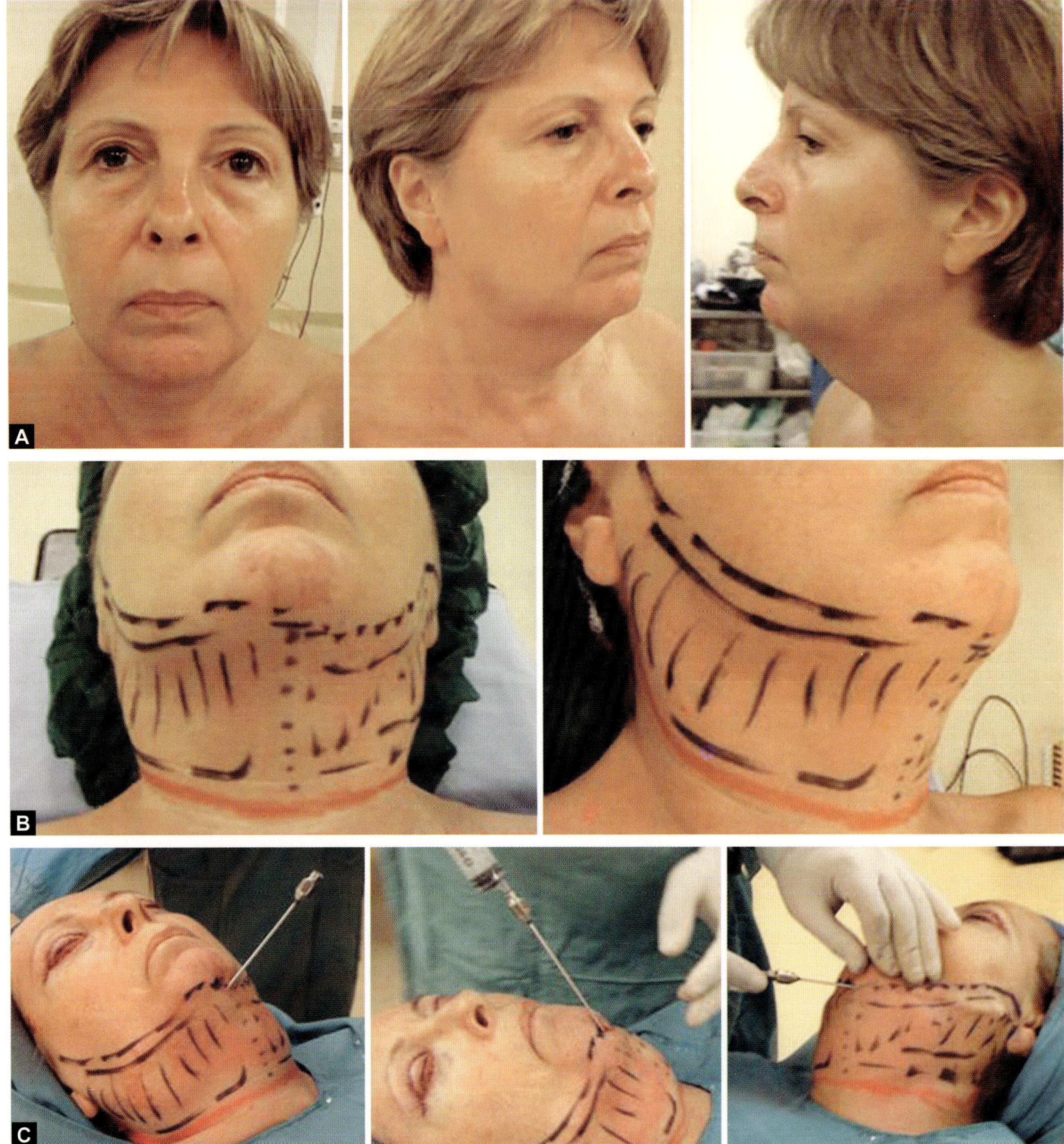

Figs. 3.7A to C: (A) Preoperative 50-year-old patient, with heavy neck, heavy chin, lack of cheek definition, neck laxity, upper and lower blepharochalasis. (B) Preoperative markings. Red lines show lower limits of neck clavicle undermining. Black lines show upper limits of Vaser undermining. Dotted lines show center of neck. (C) Tumescent infiltration with blunt needle and syringe.

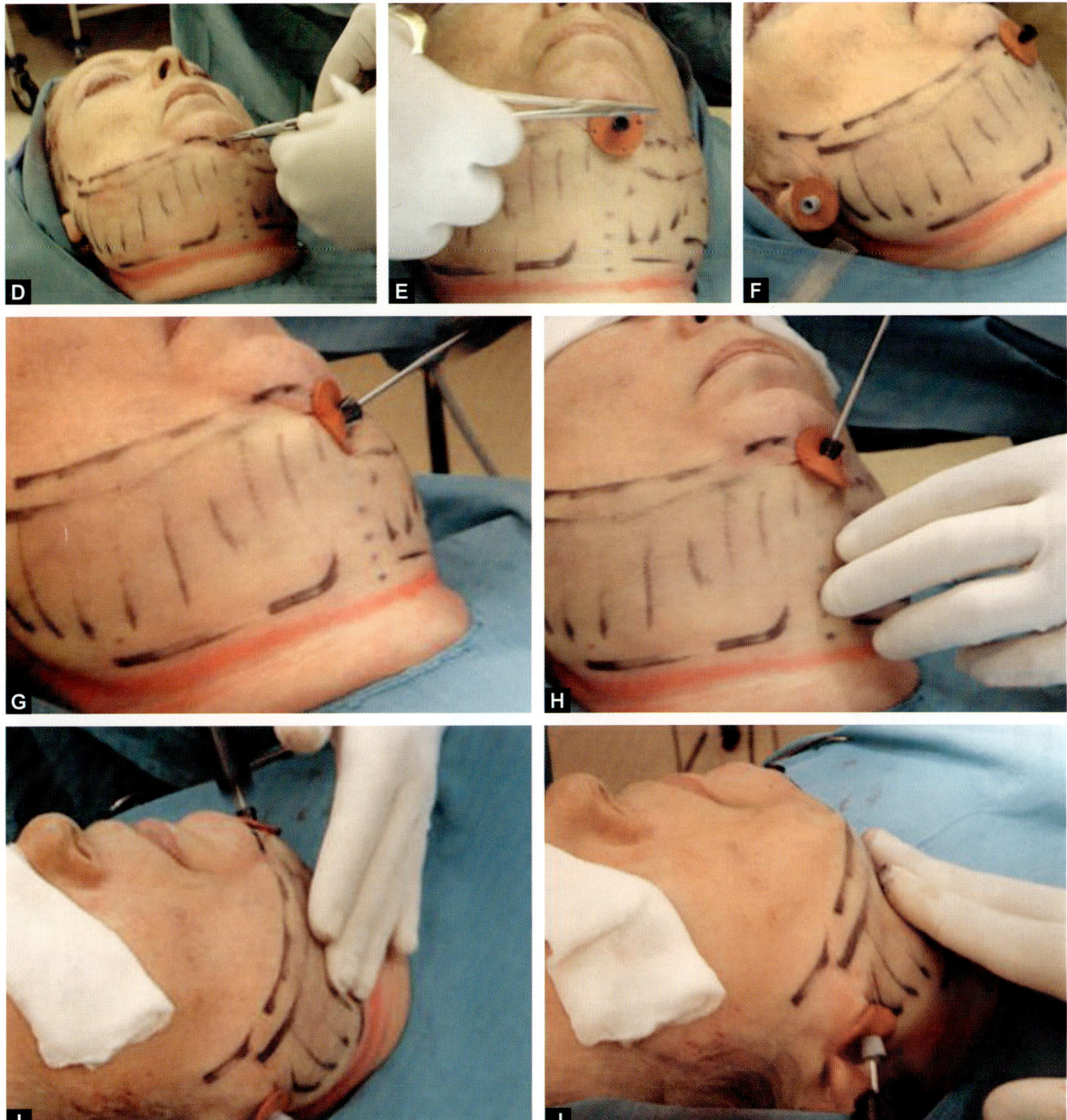

Figs. 3.7D to J: (D) Temporary suture of chin incision to avoid fluid reflow. (E) Suturing on place skin protector. (F) Other skin protector at the ear lobe incision. (G) After 11 minutes, the surgeon starts Vaser 2.2 mm probe undermining on the superficial layer. Power is set at 30% of total. (H) Vaser on action from chin incision on the deeper layer, to emulsify fat. (I) Right hand guides the probe, while left hand controls depth of action. Movements have to be gentle, avoiding too deep action. (J) Threading the lateral side.

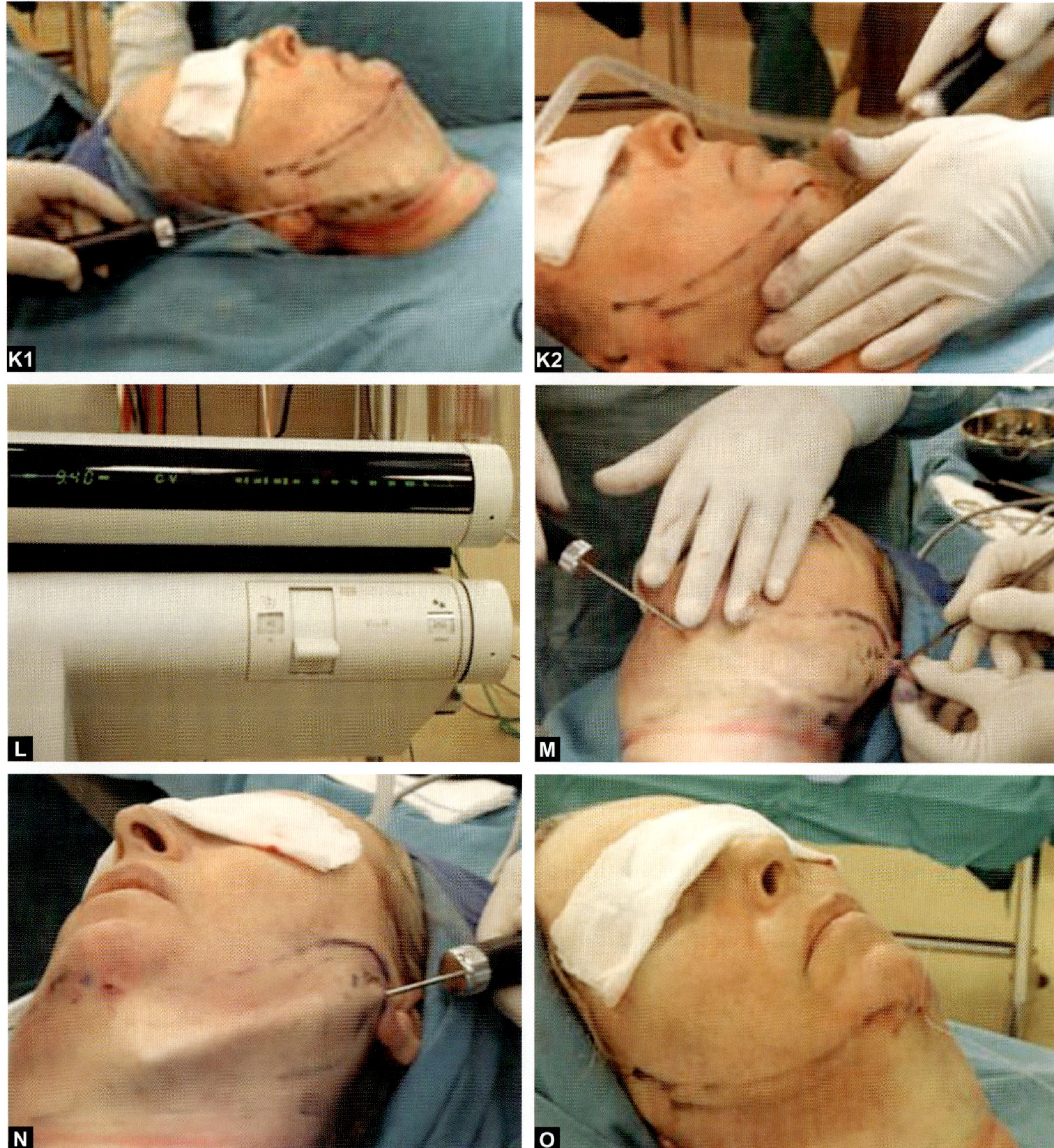

Figs. 3.7K to O: (K) Using Ventex 1.8 mm suction cannula to evacuate emulsion. (L) Vaser system. Timing: 9.40 minutes of action. (M) Completing aspiration, removing skin adhesion, checking undermining and free skin. (N) Checking thickness of the neck flap. (O) Procedure completed.

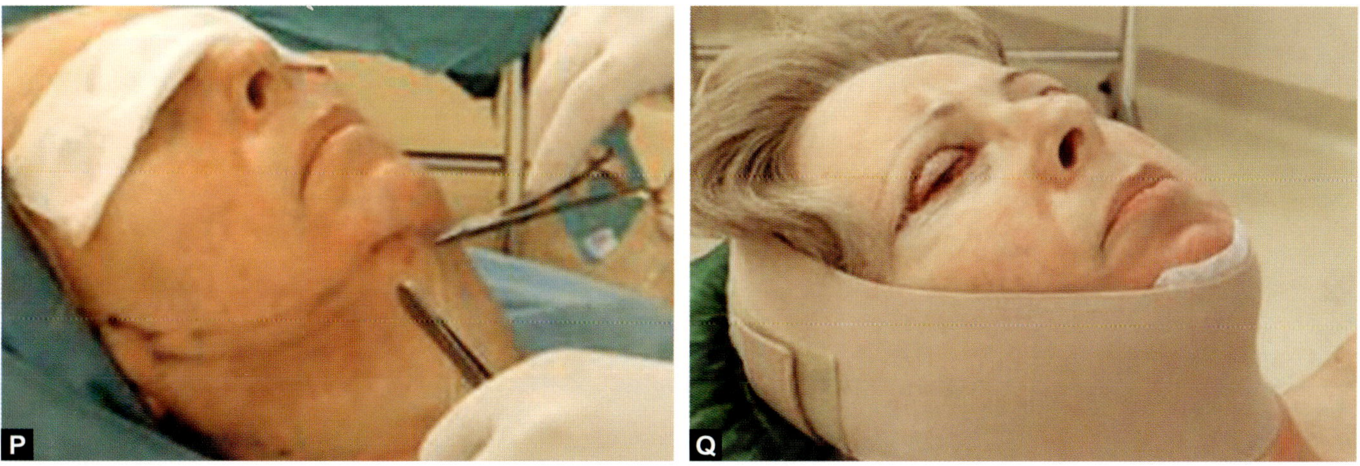

Figs. 3.7P and Q: (P) Suture of skin incision with 6-0 nylon. (Q) Postoperative garment to be worn 3 days full time and then for 2 weeks night-time.

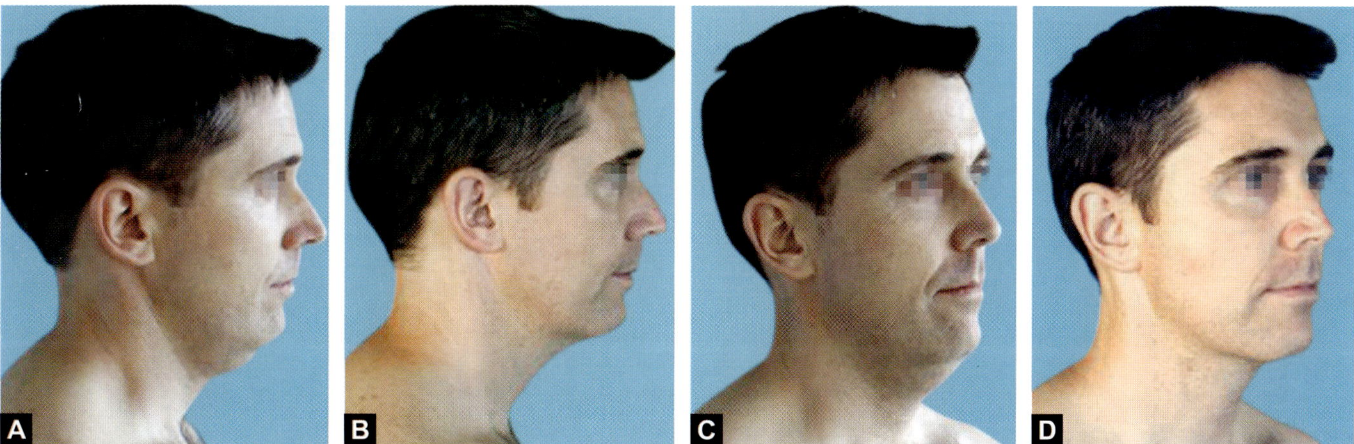

Figs. 3.8A to D: (A and C) Preoperative 38-year-old male. (B and D) Postoperative following jowl-chin-neck contouring.

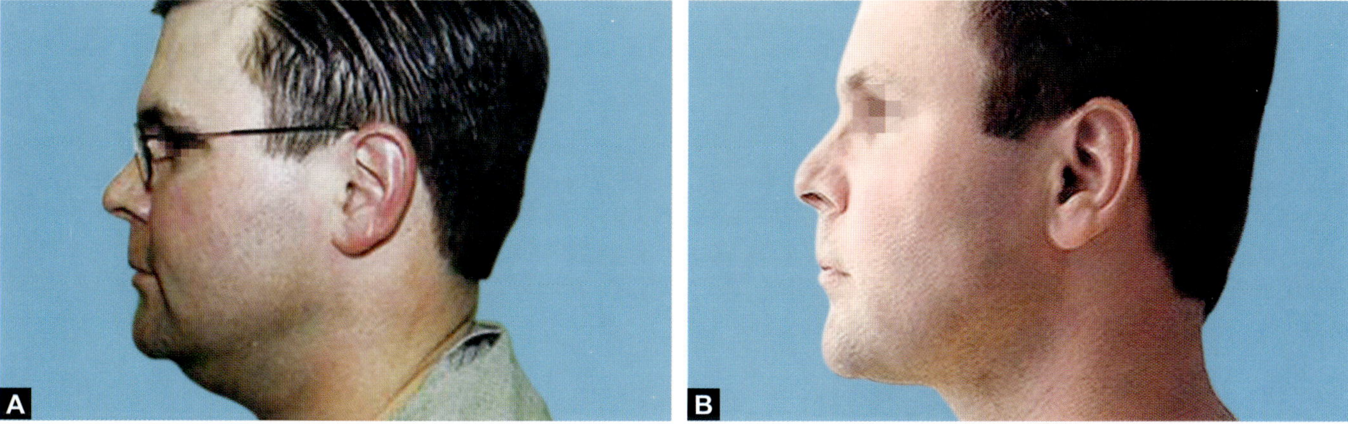

Figs. 3.9A and B: (A) Preoperative 42-year-old male. (B) Postoperative after jowl-chin-neck contouring.

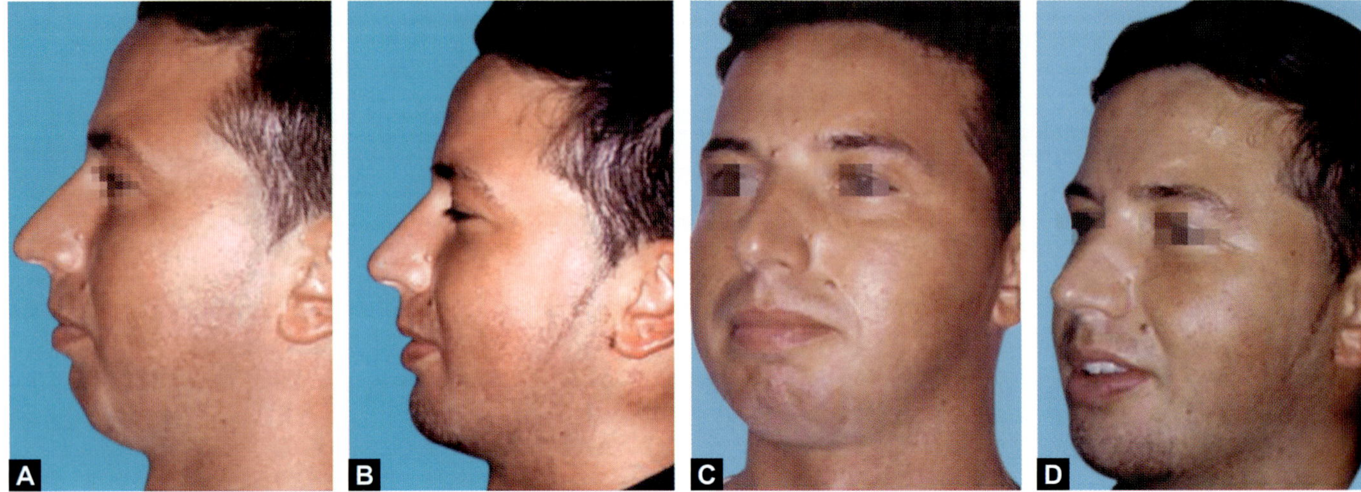

Figs. 3.10A to D: (A and C) Preoperative 27-year-old male. (B and D) Postoperative following jowl-chin-neck contouring.

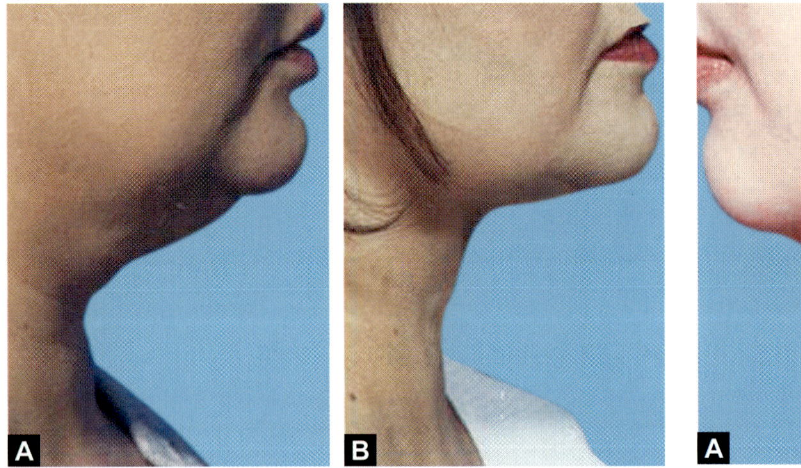

Figs. 3.11A and B: (A) Preoperative 45-year-old female. (B) Postoperative after neck-jowl-chin contouring.

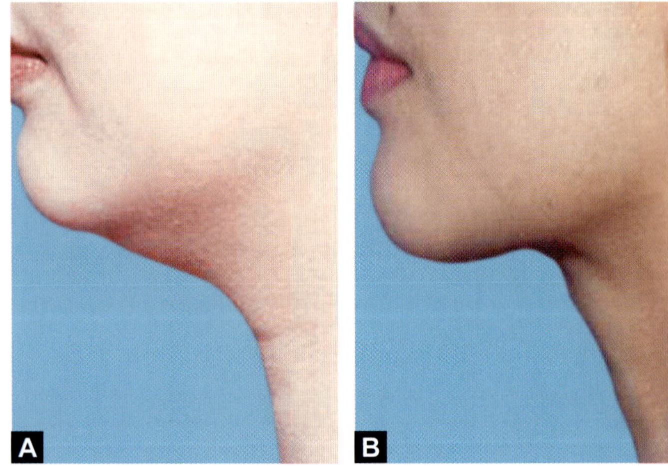

Figs. 3.12A and B: (A) Preoperative 38-year-old female. (B) Postoperative after neck Vaser.

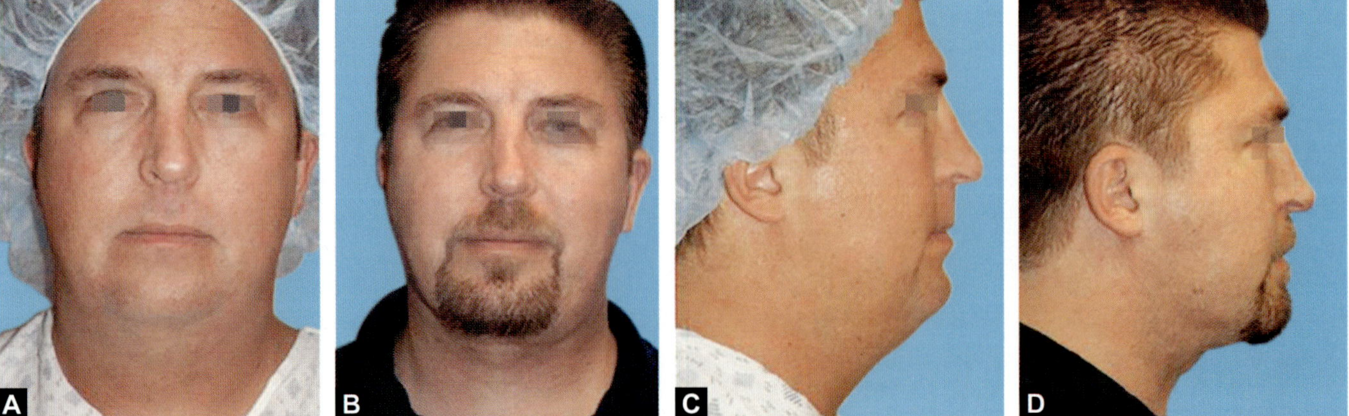

Figs. 3.13A to D: (A and C) Preoperative 50-year-old male. (B and D) Postoperative following neck Vaser.

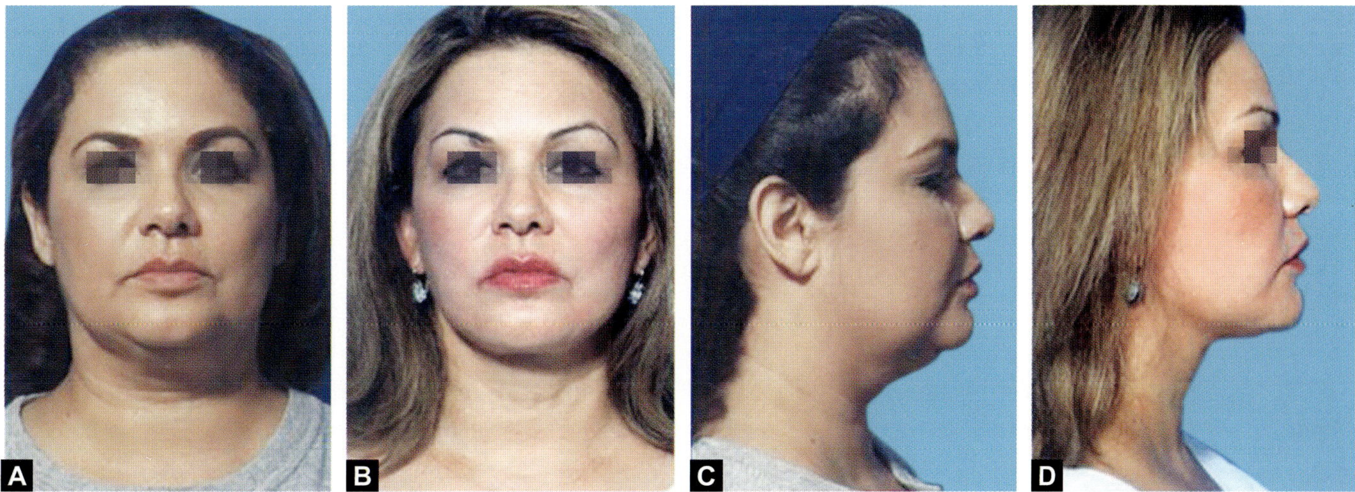

Figs. 3.14A to D: (A and C) Preoperative 46-year-old female. (B and D) Postoperative after neck Vaser.

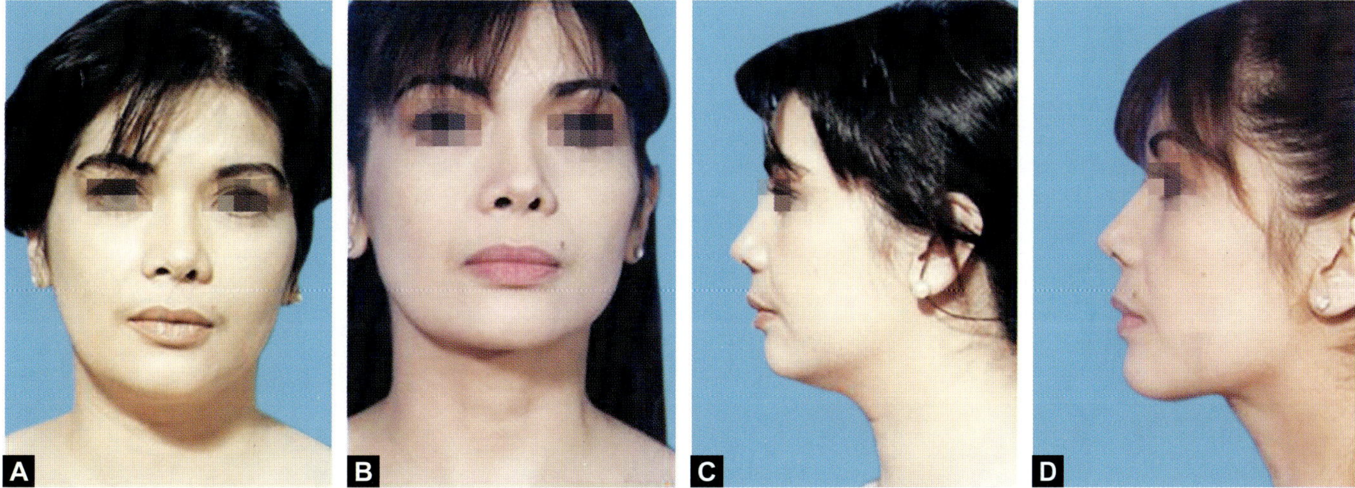

Figs. 3.15A to D: (A and C) Preoperative 35-year-old female. (B and D) Postoperative following neck Vaser.

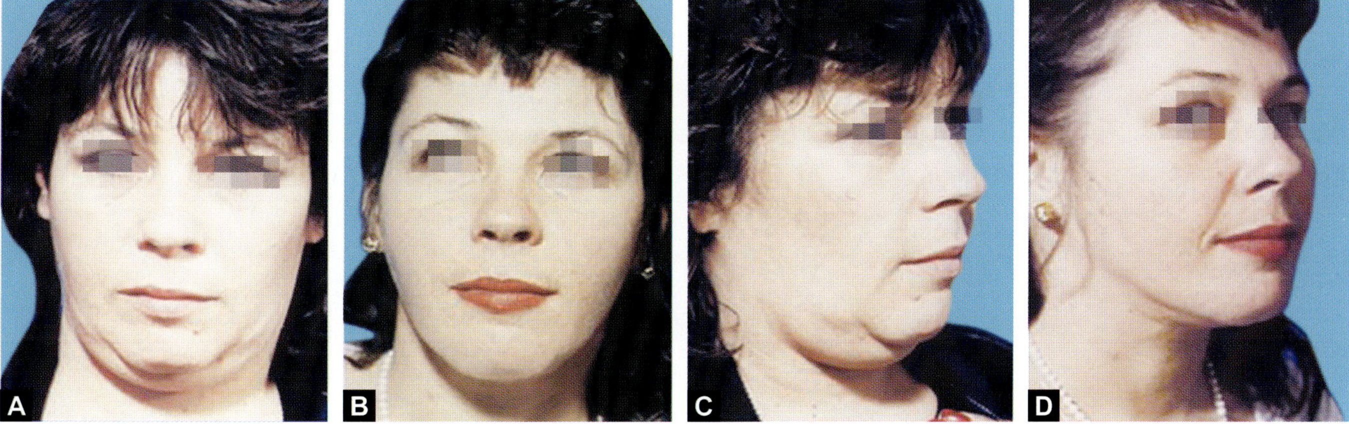

Figs. 3.16A to D

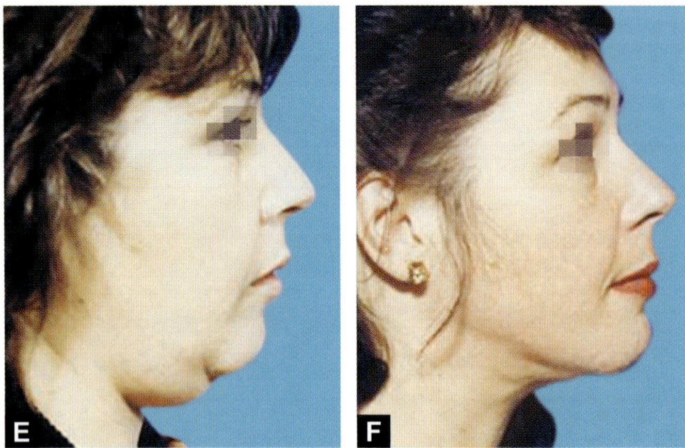

Figs. 3.16A to F: (A, C and E) Preoperative 40-year-old female. (B, D and F) Postoperative after neck Vaser.

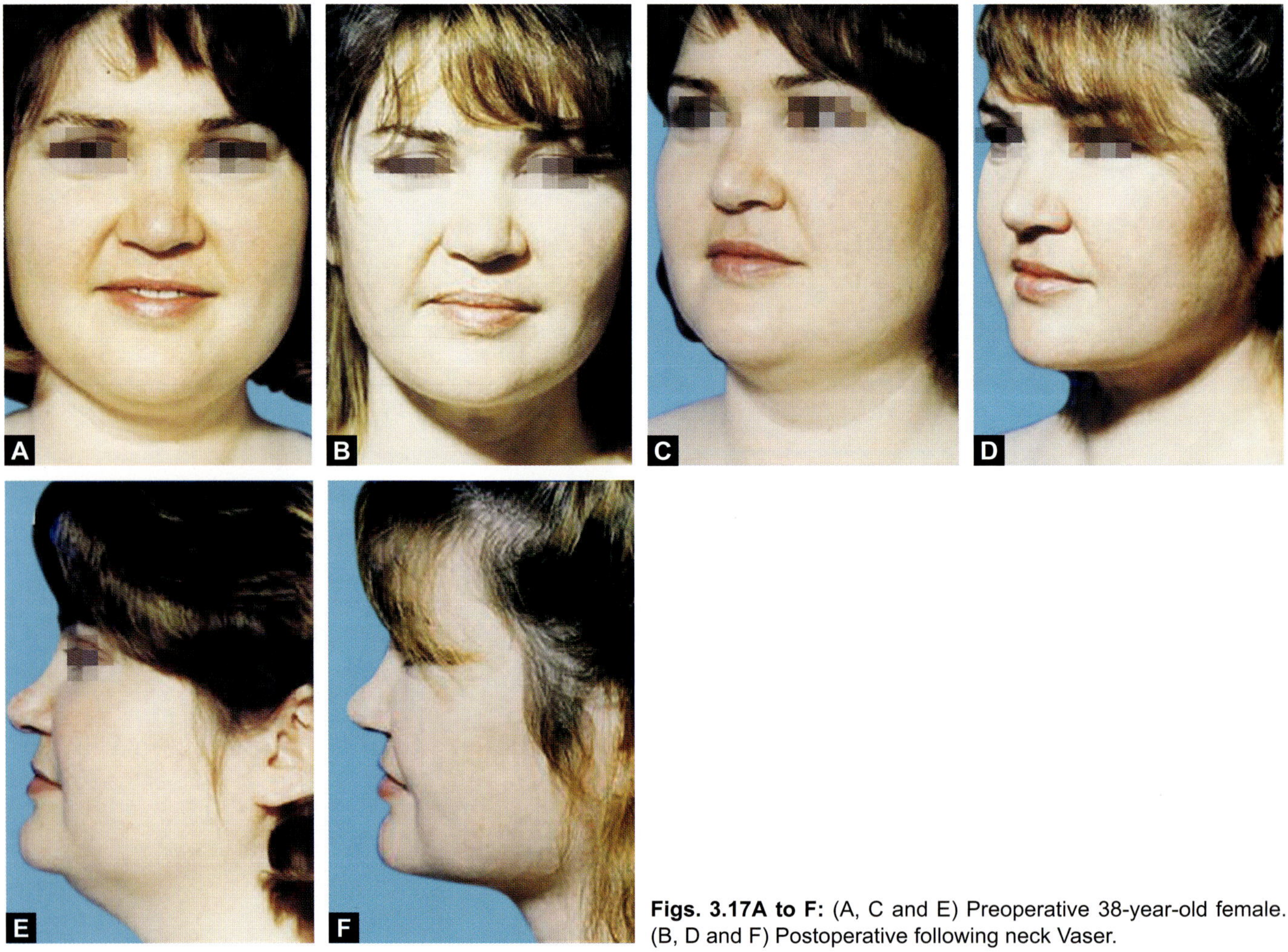

Figs. 3.17A to F: (A, C and E) Preoperative 38-year-old female. (B, D and F) Postoperative following neck Vaser.

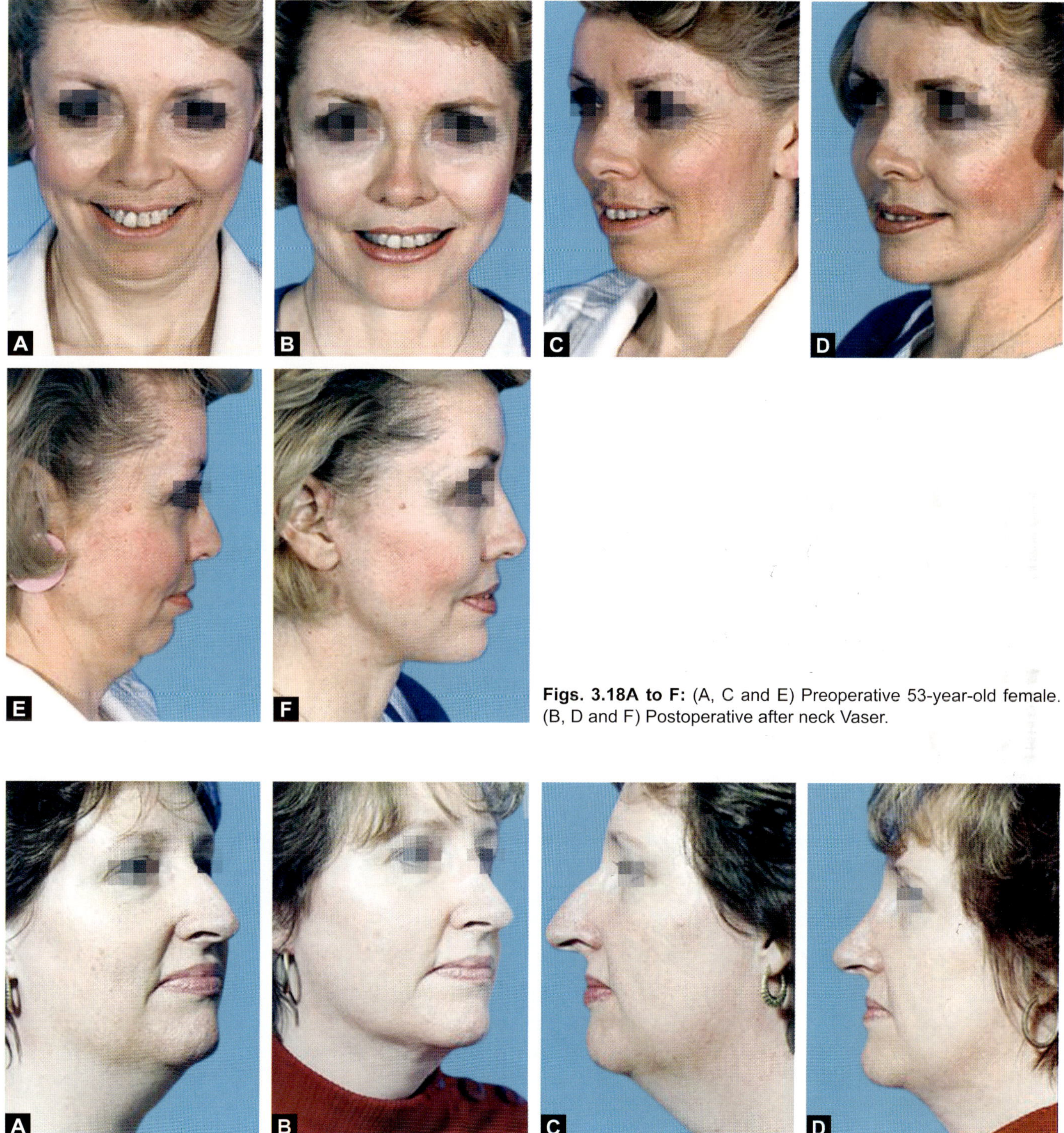

Figs. 3.18A to F: (A, C and E) Preoperative 53-year-old female. (B, D and F) Postoperative after neck Vaser.

Figs. 3.19A to D: (A and C) Preoperative 45-year-old female. (B and D) Postoperative following neck Vaser.

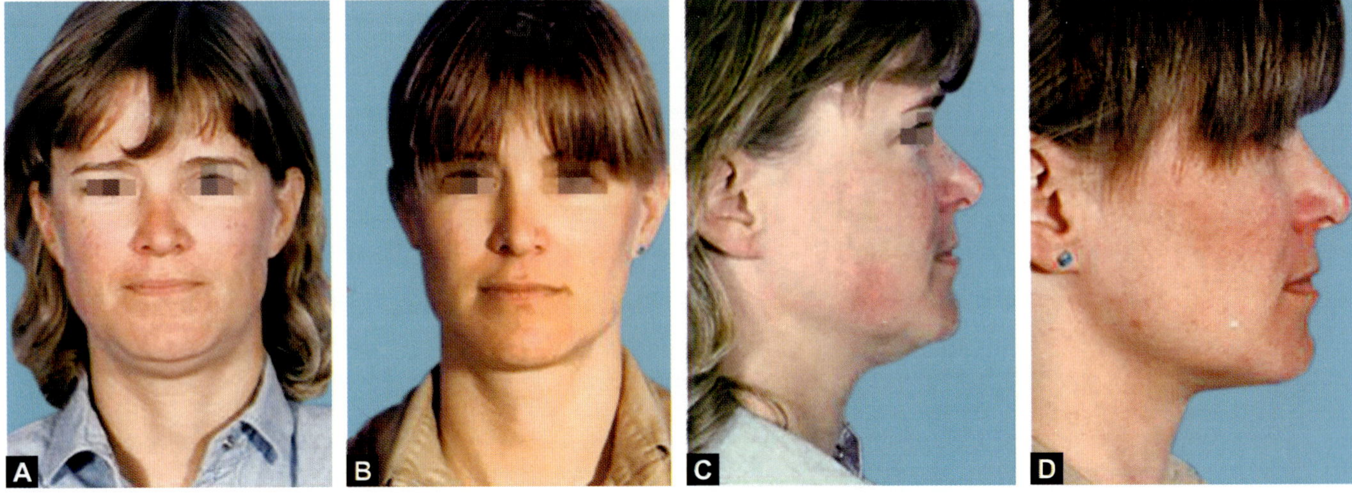

Figs. 3.20A to D: (A and C) Preoperative 42-year-old female. (B and D) Postoperative after neck Vaser.

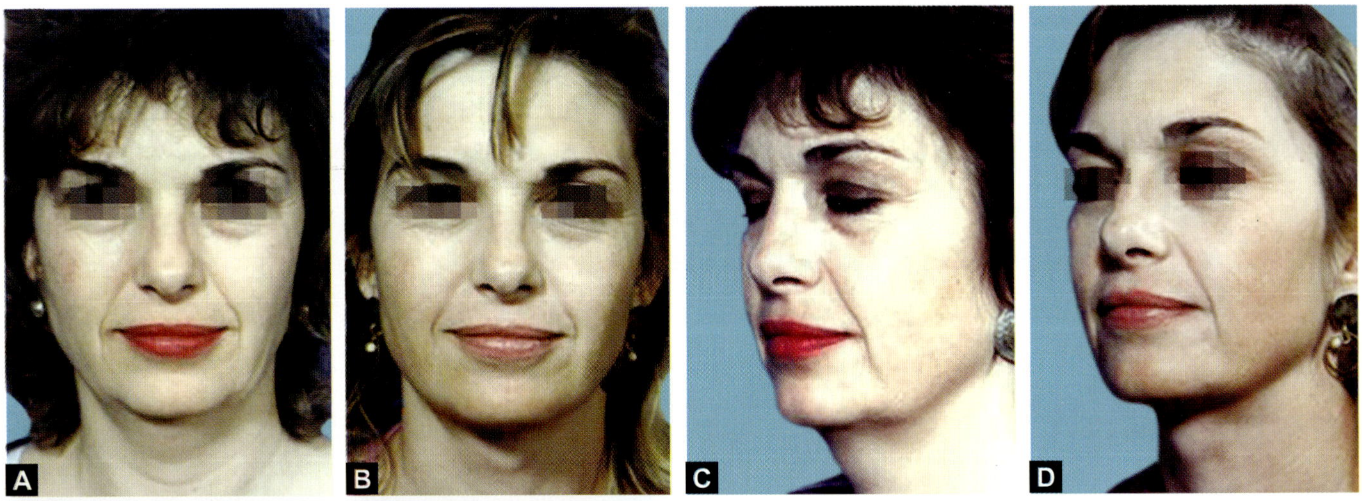

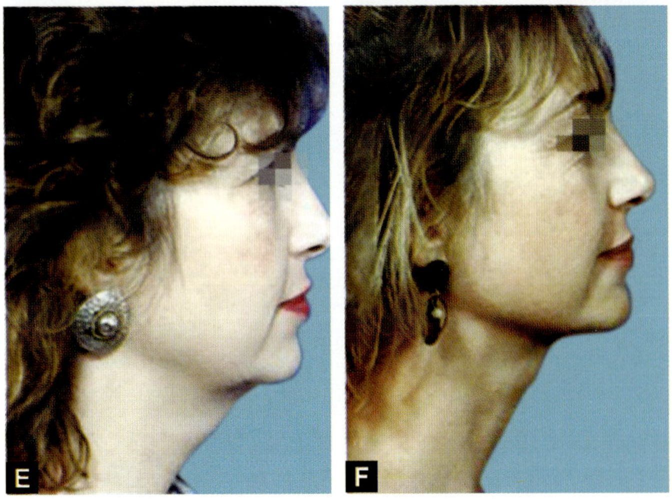

Figs. 3.21A to F: (A, C and E) Preoperative 48-year-old female. (B, D and F) Postoperative following neck Vaser.

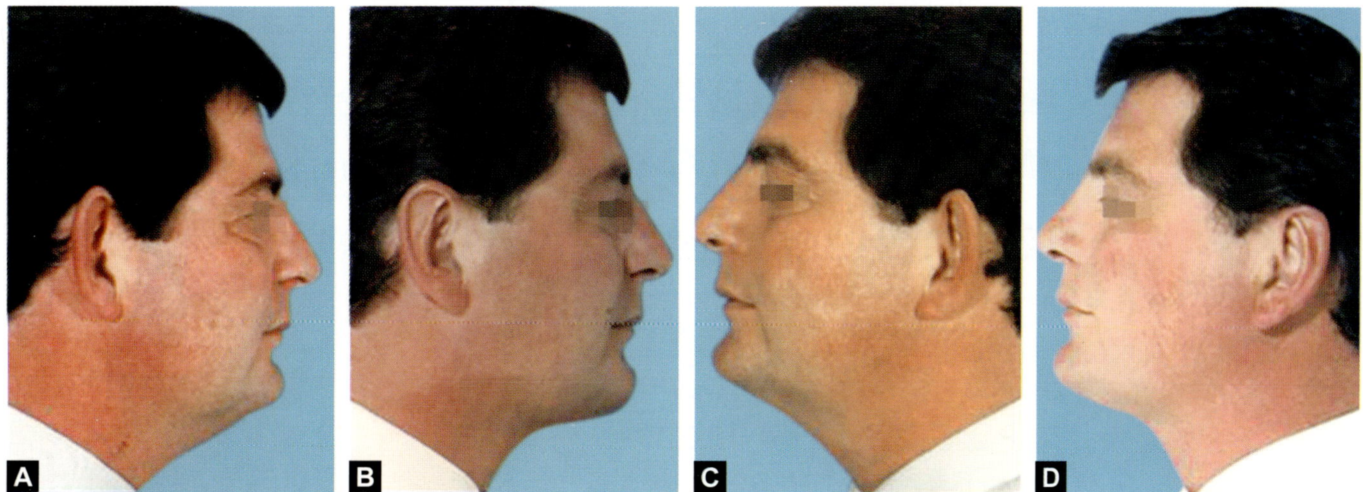

Figs. 3.22A to D: (A and C) Preoperative 58-year-old male. (B and D) Postoperative after neck Vaser.

BIBLIOGRAPHY

1. Shiffman MA, Di Giuseppe A. Body Contouring, Art, Science and Clinical Practice. Berlin: Springer; 2010.
2. Shiffman MA, Di Giuseppe A. Cosmetic Surgery, Art and Techniques. Berlin: Springer; 2013.
3. Shiffman MA, Di Giuseppe A. Liposuction, Principles and Practice. Berlin: Springer; 2006.

4 Endoscopically Assisted Temporalis Muscle Transfer Harvesting for Orbit Reconstruction

Riccardo Girotto, Marco Messi, Paolo Balercia

INTRODUCTION

The temporalis muscle flap (TMF) is a workhorse in our daily surgical practice of head and neck/reconstructive surgeons.[1-8] Its main address is to reconstruct the orbital content (where removed for oncological reasons) and the upper jaw. Some authors recommend its use in retromolar trigone cancer reconstruction, but we believe that contraindications and sequelae are worse than benefits, since mouth opening can become less and less during the time with fibrotization of the flap and muscular necrosis can increase the intraoral wound healing time.

Nowadays surgery has increased its possibilities becoming less invasive and aggressive. Endoscopy gives to the surgeon the opportunity to reach otherwise difficulty reachable anatomical structures and perform the operation with great respect to nearer anatomical structures.

It is so possible to dissect the temporalis muscle without impairment of the frontalis branch of the facial nerve, with minimal periosteum elevation, and thus respect of the facial "danger zones".

With the endotechnique there is preservation of the sensory nerves and the rate of postsurgical alopecia is less. There is less numbness, less blood loss, and less recovery time. The surgical time is also shorter and the procedure can be easily applied to bald patients.[9]

It is not possible to not considerate the disadvantages. Those are represented by a higher difficulty level; the accuracy of the operation is operator and instrument dependent. The procedure is new and requires a new understanding of the surgery itself.

ANATOMICAL BASIS

The temporalis muscle is a fan-shaped muscle on the lateral skull, filling the entire temporal fossa. It passes under the zygomatic arch to insert onto the coronoid process and the anterior aspect of the ramus of the mandible (Fig. 4.1).

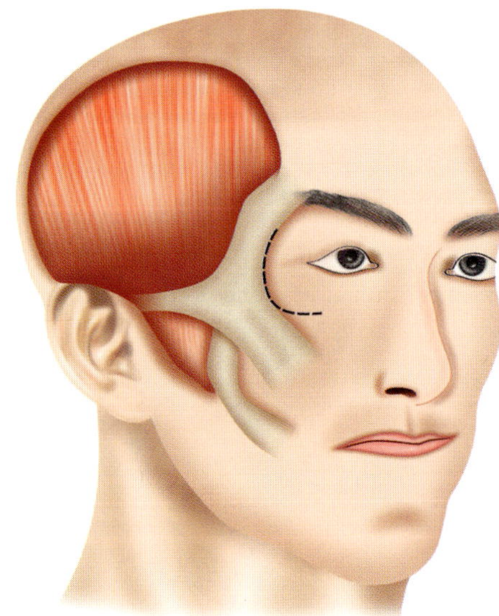

Fig. 4.1: Temporalis muscle flap.

The TMF has a type III pattern of circulation. The dominant pedicles are the anterior and posterior deep temporal arteries and venae comitantes. These arteries arise from the internal maxillary artery that is a branch of the external carotid artery. The vascular pedicle enters the muscle at its undersurface.

The average size of the temporalis muscle is approximately 10 × 20 cm and has its pivot at the level of the coronoid insertion/origin of the temporalis vessels from the maxillary artery.[10,11]

SURGICAL TECHNIQUE

Endoscopy has completely changed the approach to this surgery since it reduces damages to temporal "zones of

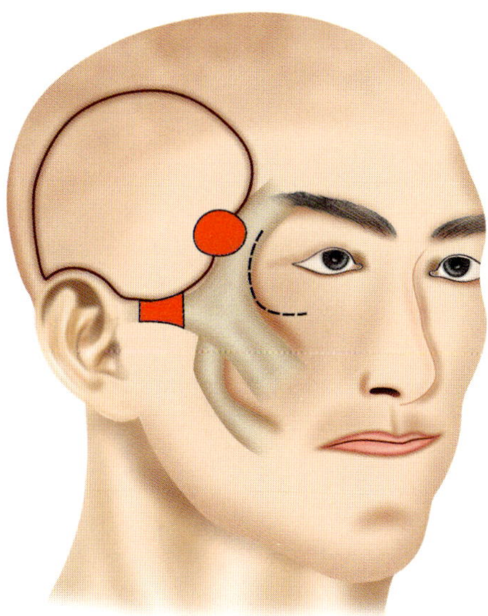

Fig. 4.2: Danger zones.

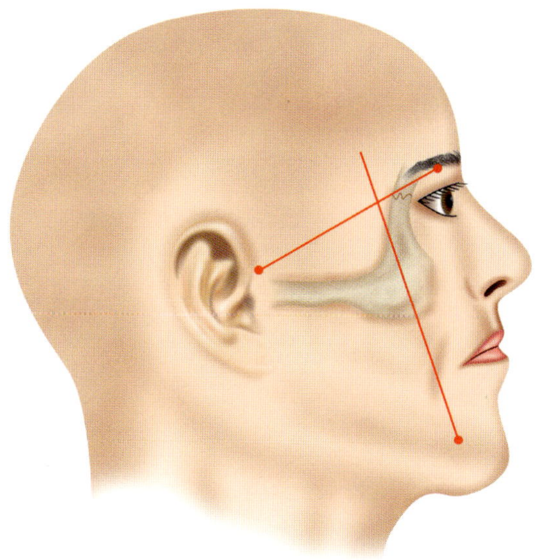

Fig. 4.3: Relationship between facial nerve and sentinel vein.

caution" (Fig. 4.2). This concept was introduced by different authors and well explained by Trinei and Nahai in 1997.[12]

The zone of caution comes from the direct dissection and visualization of a consistent relationship between the temporal branch of the facial nerve and the sentinel vein. The temporal branch comes from the main trunk immediately caudal to the zygomatic arch approximately 1.5 cm in front of the tragus, crossing the arch approximately 2.5 cm in front of the anterior border of the external auditory meatus.[12]

Hinderer et al.[13] have described the midpoint of the line between the helix and the lateral canthus as being external Landmark where the temporal branch crosses the zygomatic arch.

The temporal division courses within or immediately deep to the temporoparietal fascia and after crossing the zygomatic arch curves forward to enter the deep surface of the frontalis muscle approximately 2 cm above the level of the eyebrow.[14]

De la Plaza et al.[15] described perforating vessels in the temporal region and piercing the temporalis fascia. He named these the "sentinel vessels of the lateral wall of the orbit". This vein is located 5 mm lateral to the frontozygomatic suture line and is a tributary of the internal maxillary vein draining the temporal region. Its location relative to fixed skeletal landmarks correspond with the intersection point of a line drawn from the supraorbital notch to the base of the zygoma, and another line passing from the mental foramen to the angle formed by the superior border of the zygoma and the lateral orbital rim (Fig. 4.3).

All of these concepts reduce their importance in the case of the endoscopic approach: the dissection is deeper to any important vascular or nervous structure because performed in the virtual space between the deeper temporal fascia and superficial temporal fascia. It is recommended as the first surgical maneuver to identify immediately the deeper temporal fascia and elevate all the soft tissues lying above with a large elevator. If the surgical space is correct this action is incredibly fast and bloodless and does not require any force (Fig. 4.4).

The harvesting of the TMF is the same for orbital and maxillary reconstruction. The only difference is the transposition of the flap that is passed through a bony hole in the lateral part of the orbit for orbital reconstruction or below the zygomatic arch if used for maxillary reconstruction. The infiltration of a solution of lidocaine 2% with adrenaline 1:100.000 only on the incision site that are limited to two 2 cm incision, the first in the parietal region, approximately 2–3 cm behind the hairline in a vertical fashion, and a second one 3 cm long in the temporal region, above the auricle and above the zygomatic arch, as a prosecution of a preauricular incision (Fig. 4.5). After the injection of anesthetic solution it is advisable to wait a few minutes to allow the adrenaline to act.

The first incision is the temporal one and the skin is done with a no. 15 steel blade in the way to preserve the hair follicles. The subcutaneous tissue is dissected with

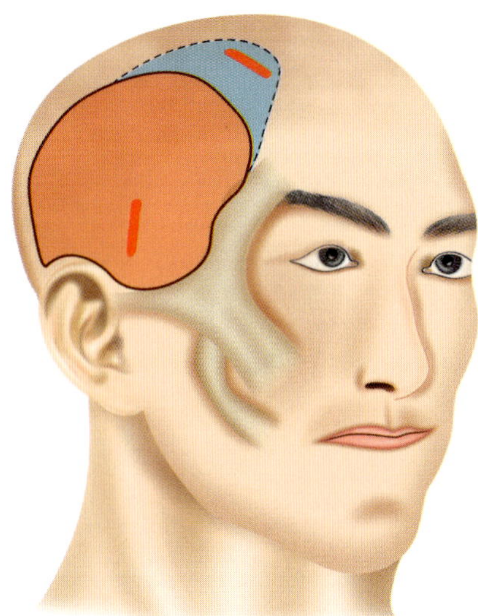

Fig. 4.4: Entity of periosteal elevation (blue) and superficial temporoparietal fascia elevation (red).

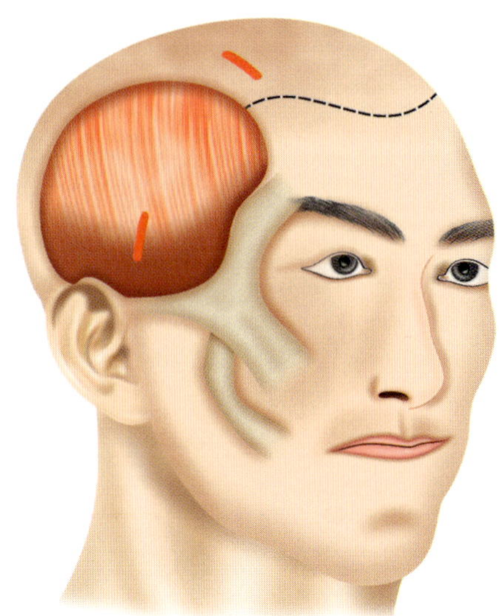

Fig. 4.5: Surgical incisions.

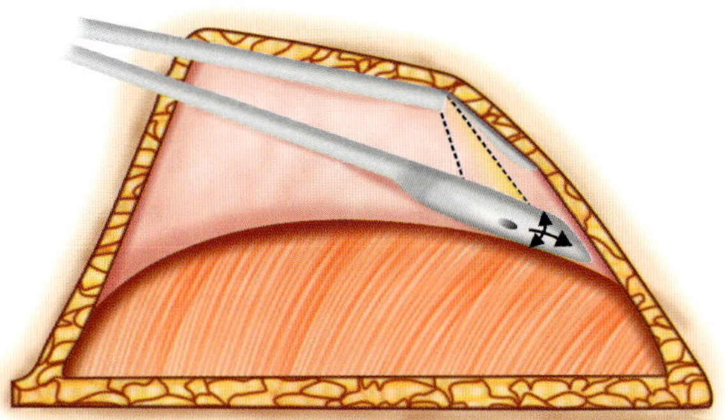

Fig. 4.6: Endoscopic dissection above deep temporal fascia.

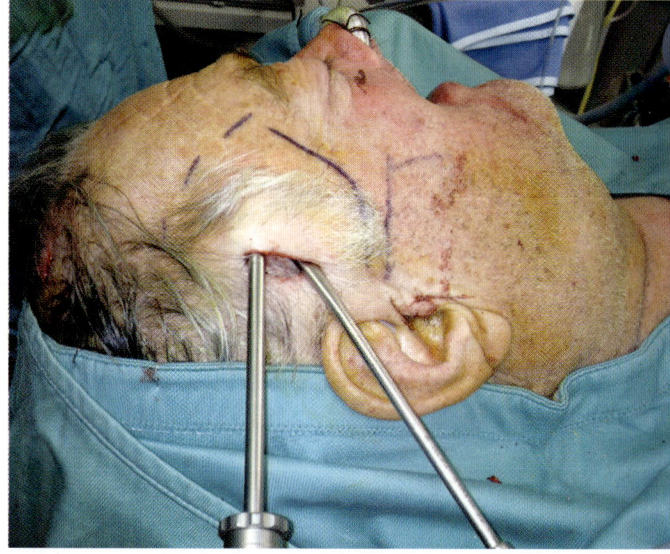

Fig. 4.7: For anterior and upper dissection both instruments are introduced from the same access.

electrocautery to reduce the bleeding since the superficial temporalis fascia is reached. One 5 mm double skin hook is position on each edge of the wound and retracted to enlarge the wound and elevate the skin from the deeper structures. The superficial temporal fascia is incised with a tenotomy scissor, since the deep temporal fascia is encountered. The deep fascia has to be preserved and represent the guide for the first phase of endoscopical dissection. Using a large elevator a blind dissection of the deep temporalis fascia is performed until the temporal crest is identified (Fig. 4.6).

Now the incision in the parietal region is carried out with a no. 15 blade to preserve the hair follicles and electrocautery is used until the bone is identified. The elevator is used to detach the periosteum laterally. A 4-mm 30° endoscope is positioned through the temporal incision.

At this point, it is mandatory to create a unique optical cavity, thus detaching the tissues along the temporal crest. A suction-elevator, like the one used in endoscopic surgery for mandibular condylar fracture, is used to sharply detach the temporalis muscle from its upper and posterior insertion under endoscopic control. The endoscope is positioned through the same temporal hole of the elevator (Fig. 4.7).

The endoscope is then retracted and passed through the parietal access looking downward to the zygomatic

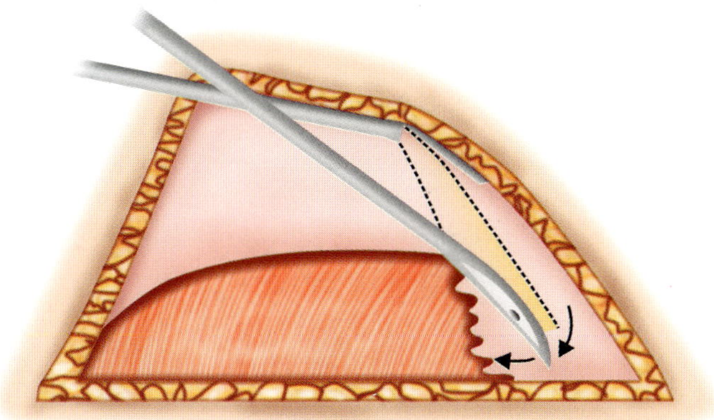

Fig. 4.8: After dissection of the outer part of the temporalis muscle, the elevator detach the temporalis muscle from the temporal bone.

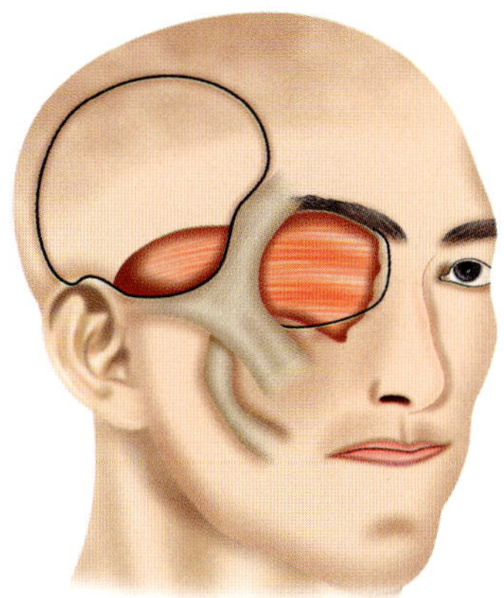

Fig. 4.9: The temporalis flap is passed in the orbit through a hole in the lateral orbital wall drilling the greater sphenoid wing, the muscle is the sutured to five to six holes made in the orbital rim and secured with resorbable sutures.

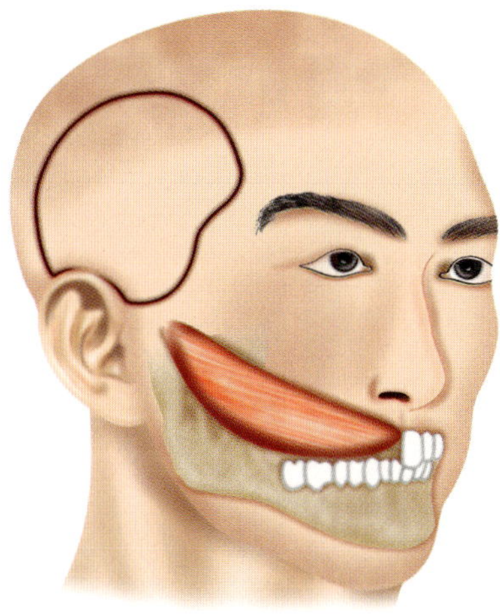

Fig. 4.10: The temporalis flap is passed below the zygomatic arch through the infratemporal fossa in the oral cavity to reconstruct the intraoral defect.

arch. With the same elevator the periosteum is incise over the upper edge of the zygomatic arch and the temporalis muscle is detached from the deeper surface of this bone until the posterior part of the body of the zygoma is exposed (Fig. 4.8). The dissection proceeds then on the anterior part of the muscle. The sentinel vein is identified and coagulated with bipolar forceps. Elevation of the temporalis muscle now can be performed easily in all its length down to the zygomatic arch.

If the muscle is used to reconstruct the orbit, from the orbital side, all the lateral orbital wall/greater sphenoid wing is removed with a drill. The TMF is passed into the orbit piercing its fascia with a Mosquito clamp and pulling it anteriorly with a gentle maneuver. The muscular part is the sutured to five to six bony holes already prepared at the level of the superior and inferior orbital rim (Fig. 4.9).

For maxillary reconstruction, after the maxillectomy is performed, a long Klemmer clamp is introduced from the mouth and driven superiorly passing in between the temporalis muscle and the zygomatic bone. Under direct vision, the deep temporalis fascia is grabbed with the clamp and pulled gently in the mouth while a large elevator push the muscle downward in the infratemporal fossa. Direct suture is performed between the muscle and the mucosal edges (Fig. 4.10).

Endoscopic surgery represents a good option of surgical improvement for several reasons:

- Requires precise anatomical knowledge and thus surgical basis
- Reduces surgical dissection and operating time
- Reduces bleeding and thus blood loss
- There is less recovery time
- Reduces local complications, i.e. local alopecia and numbness and facial soft tissues swelling.

Obviously, like any surgical advanced technique, endoscopic surgery requires longer training for understanding the goal of the surgery, how to manage the instruments and endoscope. The harvest of the temporalis muscle requires only a few instruments but, other than the endoscope, one is crucial in a safer and faster surgery and is the suction/elevator. Certainly the bleeding along this procedure is minimal but if the optical cavity is small, like in this case, even a few collected blood retained in this space can represent a problem for endoscopic view.

Figures. 4.11 and 4.12 are clinical cases.

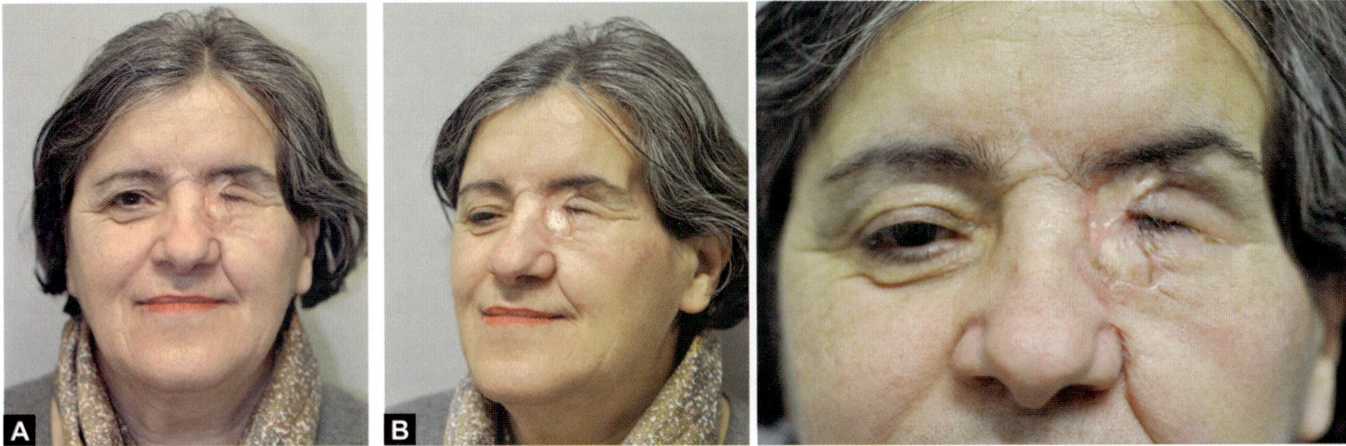

Figs. 4.11A and B: (A) Female patient operated on for skin cancer involving the left inner canthus, lacrimal sac, and operated with orbital exenteration "en bloc" with the inner canthus and medial part of upper and lower eyelids. (B) Postoperative pictures show a good external cutaneous lining with minimal orbital retraction. A depression is still present in the temporal area probably because of extended periosteal elevation being our first endoscopic case.

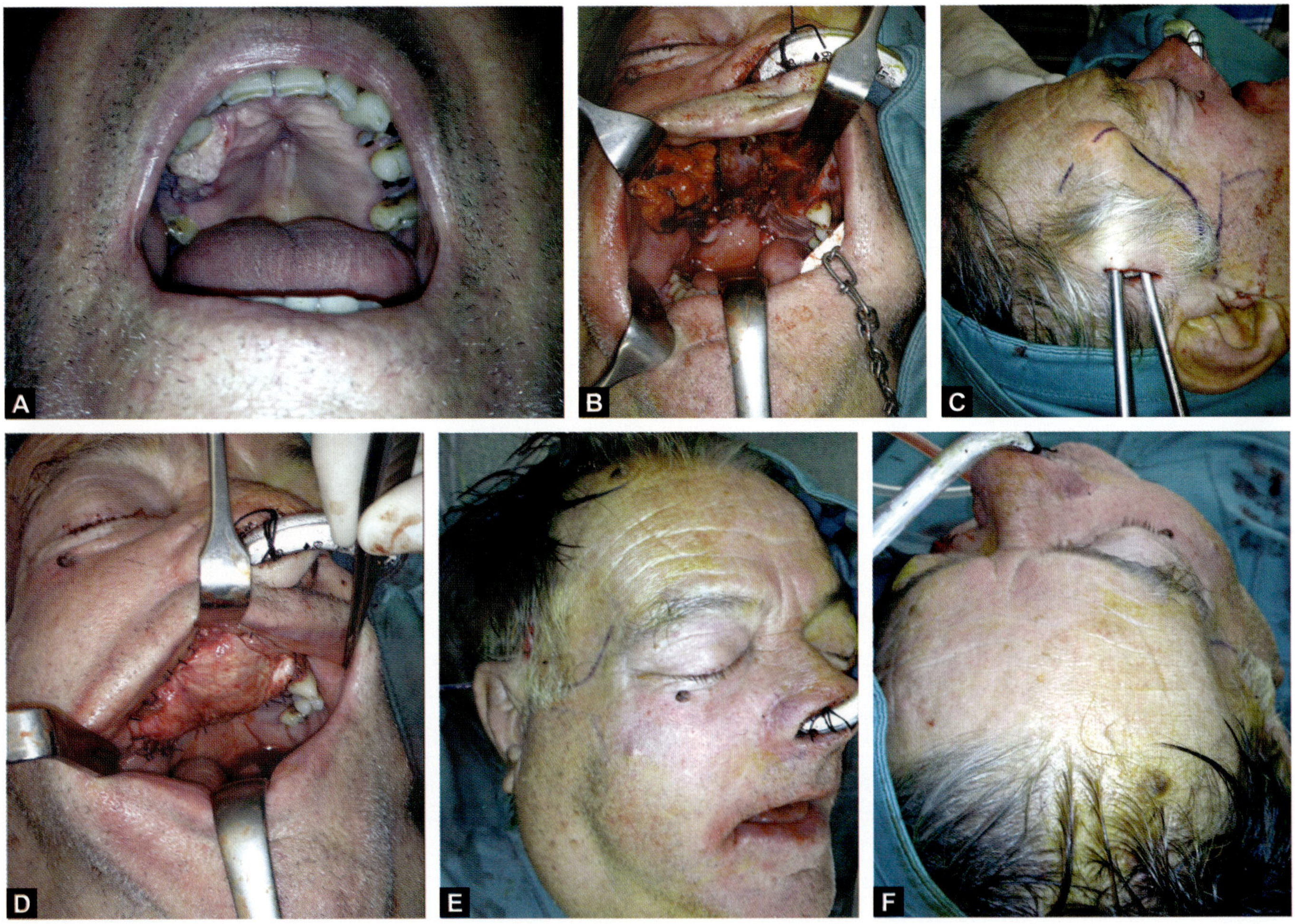

Figs. 4.12A to F: (A) Male patient operated on for oral maxillary cancer involving the right maxilla up to the lower orbital rim that was preserved from resection. (B) The surgical incisions in the temporal and parietal region are made in blue. (C) Surgical incisions. (D) Right maxillectomy. (E) Dissection of the danger zone. (F) Postoperative.

REFERENCES

1. Clauser L, Curioni C, Spanio S. The use of the temporalis muscle flap in facial and craniofacial reconstructive surgery: a review of 182 cases. J Craniomaxillofac Surg. 1995; 23(4):203-14.
2. Pia F, Aluffi P, Crespi MC, et al. Intraoral transposition of pedicled temporalis muscle flap followed by zygomatic implant placement. J Craniofac Surg. 2012;23(5):e463-5.
3. Michaelidis IG, Hatzistefanou IM. Functional and aesthetic reconstruction of extensive oral ablative defects using temporalis muscle flap: a case report and a sort review. J Craniomaxillofac Surg. 2011;39(3):200-205.
4. Koranda FC, McMahon MF. The temporalis muscle flap for intraoral reconstruction: technical modifications. Otolaryngol Head Neck Surg. 1988;98(4):315-18.
5. Assael LA. Maxillary intraoral reconstruction with regional flaps. Atlas Oral Maxillofac Surg Clin North Am. 1995;3(1): 63-73.
6. Koranda FC, McMahon MF, Jernstrom VR. The temporalis muscle flap for intraoral reconstruction. Arch Otolaryngol Head Neck Surg. 1987;113(7):740-43.
7. Abubaker AO, Abouzgia MB. The temporalis muscle flap in reconstruction of intraoral defects: an appraisal of the technique. Oral Surg Oral Med Oral Pathol Oral Radiol Endod. 2002;94(1):24-30.
8. Pinto FR, de Magalhães RP, Capelli Fde A, et al. Pedicled temporoparietal galeal flap for reconstruction of intraoral defects. Ann Otol Rhinol Laryngol. 2008;117(8): 581-6.
9. Ramirez OM. Why I prefer the endoscopic forehead lift. Plast Reconstr Surg. 1997;100(4):1033-9.
10. Squaquara R, Kim Evans KF, Spanio di Spilimbergo S, et al. Intraoral reconstruction using local and regional flaps. Semin Plast Surg. 2010;24(2):198-211.
11. Clauser L, Curioni C, Spanio S. The use of the temporalis muscle flap in facial and craniofacial reconstructive surgery. A review of 182 cases. J Craniomaxillofac Surg. 1995; 23(4):203-14.
12. Trinei FA, Januszkiewicz J, Nahai F. The sentinel vein: an important reference point for surgery in the temporal region. Plast Reconstr Surg. 1998;101(1):27-32.
13. Hinderer UT, Urriolagoitia F, Vildósola R. The blepharo-periorbitoplasty: anatomical basis. Ann Plast Surg. 1987;18 (5):437-53.
14. Lettieri S. Frontal branch of the facial nerve: galeal temporal relationship. Aesthet Surg J. 2008;28(2):143-6.
15. De La Plaza R, Valiente E, Arroyo JM. Supraperiosteal lifting of the upper two-thirds of the face. Br J Plast Surg. 1991; 44(5):325-32.

5 Augmentation Rhinoplasty

José Guerrerosantos

INTRODUCTION

In the sixties, aesthetic rhinoplasty was almost always performed as a reduction surgical procedure. Although good results were obtained, the amount of bone and cartilage removed from the nasal dorsum tended to be huge, producing a "ski slope" nose appearance. Over time, augmentation rhinoplasty came on the scene with apparently remarkable results. To give the nasal dorsum or bridge of the nose the desired height, bone grafts were used for years. Oftentimes they were slowly absorbed. As a result, many plastic surgeons started using cartilage grafts. I myself used strips of cartilage for nose jobs with optimal results. In the case of skinny patients though, the sharp edges of the cartilage were notorious postoperative. In order to avoid this, fascia grafts started to be used as a cover for cartilage grafts; the procedure yielded excellent results. Later and still the preferred method today—the use of fragmented cartilage grafts coated with fascia became the trend.

To meet aesthetic nose goals, plastic surgeons must maneuver to reduce both contour and volume of the tissues, especially bone and cartilage. At times, plastic surgeons perform either primary or secondary rhinoplasty to increase contour and nasal volume. For an increased nasal dorsum, bone grafts were used in the 50s and 60s. The practice ceased to be used due to partial absorption of the grafts that caused the aesthetic aspect of the nasal dorsum not to look its best. In my personal experience, I have used cartilage grafts and fascia grafts using various techniques that will be included in this paper.

CARTILAGE GRAFTS IN RHINOPLASTY

Some of the surgeons who initially reported the advantages of the use of cartilage in rhinoplasty were Stark,[1] Ortiz-Monasterio,[2,5] Gurrerosantos,[3] Sheen,[4] and Gunter.[6] They all mentioned the improvement achieved with cartilage grafting in augmentation nose corrections.

Cartilage grafts can be obtained from the nasal septum, from the auricular shell, or from the cartilaginous portion of the rib cage.

The preferred method was to use cartilage strips wrapped with fascia[3] taken off either from the nasal septum (Fig. 5.1) or the pinna (Fig. 5.2). Good results for the nasal dorsum were seen. However, for thin-skinned patients with little subcutaneous tissue, edges of grafted cartilage were visible 16 months following surgery when postoperative edema disappeared. To overcome this obstacle, use of cartilage graft strips coated with fascia have proved to be an effective practice. The method was modified by using stiff and nonabsorbable deep temporal fascia, instead of thin and absorbable superficial temporal fascia. I have used temporal fascia for over 35 years with excellent results.

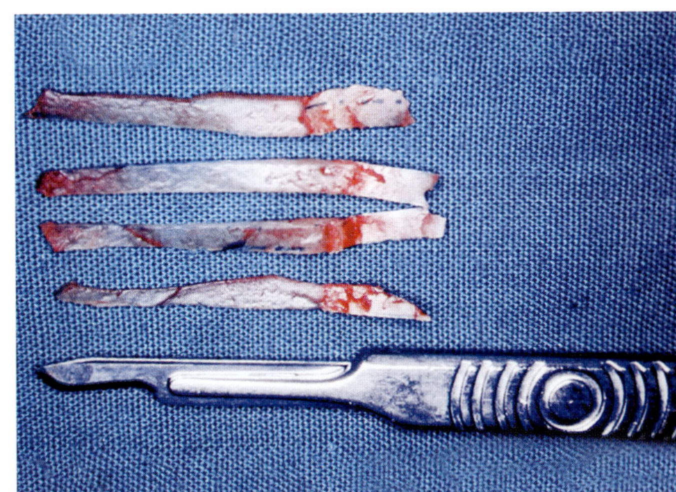

Fig. 5.1: Cartilage grafts taken from the nasal septum before being implanted on the dorsal roof of the nasal cavity.

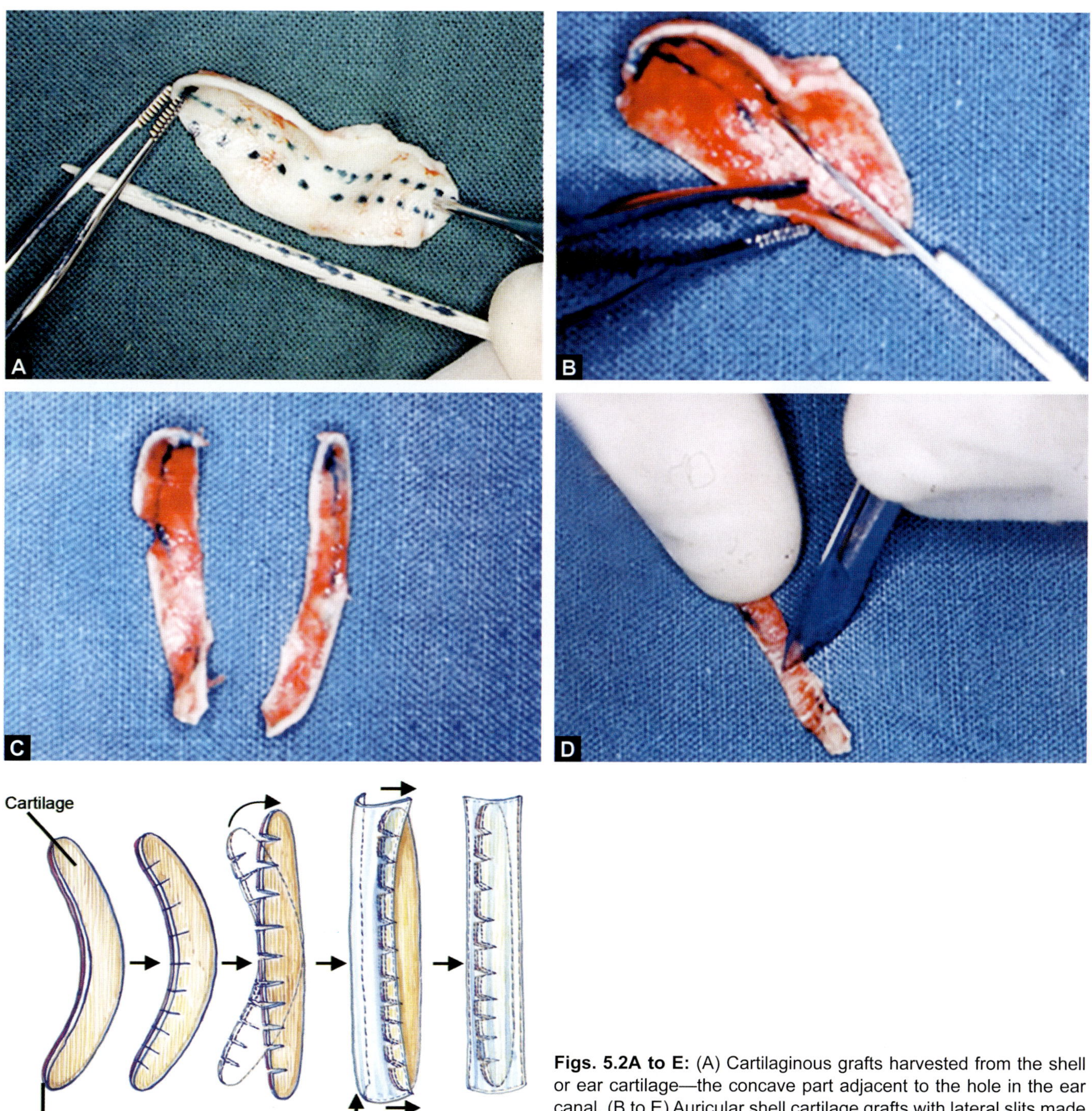

Figs. 5.2A to E: (A) Cartilaginous grafts harvested from the shell or ear cartilage—the concave part adjacent to the hole in the ear canal. (B to E) Auricular shell cartilage grafts with lateral slits made to cause them lose "memory" and remain straight after being placed in the recipient area.

Cartilage grafts are obtained from the entire auricular shell of the pavilion of the ear (Fig. 5.2). One auricular shell will usually do. Only when the depression of the nasal dorsum is deeply pronounced, auricular shells from both ears become necessary.

To make the straight cartilage grafts, perform as follows: draw lines to give rightness to the graft and to make straight cuts. In spite of this, cartilage grafts have the tendency to warp. Generally, two or three strips can be obtained from each auricular cartilage. For grafts to be placed in straight fashion when introduced into the nasal cavity above the bone and cartilaginous septum, make small lateral cuts to the cartilage for it to lose memory and avoid bending (Fig. 5.2). The recipient bed on the dorsum must be made as flat, deep, narrow and smooth as possible to accommodate the cartilage grafting. The carving of the recipient bed is routinely performed in the hospital (Fig. 5.3A). Detachment of the skin and subcutaneous tissue is made with a 4-mm needle-holder, not scissors (Fig. 5.3B); bone scraping is made with an instrument 3 mm in width (Fig. 5.3C).

If a wide recipient bed is carved, the graft material will not remain straight and the nasal dorsum will be deviated. The amount of necessary cartilage for dorsum augmentation is calculated so that a proper nose correction is obtained. Also the decision of using one or more strips is made (Figs. 5.4A and B).

Fascia graft is mostly obtained from the temporal area through a straight incision usually 3 cm in length (Fig. 5.3C). This must be done by inclining the scalpel blade so as not to damage the hair follicles and avoid alopecic areas. After dissection of the superficial temporal fascia in the deep temporal fascia, an incision is made to the appropriate depth in order to obtain a fascia graft of an adequate size to thoroughly cover the cartilaginous graft, connected with absorbable suture (Figs. 5.5 and 5.6). The combined graft is then carefully placed on the nasal dorsum. Augmentation may be achieved with no osteotomy rhinoplasty; though sometimes osteotomy rhinoplasty is the only solution at hand (Figs. 5.7A and B). In special cases, fascia grafts with no cartilage are placed. They will be described herein (Figs. 5.7C and D).

CLINICAL CASES

The comment was already made that this procedure increases the height of the nasal dorsum in patients in whom a previously primary rhinoplasty has been performed. There are also cases where the dorsum is congenitally depressed with no rhinoplasty involved. Some of these cases will also be shown.

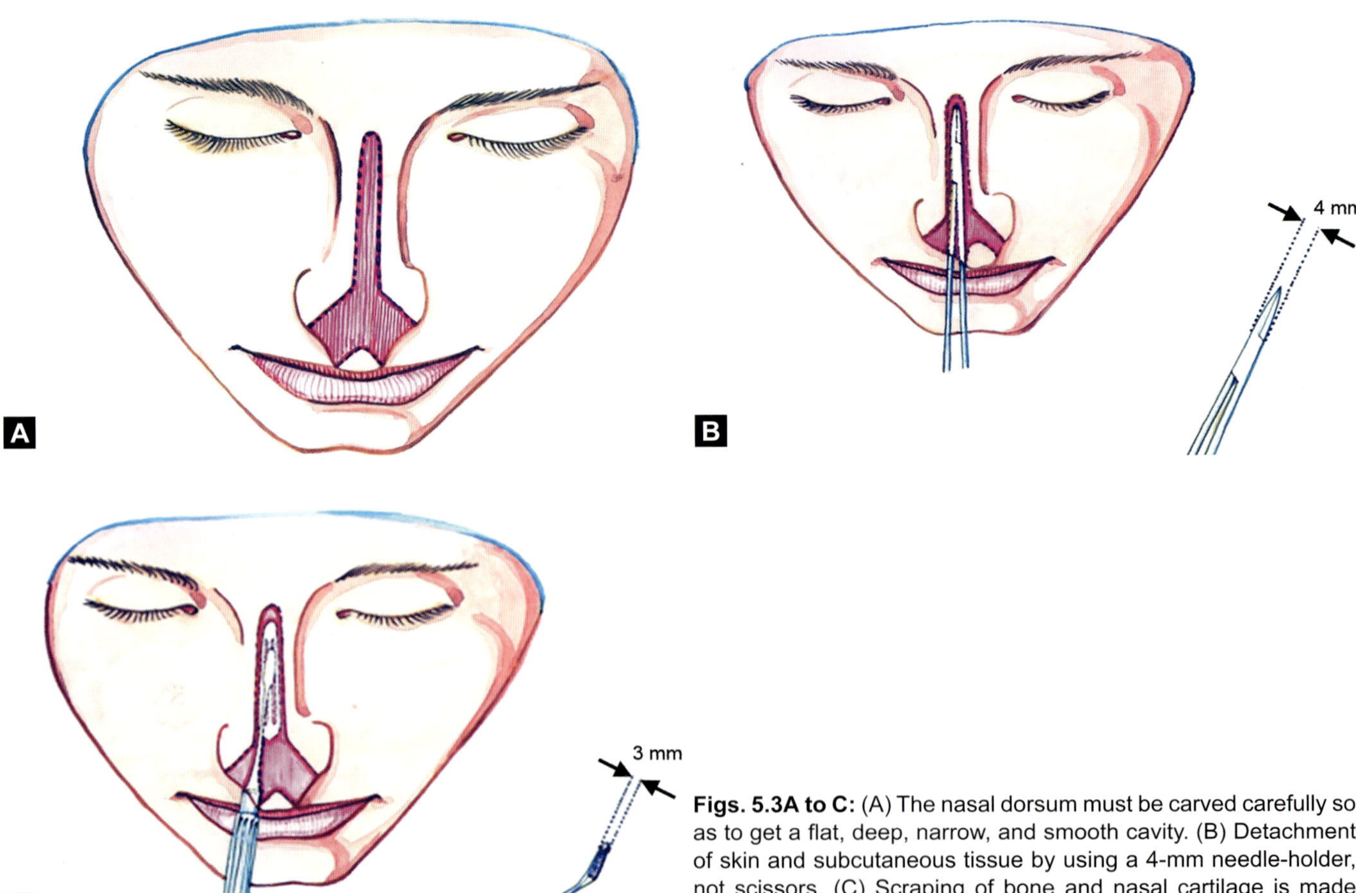

Figs. 5.3A to C: (A) The nasal dorsum must be carved carefully so as to get a flat, deep, narrow, and smooth cavity. (B) Detachment of skin and subcutaneous tissue by using a 4-mm needle-holder, not scissors. (C) Scraping of bone and nasal cartilage is made with an instrument 3 mm in width.

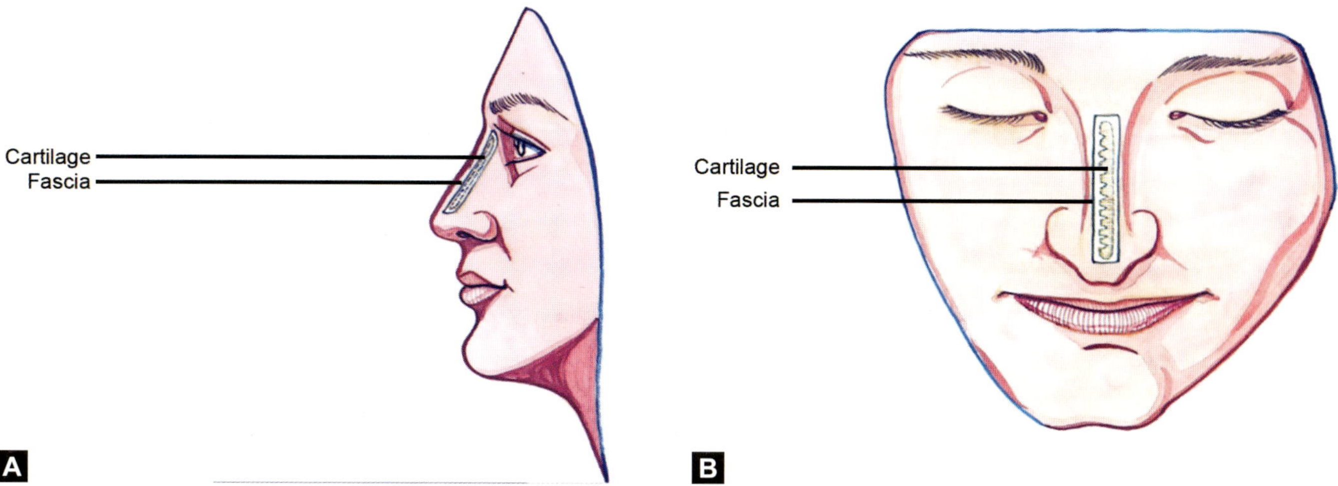

Figs. 5.4A and B: Placing of the fascia-wrapped cartilage grafting. If more than one strip is used, they are closed with absorbable suture material.

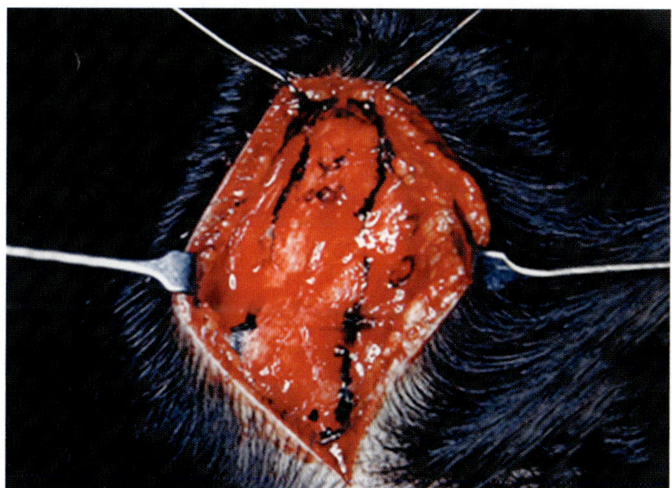

Fig. 5.5: After the incision is made in the temporal region, the superficial temporal fascia is discarded and the deep temporal material used.

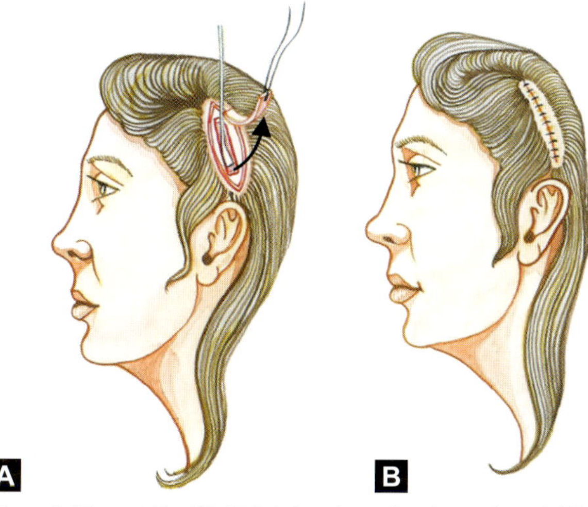

Figs. 5.6A and B: (A) Obtaining deep fascia graft and (B) closing of the donor area.

Case 1. ASM is a 25-year-old patient with depressed congenital dorsum (Figs. 5.8A and C). An aesthetic rhinoplasty was performed to increase nasal dorsum height, combined with cartilage graft and fascia grafts in the nasal tip, and preseptal cartilage graft with acceptable results as seen 10 years after surgery (Figs. 5.8B and D).

Case 2. LAG is an 18-year-old patient with congenital depressed dorsum (Figs. 5.9A and C). Outcome of aesthetic rhinoplasty with an increase in dorsal height with fascia and cartilage grafting as observed 1 year after surgery (Figs. 5.9B and D).

Case 3. AMG is a 22-year-old female patient with depressed nasal dorsum, broad nasal tip, large nasal pores, and hypertrophic nasal wings (Figs. 5.10C and E). Rhinoplasty with an increase in dorsum with fascia and cartilage graft, cartilage thinning of nasal tip and nasal wings, Sheen-type shield graft for the nasal tip, reduction of nasal pore, and thinning of the wings (Figs. 5.10A and B). Patient shown 1 year after surgery (Figs. 5.10D and F).

Case 4. A 42-year-old patient with highly depressed dorsum and retraction of nasal tip who underwent aesthetic

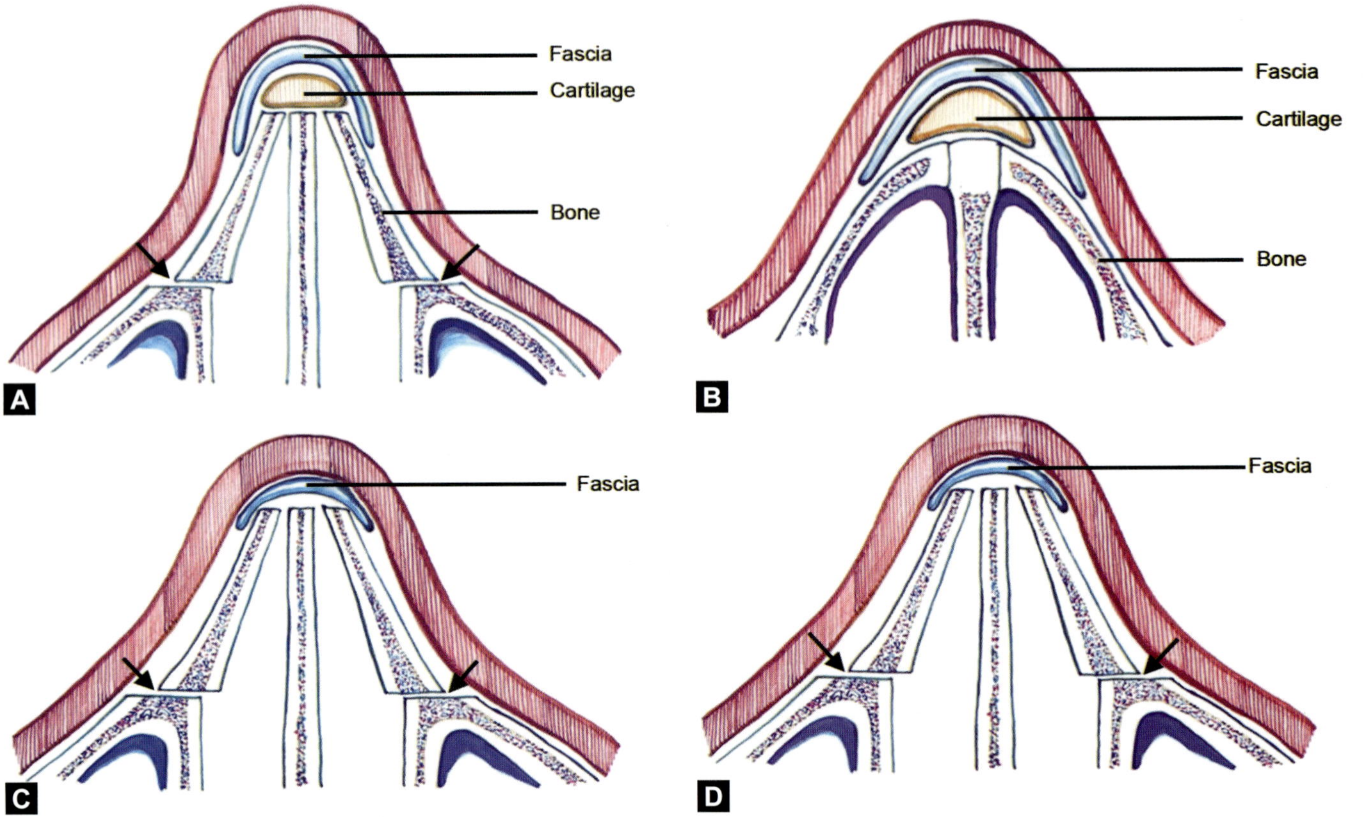

Fascia
Cartilage
Bone
A

Fascia
Cartilage
Bone
B

Fascia
C

Fascia
D

Figs. 5.7A to D: (A and B) Schematic of the positioning of cartilage grafts wrapped with fascia in rhinoplasty with and without osteotomy. (C and D) Schematic placing of fascia-only grafts.

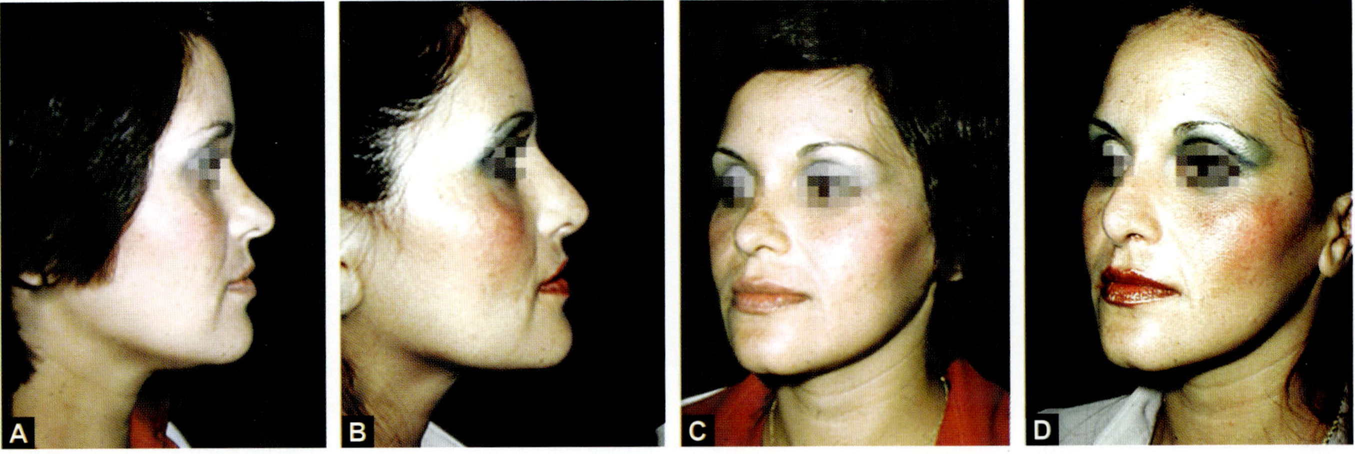

Figs. 5.8A to D: (A and C) ASM is a patient with underdeveloped congenital nasal dorsum. (B and D) ASM is a female patient in whom augmentation rhinoplasty was performed.

rhinoplasty in the early 50s (Figs. 5.11C and E). A secondary rhinoplasty was performed applying cartilage graft and deep temporal fascia in the dorsum, tip nasal cartilage graft, and preseptal cartilage graft (Figs. 5.11A and B). One-year picture following secondary rhinoplasty (Figs. 5.11D and F).

MULTIPLE WAYS TO USE FASCIA GRAFT IN AESTHETIC RHINOPLASTY

Due to its anatomical characteristics, the fascia can be used in varied ways in aesthetic rhinoplasty, a few will be mentioned: for heightening the radix and nasal dorsum,

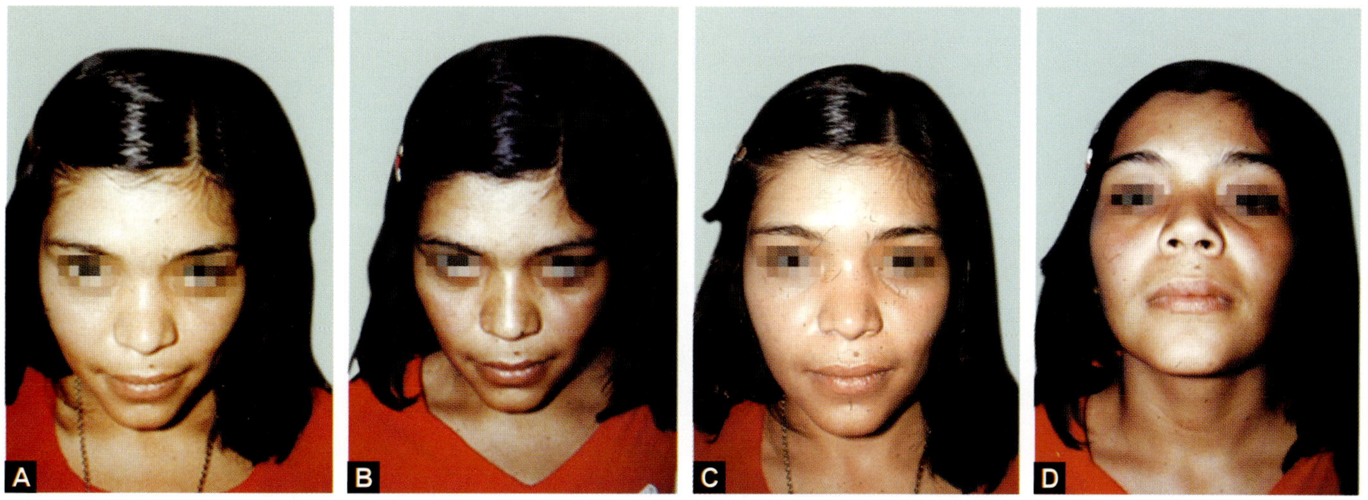

Figs. 5.9A to D: LAG is a patient with congenital depressed dorsum before and after aesthetic surgery.

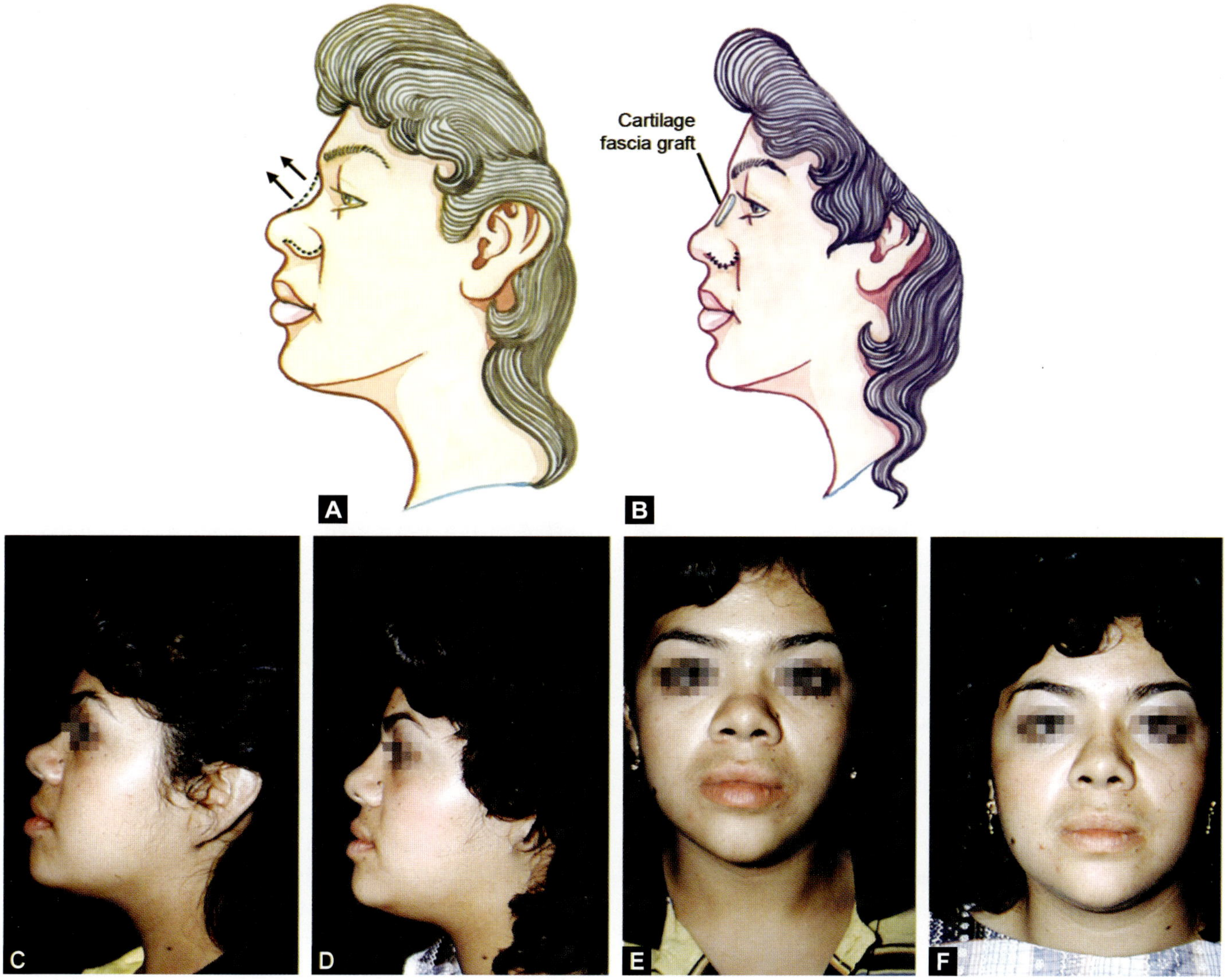

Cartilage fascia graft

Figs. 5.10A to F: (A and B) Schematic treatment of patient. (C to F) Before and 1-year after aesthetic correction.

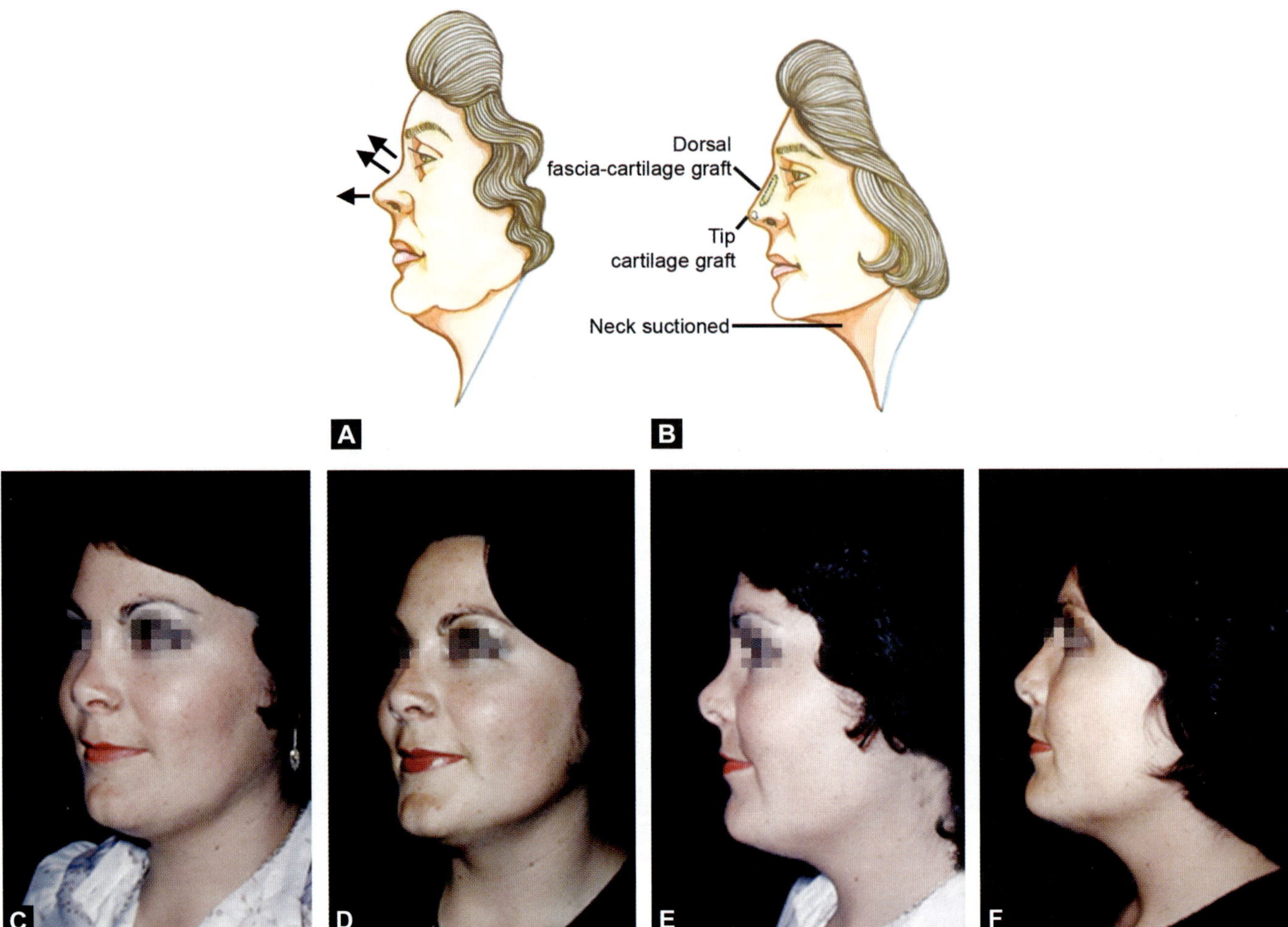

Figs. 5.11A to F: (A and B) Schematic of treatment used. (C to F) LLD is a patient before treatment and 1 year after corrective surgery.

as spreader graft, or for improving the nose tip where hypertrophy of cartilages is notorious. It is also for improving the nasal height, along with cartilage, in the paranasal region. In thin-skinned patients with little subcutaneous tissue and a slight depression of the nasal dorsum, fascia graft proves to be very advantageous.

Some clinical cases are shown here which clearly indicate when fascia grafting can produce excellent results.

Case 5. JCL is a 24-year-old patient with a moderate depression of the nasal dorsum (Figs. 5.12A, C, and E). An aesthetic rhinoplasty was performed by scraping and applying fascia graft in the dorsum, tip nasal cartilage graft from the auricular shell, and preseptal cartilage graft (Figs. 5.12A and B). Picture of patient taken 1 year postoperative showed a noticeable aesthetic improvement (Figs. 5.12B, D, and F).

Case 6. PBM is a 26-year-old patient with deviated nasal septum, ultra-thin skin, and little subcutaneous tissue (Figs. 5.13A and C). An aesthetic nasal correction was performed using fascia graft in the dorsum, along with a septoplasty to correct the deviation of the nasal septum (Fig. 5.13). Patient 18 months after rhinoplasty showed excellent results with combination treatment (Figs. 5.13B and D).

Case 7. OMZ is a 43-year-old patient with a nasal hump (Figs. 5.14C and E) in whom the Skoog rhinoplasty method involving removal of the nasal hump followed by molding it and applying it back in the nasal dorsum was performed. The technique was applied on this patient where the molded dorsum was wrapped with fascia (Figs. 5.14 and 5.15). The outcome was satisfactory, as seen in this picture 1 year after surgery (Figs. 5.14A and F).

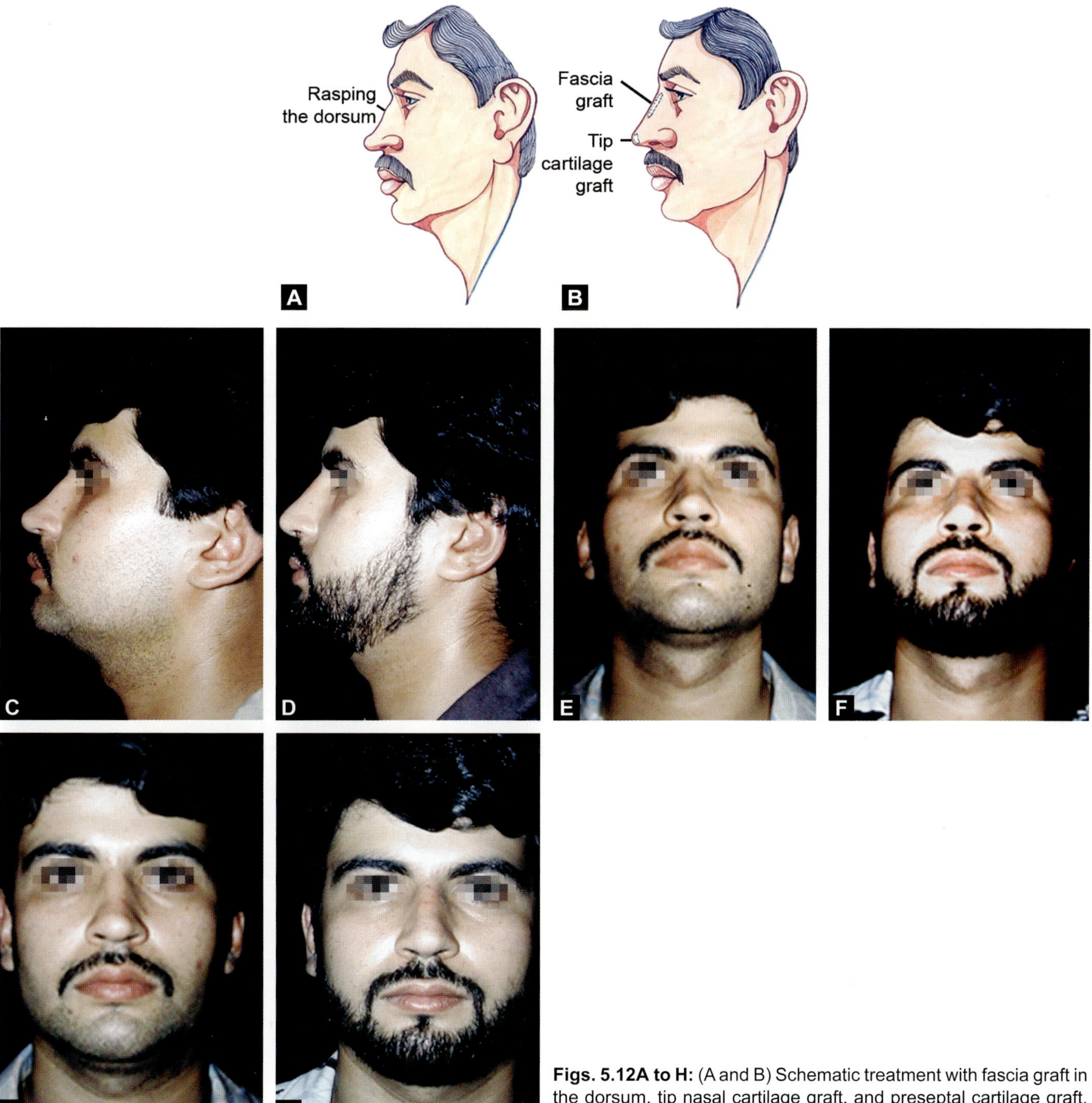

Figs. 5.12A to H: (A and B) Schematic treatment with fascia graft in the dorsum, tip nasal cartilage graft, and preseptal cartilage graft. (C to H) Patient before and after 1 year following corrective surgery.

ROLLED FASCIA GRAFT

To improve a depressed nasal dorsum rolled fascia grafts with no cartilage can be used with an acceptable cosmetic result (Figs. 5.15A and B). The technique involves rasping of the bony dorsum and deep detaching of skin and subcutaneous tissue to apply a roll-shaped fascia graft. Care must be taken not to over detach the skin and subcutaneous tissue when carving the recipient bed where the graft will be placed so as to avoid deviations.

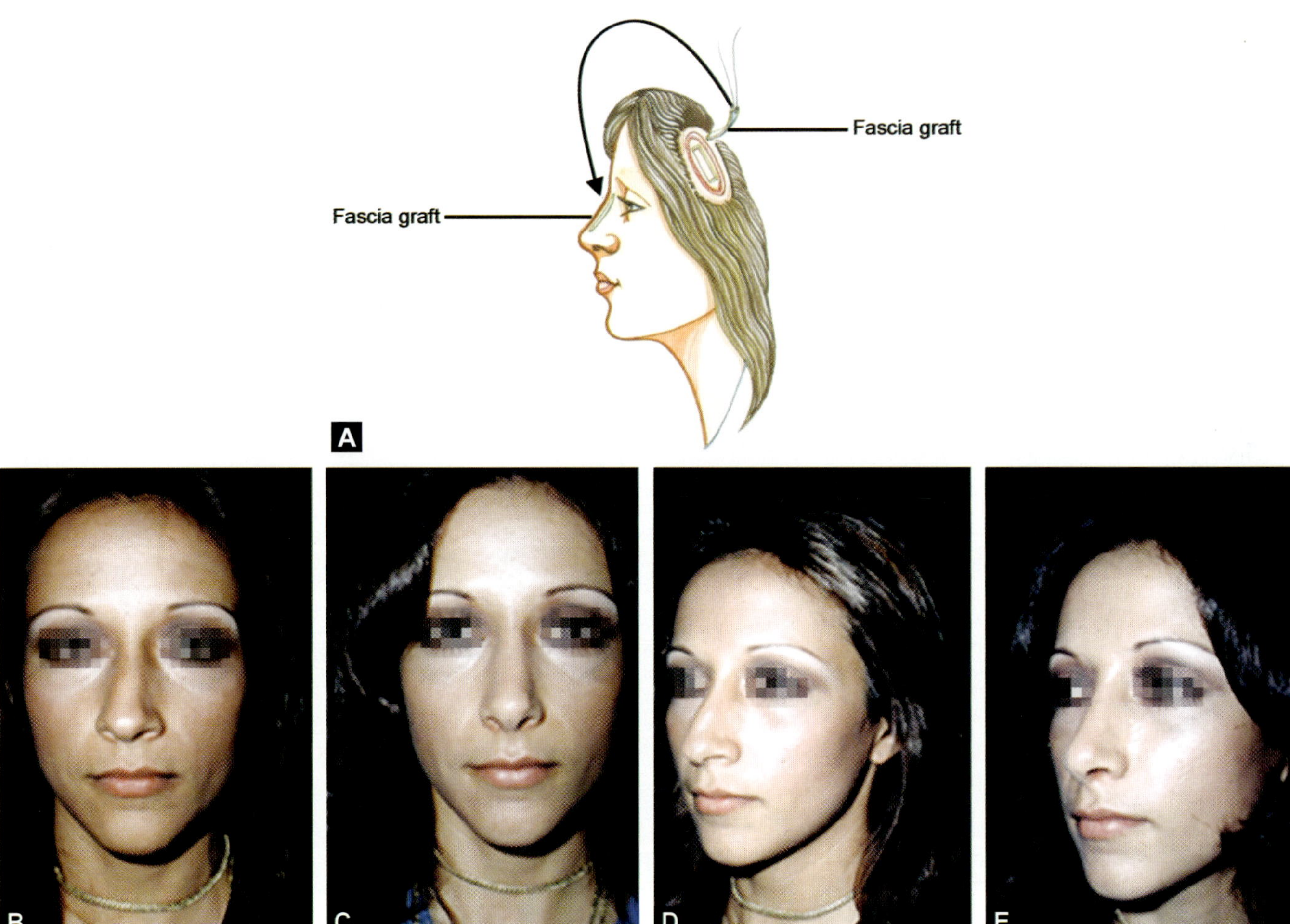

Figs. 5.13A to E: (A) Schematic treatment of fascia graft in the nasal dorsum and septoplasty to correct a deviated nasal septum. (B to E) PBM is a thin-skinned patient with little subcutaneous tissue and deviated nasal septum before rhinoplasty. Patient 18 months after surgery showing favorable aesthetic results.

CLINICAL CASES

Case 8. RBP is a 47-year-old patient with depressed nasal dorsum (Figs. 5.16C and E). An open-tip technique without skin-columella incision involving preparation of the cavity in the nasal dorsum, along with bone and cartilage rasping followed by the introduction of a roll-shaped fascia graft was performed. Also, cartilage grafting and preseptal cartilage grafting material was applied (Figs. 5.16A and B). Result 18 months postoperative was very satisfactory (Figs. 5.16D and F).

Case 9. JAE is a 38-year-old patient with a depression of the radix of the nose, nasal dorsal hump, droopy nasal tip, and columellar retraction (Figs. 5.17C to E). A nasal hump resection, augmentation of the radix and nasal dorsum with rolled fascia graft material, cartilage graft at the nose tip, and suturing the lower portion of the columellar vertical cartilages was performed (Figs. 5.17A and B). Patient satisfaction was achieved 8 months after surgery (Figs. 5.17F to H).

Some patients present localized depressions in nasal contouring caused by either a previous surgical procedure or trauma. In these cases, application of fascia strips may be the solution.

Case 10. AGV is a patient of 22 years who underwent rhinoplasty and presented a depression in the lateral dorsum behind the left nasal wing, as an after-effect of surgery (Figs. 5.18C and E). For reconstruction, deep temporal

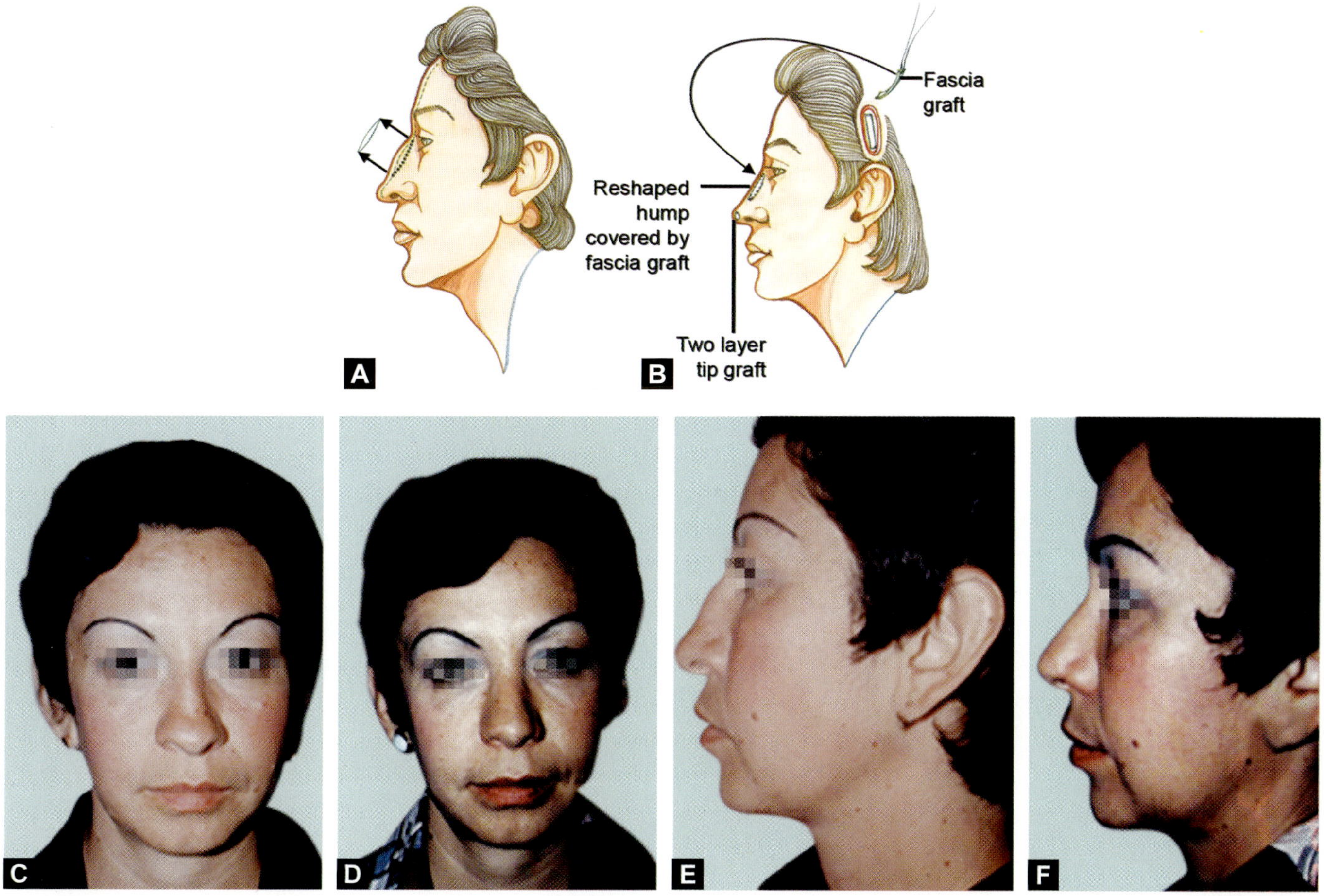

Figs. 5.14A to F: (A and B) Schematic treatment of the Skoog technique and fascia graft used. (C to F) OMZ is a patient before and after treatment.

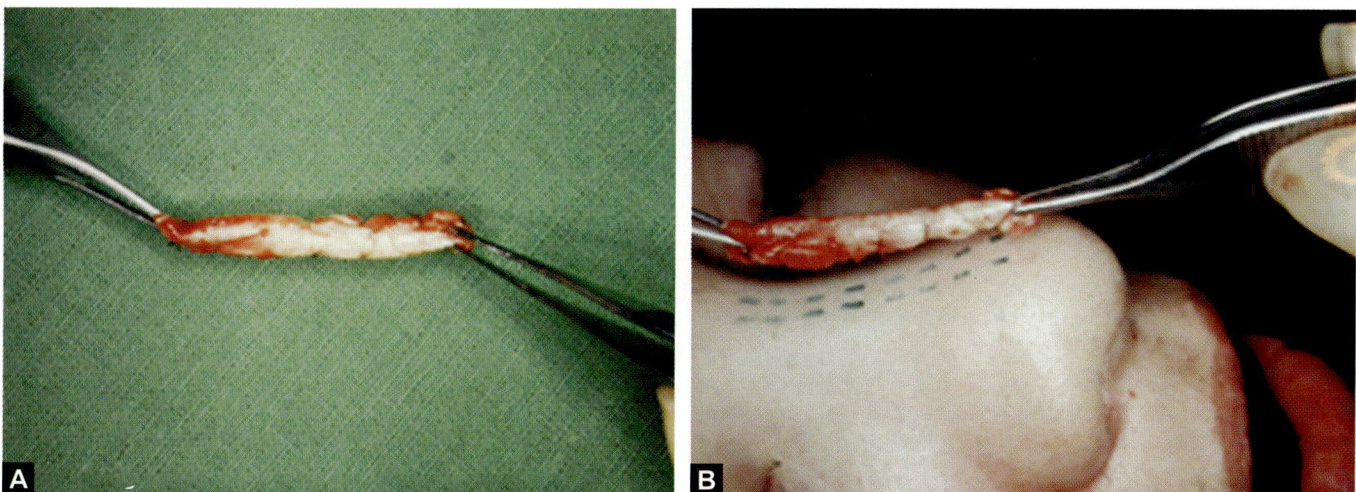

Figs. 5.15A and B: Fascial graft.

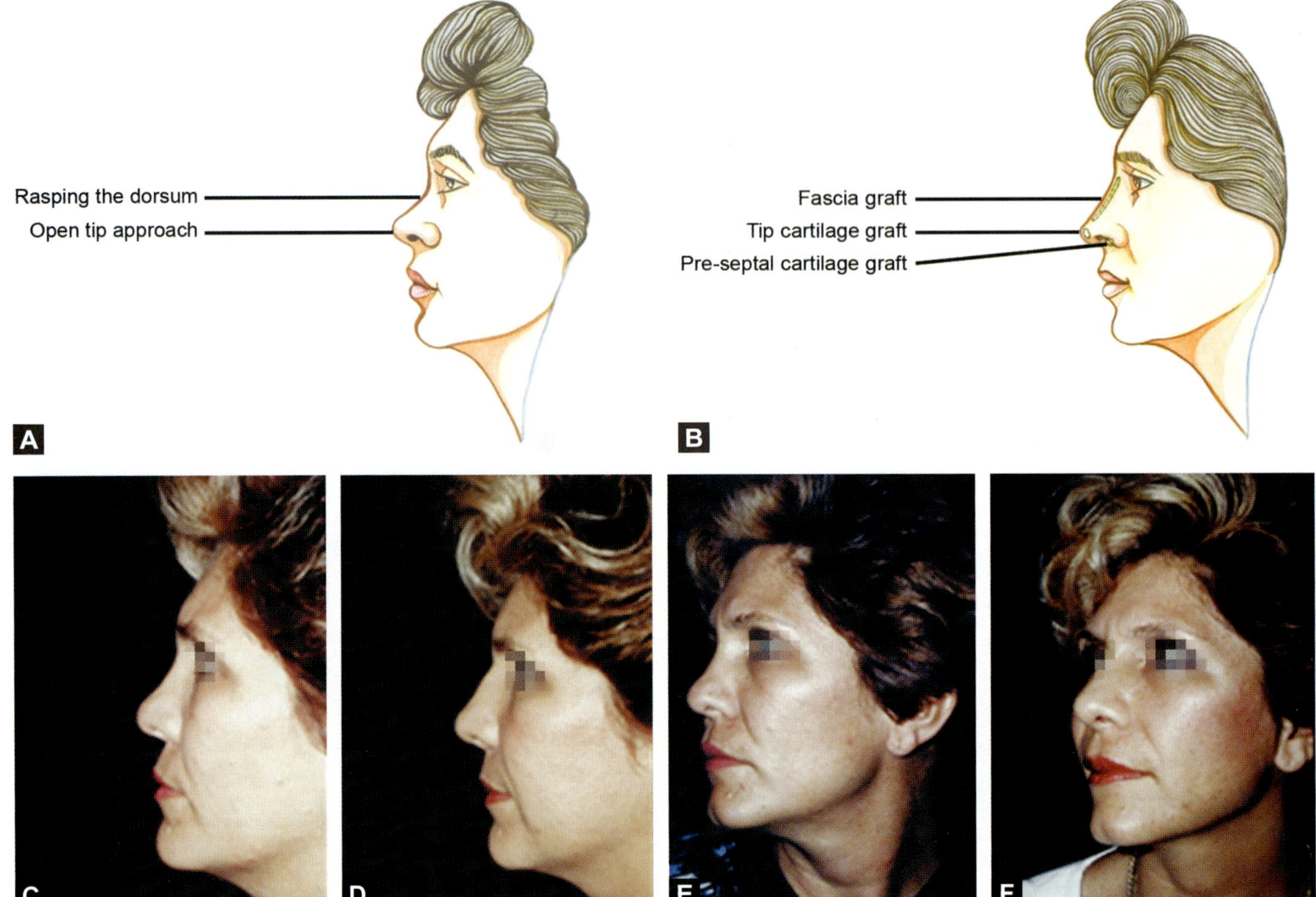

Figs. 5.16A to F: (A and B) Schematic of treatment. (C to F) RBP is a patient for whom I performed a rhinoplasty to increase the dorsum height with rolled fascia graft.

fascia graft material of an appropriate size was obtained (Figs. 5.18A and B). Preparation of the cavity through an intranasal incision was made previous to the introduction of the graft. The surgical procedure yielded an excellent outcome after 1 year (Figs. 5.18D and F).

Fascia grafts can also be used as spreaders. The vast majority of plastic surgeons use cartilage spreader grafts. A good alternative is the deep temporal fascia graft.

Case 11. AIG is a 42-year-old patient who underwent rhinoplasty in whom I used fascia grafts as spreaders (Figs. 5.19A and B). On physical examination, there was a moderate nasal deformity (Figs. 5.19C, E, and G). Patient a year and a half later had an excellent cosmetic result (Figs. 5.19D, F, and H).

Case 12. LGU is a 35-year-old patient with depressed radix, moderate dorsal hump, and lack of nasal tip projection (Figs. 5.20B, D, F, and M). Rhinoplasty consisted of a fascia graft to increase the radix, removal of the nasal hump, deep temporal fascia grafts to be applied as spreaders, and tip nasal cartilage graft (Fig. 5.20A). The cosmetic result was excellent, as shown by the patient a year after (Figs. 5.20C, E, G, and I).

Case 13. MLG is a 26-year-old patient who had a nasal hump at the area of the nasal septum, as well as a depressed radix (Figs. 5.21C and E). Excess of dorsal cartilage was removed. From the removed cartilage, preseptal grafting material was obtained. A fascia graft was applied to the radix (Figs. 5.21A and B). The result achieved after 1 year of surgical procedure is seen in this picture (Figs. 5.21A and F).

Case 14. MFG is a 27-year-old patient who presented a nasal dorsal hump, depressed radix, and lack of definition of nasal tip (Fig. 5.22B). A hump reduction rhinoplasty, deep temporal fascia graft to the radix and cartilage graft to nasal tip (Fig. 5.22A). The result after 1 year was satisfactory (Fig. 5.22C).

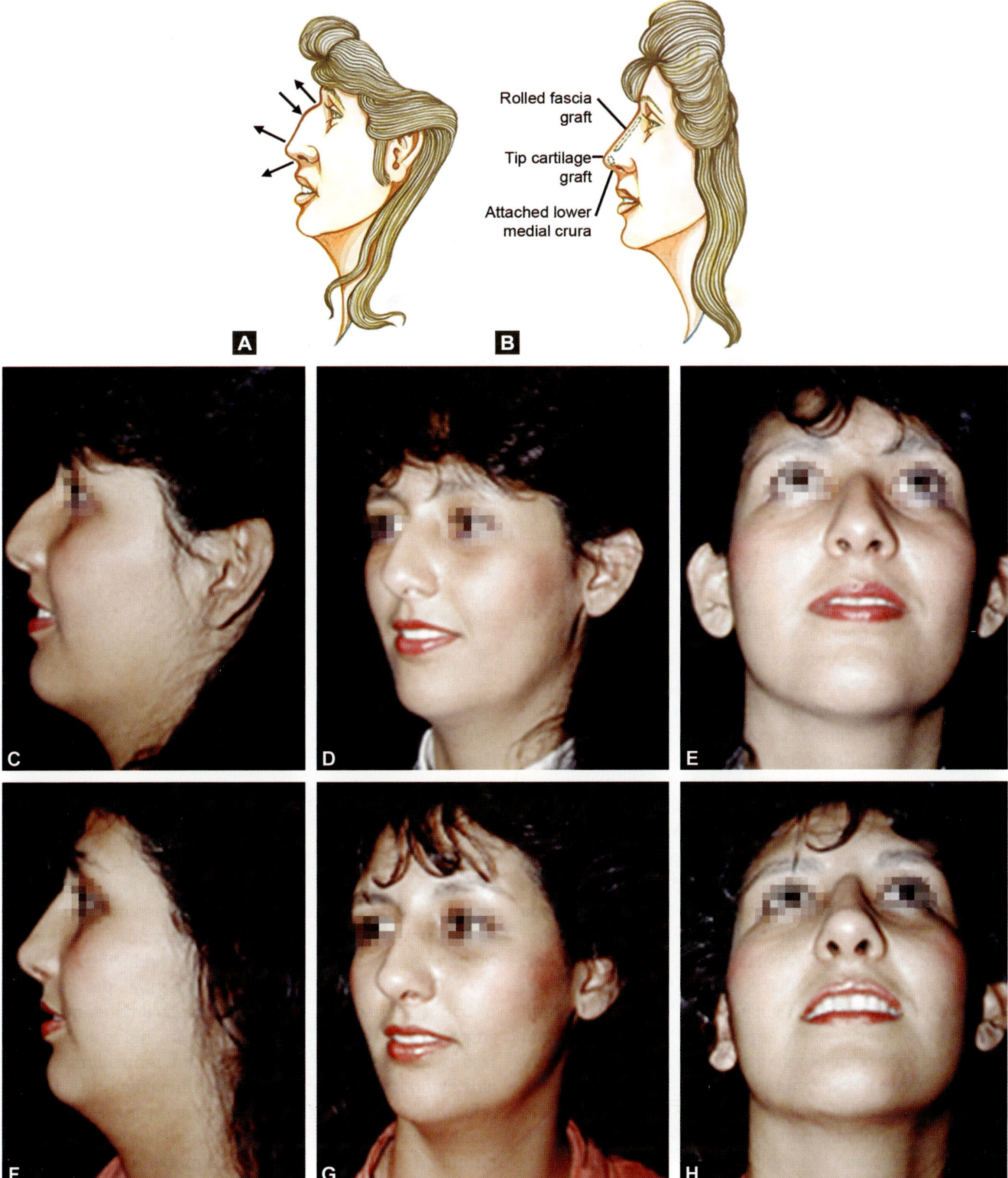

Figs. 5.17A to H: (A and B) Schematic treatment described. (C to H) Preoperative management of the patient and cosmetic results eight months after surgery.

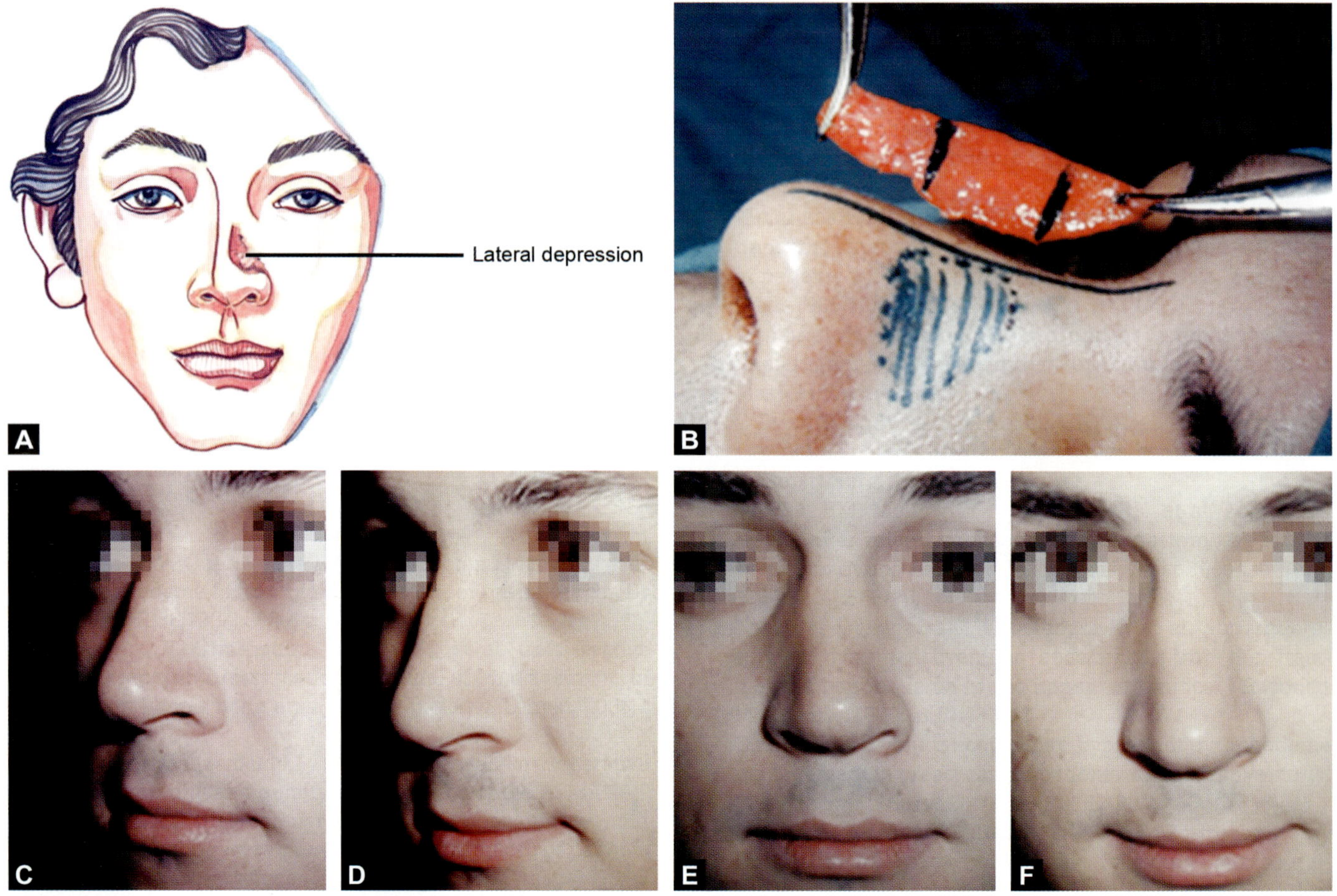

Figs. 5.18A to F: (A and B) Schematic of a depressed area and fascia graft used to correct it. (C to F) Pictures of patient before and after 1 year of fascia graft material application.

Case 15. BS is a 55-year-old patient with thick-skinned nose, retracted columella, nasal tip fall, depressed radix and nasal hump (Figs. 5.23C and E). An aesthetic rhinoplasty was performed to increase nasal dorsum height, combined with deep fascia graft in the radix, nasal hump correction, cartilage graft in the nasal tip, and preseptal cartilage graft (Figs. 5.23A and B). Acceptable results, as seen 1 year after surgery (Figs. 5.23D and F).

Case 16. AR is a 45-year-old patient with thin skin and little subcutaneous tissue, bulbous nasal tip due to thickening of overly convex cartilage at nose tip and wings (Figs. 5.24A and B). Treatment consisted of removal of excess cartilage and addition of fascia-wrapped cartilage graft to the nose tip (Figs. 5.24C to J). Aesthetic correction produced a very positive result, as seen in the patient 1 year after surgery (Figs. 5.24F and N).

CARTILAGINOUS SPREADER GRAFTING

Spreader grafts may be employed during primary or secondary cosmetic rhinoplasty in selected situations. Cartilage spreader grafts are indicated for depressed areas behind the nasal tip. Although they may be unilateral or bilateral, they are mostly unilateral.

Case 17. MTV is a 26-year-old patient with irregular nasal dorsum, lateral depression of the middle third of the nasal dorsum, slightly drooped nasal tip, and columellar

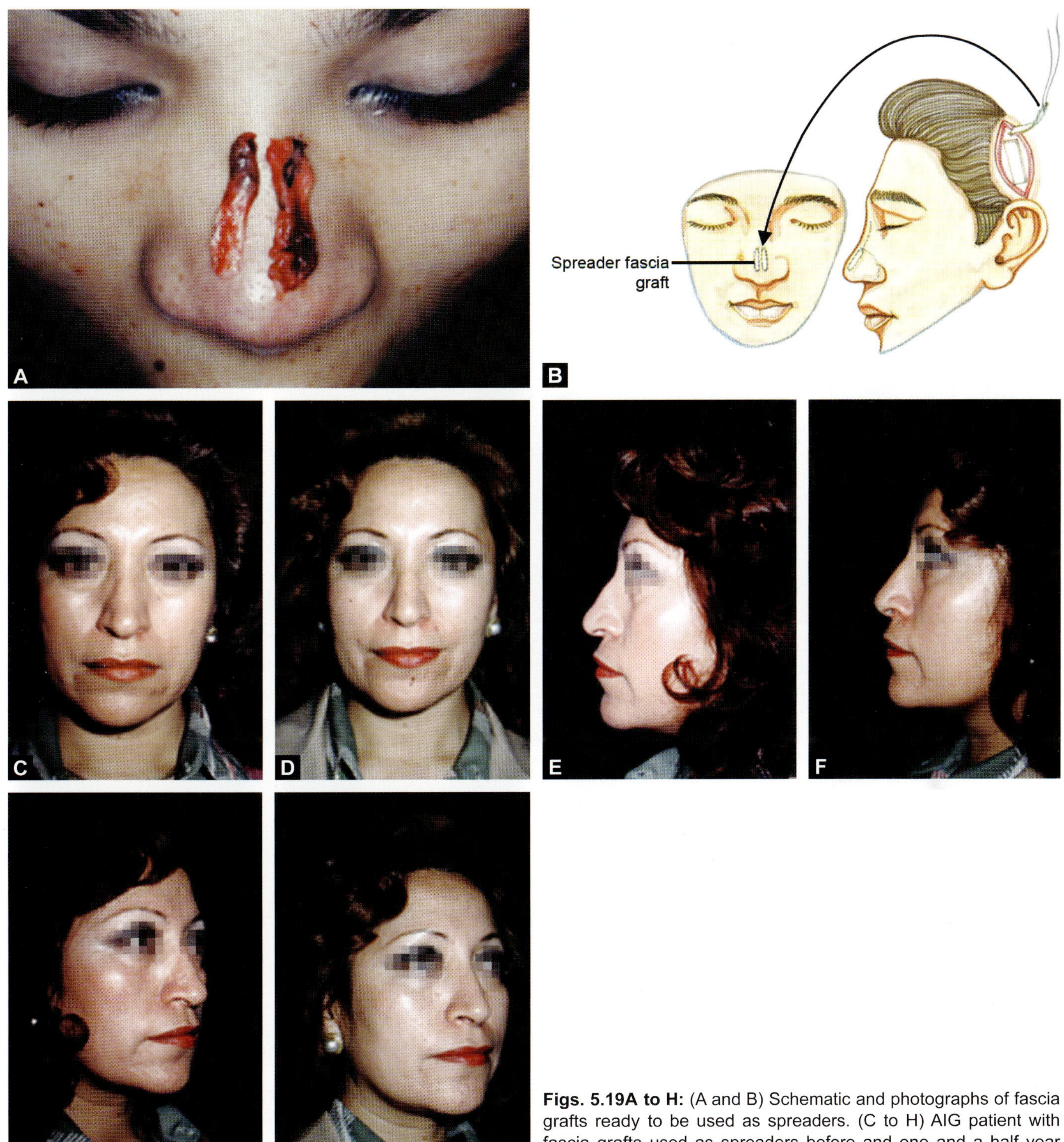

Figs. 5.19A to H: (A and B) Schematic and photographs of fascia grafts ready to be used as spreaders. (C to H) AIG patient with fascia grafts used as spreaders before and one and a half year after surgical procedure.

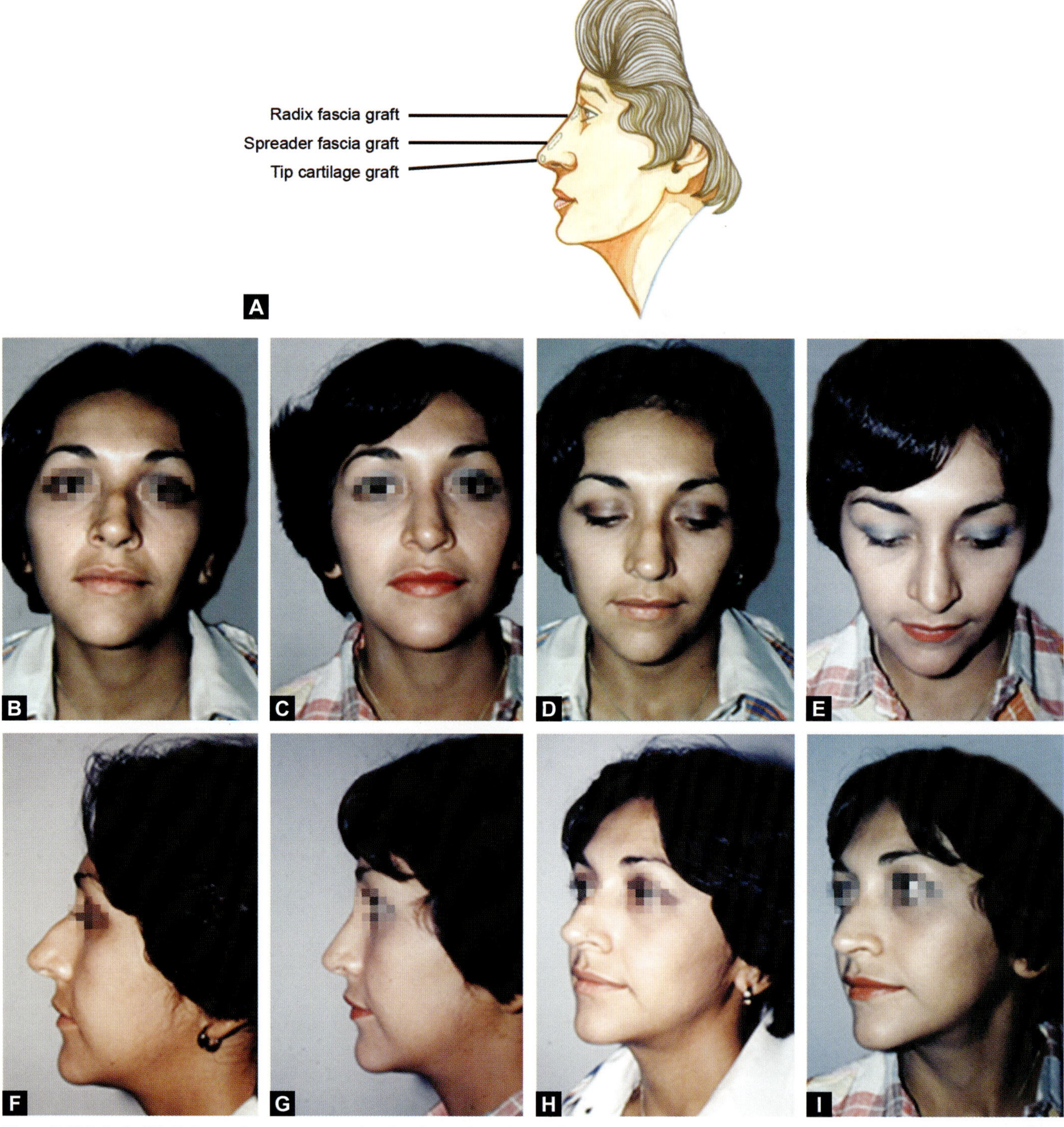

Figs. 5.20A to I: (A) Schematic treatment using fascia graft to the radix as spreader and tip nasal cartilage graft. (B to I) The patient before and after 1 year following rhinoplasty.

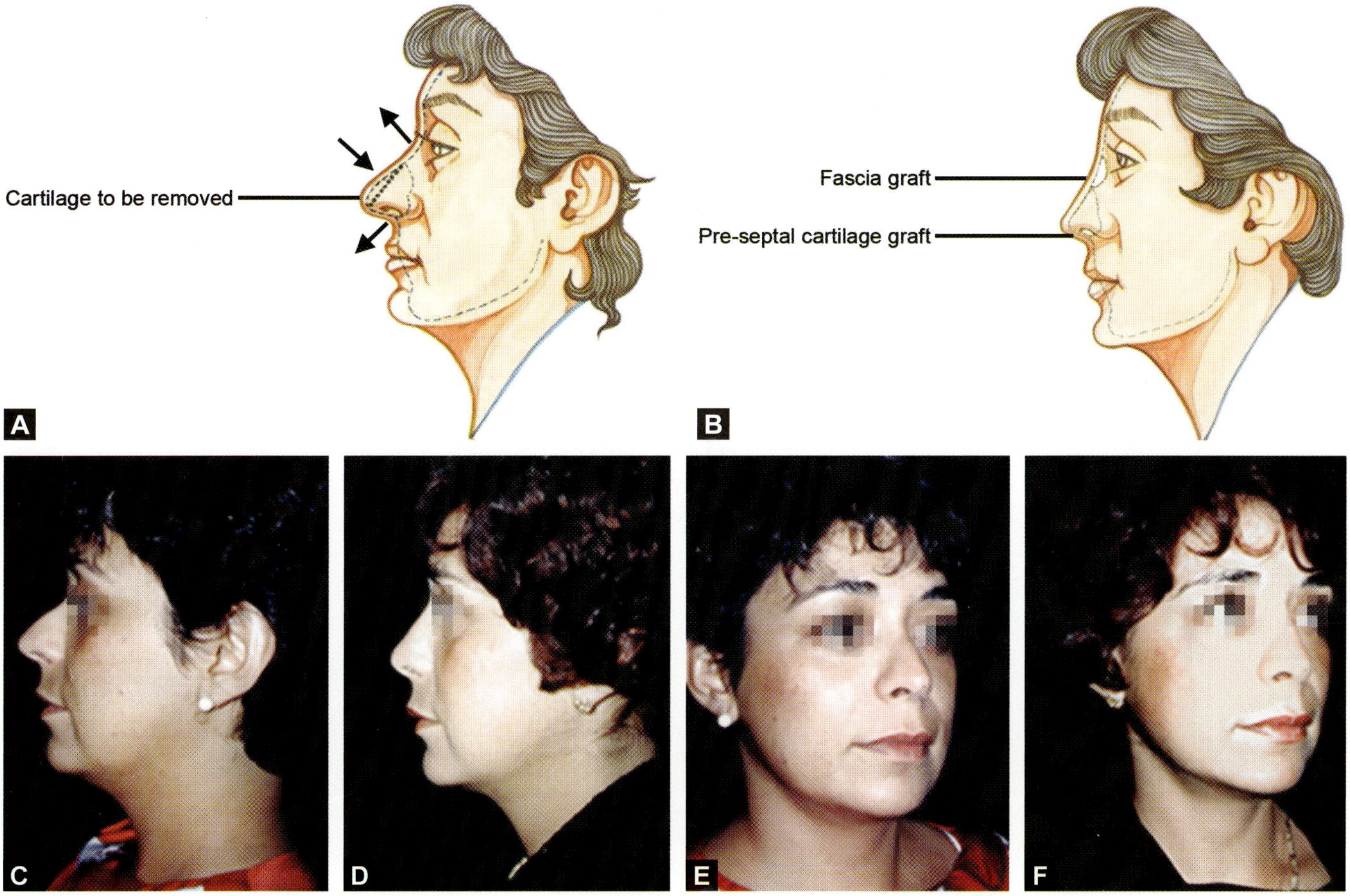

Cartilage to be removed

Fascia graft

Pre-septal cartilage graft

Figs. 5.21A to F: (A and B). Schematic treatment: (A) Resection of excess of dorsal cartilage and (B) Application of fascia graft to the radix and preseptal cartilage graft. (C to F) MGL is a patient before and after 1 year after rhinoplasty.

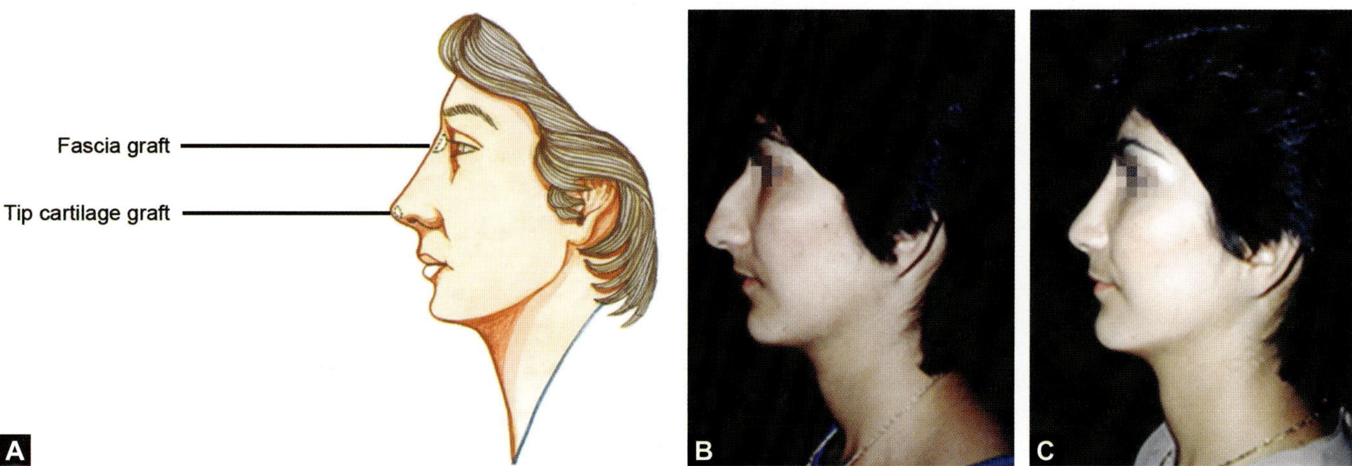

Figs. 5.22A to C: (A) Treatment scheme. (B and C) MFG is a patient before and 1 year after surgery.

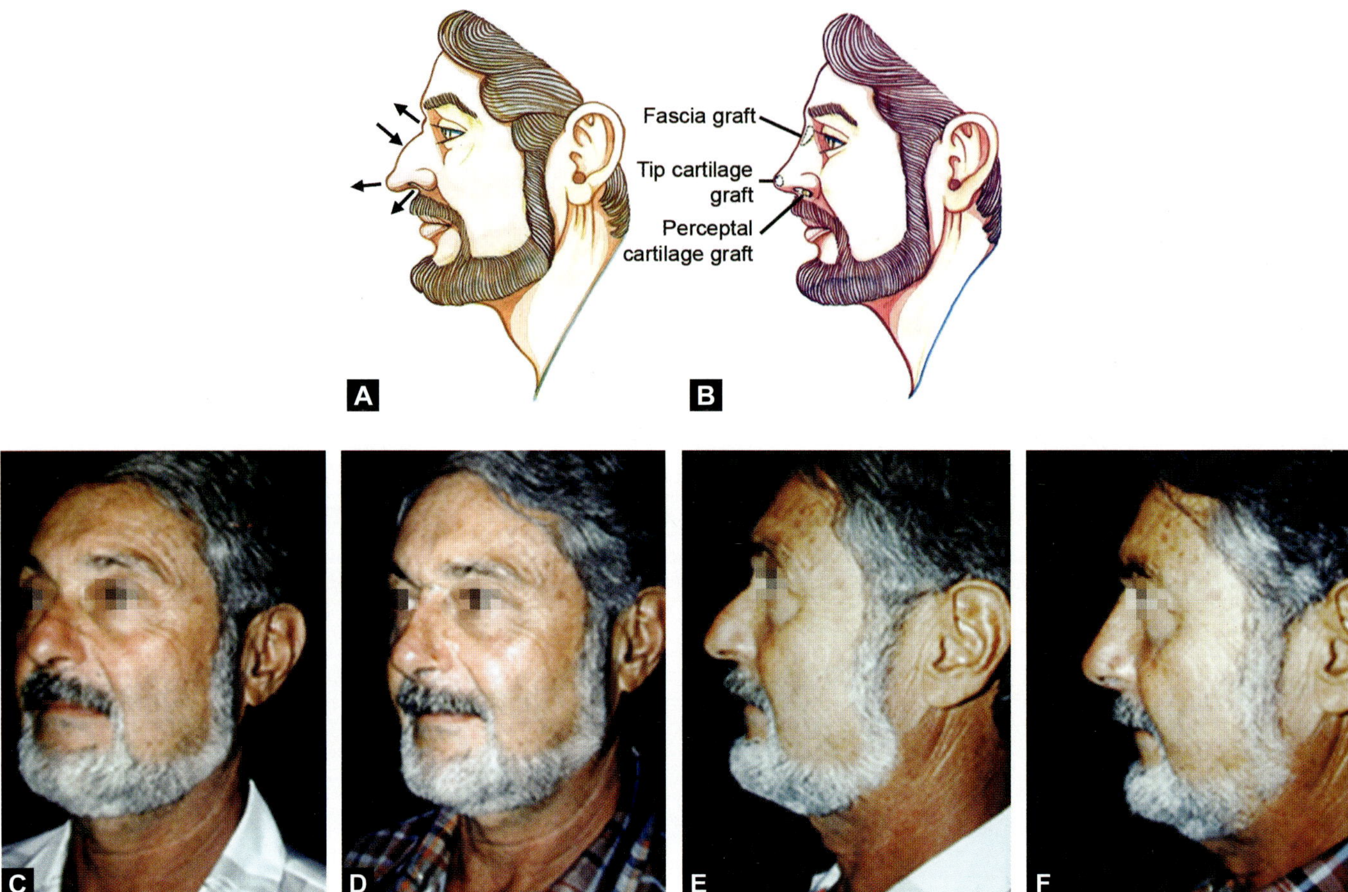

Figs. 5.23A to F: (A and B) Schematic of treatment. (C to F) BS is a patient before and after 1 year following aesthetic treatment.

retraction (Figs. 5.25C and E). A carefully scraping of the nasal dorsum, cartilage graft to the nasal, preseptal cartilage graft, and suturing of the columellar lower cartilages was performed (Figs. 5.25A and B). Highly satisfactory results 1 year after surgery (Figs. 5.25A and F).

Case 18. LJC is a 19-year-old patient operated on for primary rhinoplasty at another medical unit. She came to our clinic with a depressed middle third of the right side of the nasal dorsum (Figs. 5.26E, G, I, and K). Secondary rhinoplasty was performed by placing crushed cartilage graft to the depressed area, scraping of the dorsum and application of a cartilage graft to nasal tip (Figs. 5.26A to D). Result after 1 year of surgical nose correction (Figs. 5.26F, H, J, and L).

FRAGMENTED CARTILAGE GRAFT WRAPPED WITH FASCIA IN PRIMARY RHINOPLASTY

The Erol report was received by ISAPS in 1990[7] and presented at its 1992 congress. Dr Erol was a pioneer in the use of fragmented cartilage grafts covered with surgicel. I personally have always favored autologous grafts. A study using fragmented cartilage wrapped with autologous fascia was conducted at the Jalisco Institute of Reconstructive Surgery.[8] Results of this initial study proved highly satisfactory to us all. Consequently, it was decided to use this procedure as a preferred method of choice. Advantages are that both palpation as well as postoperative results feel and are natural looking. Daniel[9,10] also reports favorable outcomes on the use of fragmented cartilage graft covered with fascia.

Surgical Technique

Reduce the auricular or ear cartilage into small cartilaginous fragments (Figs. 5.27A to D). Place them on a strip of temporal fascia closed with a running absorbable monofilament suture in the shape of a fascia cylinder, with the crushed cartilage grafts inside. The combined graft is then placed on the nasal dorsum in a recipient bed carefully carved (Figs. 5.27E to G). On setting the combined graft

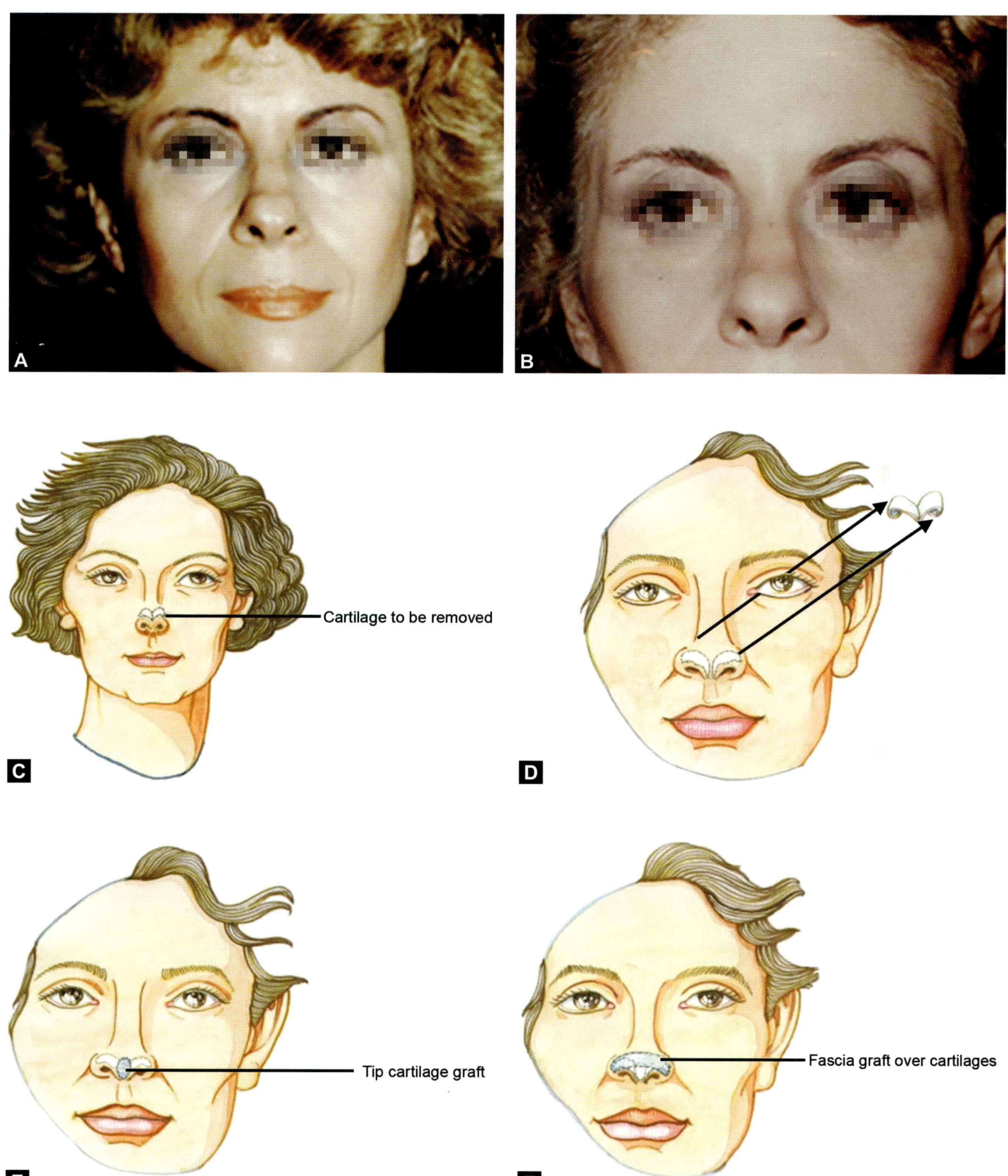

Figs. 5.24A to F: (A and B) Patient with bulbous nose tip. (C) Cartilage to be removed. (D) Cartilage removed. (E) Cartilage graft placement. (F) Fascial graft over cartilage.

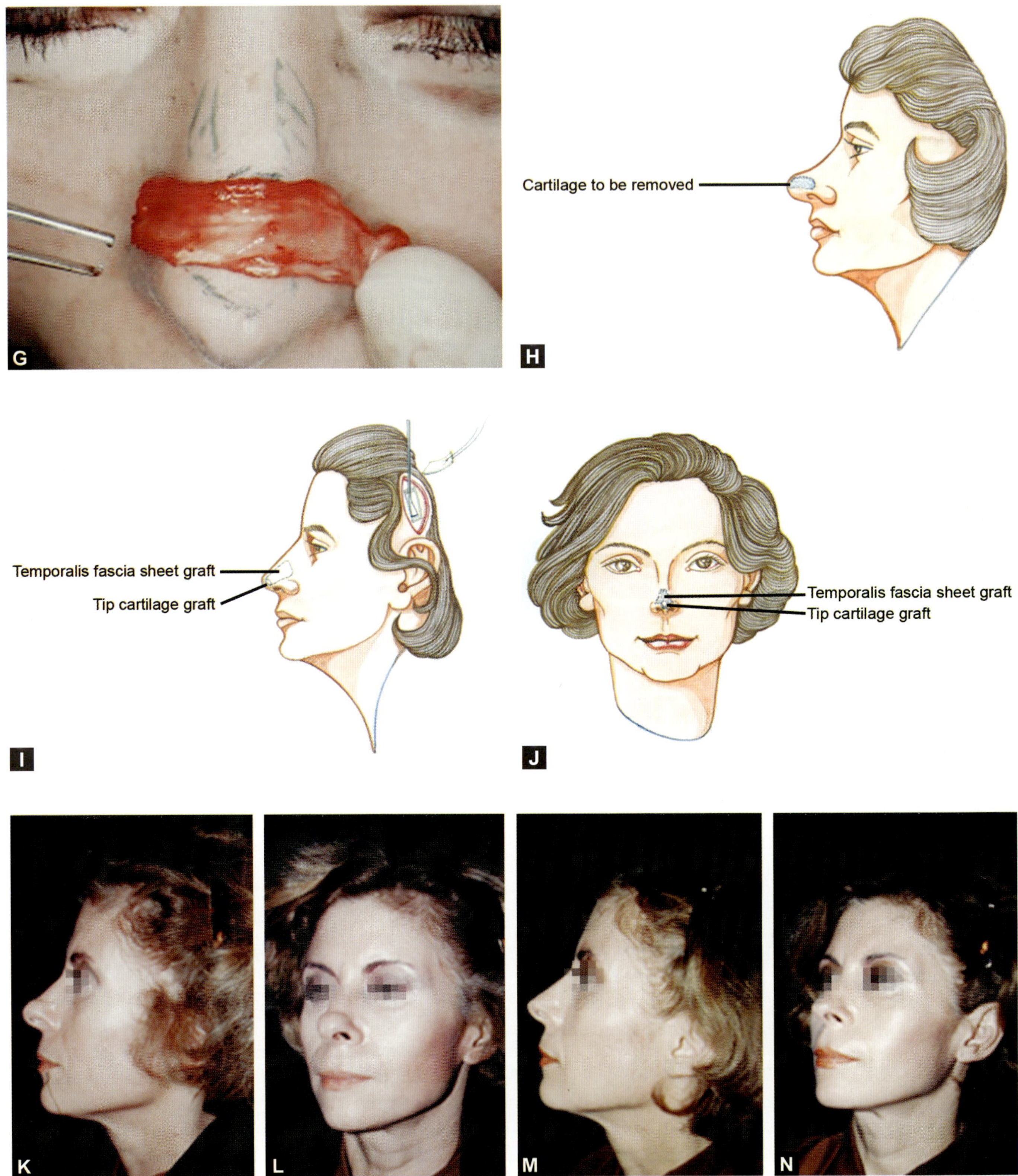

Figs. 5.24G to N: (G to J) Rhinoplasty where excess cartilage was removed, a cartilage graft to the nasal tip was applied, a cartilage graft was added to the nose tip, and where the nasal alar cartilages were wrapped with fascia graft material. (K to N) AR Patient 1 year after surgery had a positive aesthetic correction outcome.

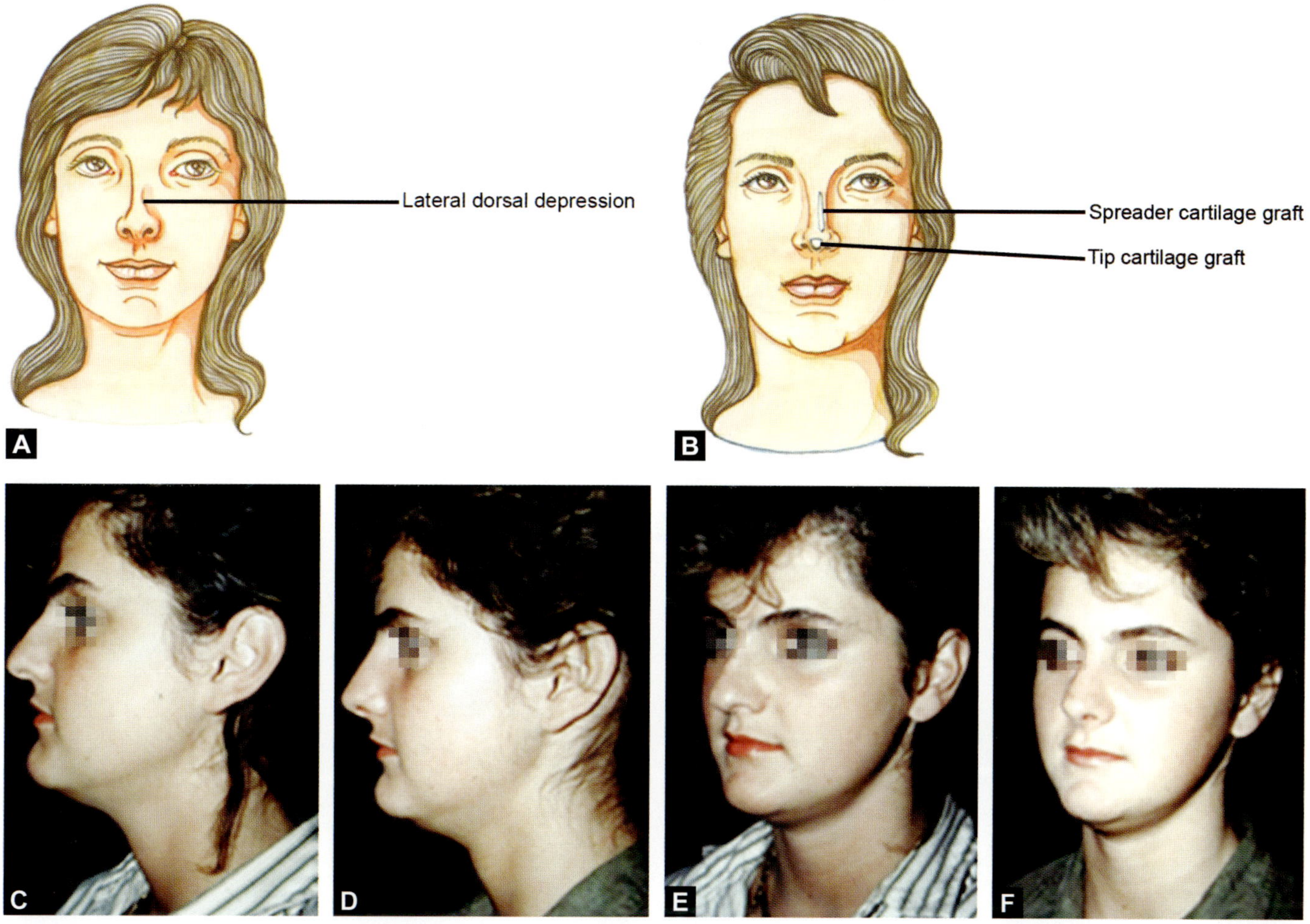

Figs. 5.25A to F: (A and B) Treatment included thorough scraping of the nasal dorsum, cartilage graft in the nasal tip, preseptal cartilage graft and of suture of the columella lower cartilages. (C to F) In the preoperative management the patient had an irregular dorsum, lateral depression of the middle third of the nasal dorsum, droopy nasal tip, and columellar retraction. A year after cosmetic correction yielded a satisfactory result, as shown.

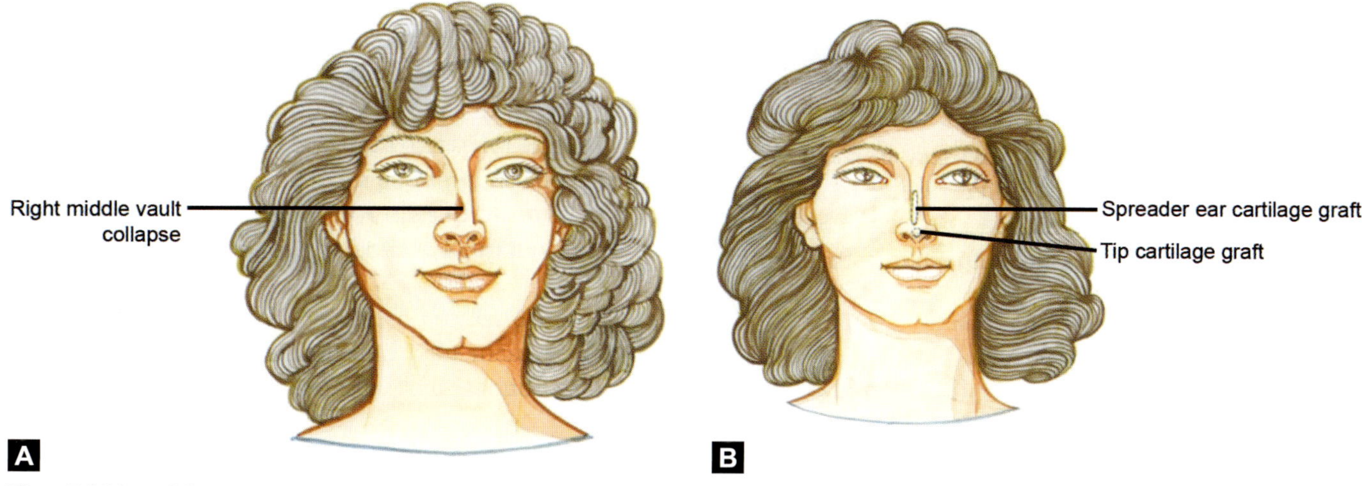

Figs. 5.26A and B

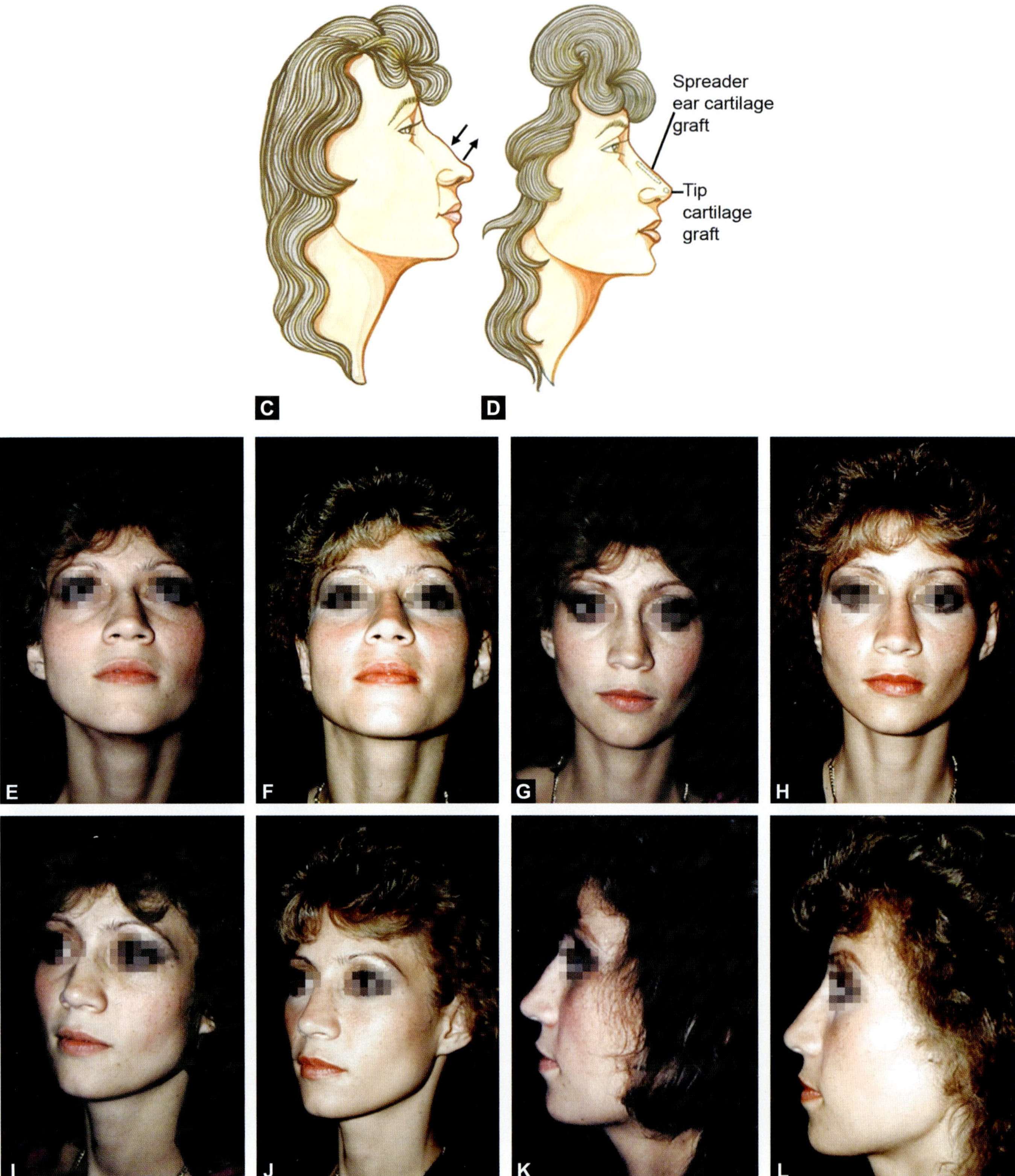

Figs. 5.26A to L: (A to D). Schematic treatment in secondary rhinoplasty where crushed cartilage graft to the depressed area, and cartilage graft to the nasal tip were applied. (E to L) Patient in preoperative management had depression of the middle third of the right side of the nasal dorsum E, G, I, K. Aesthetic result after 1 year.

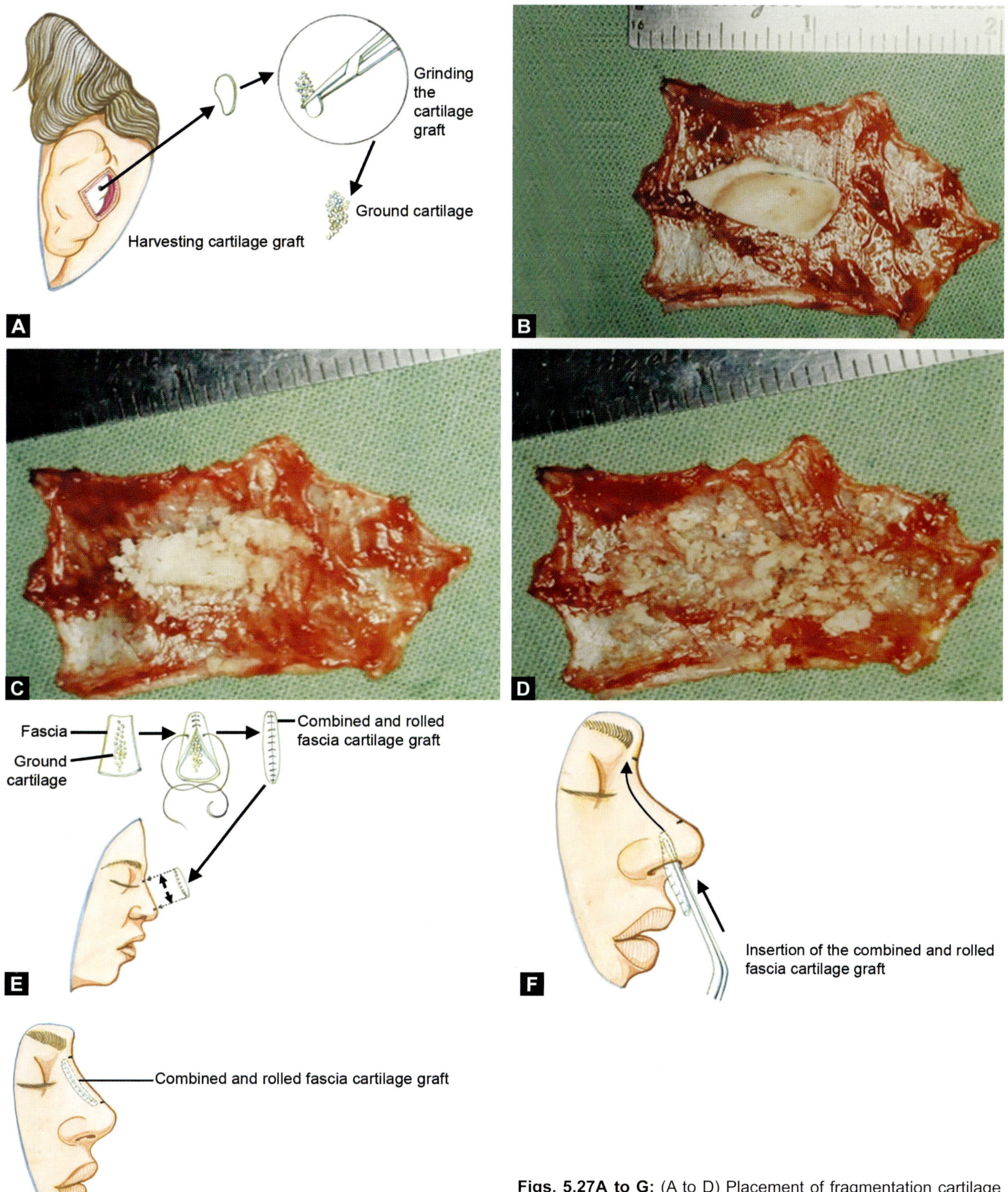

Figs. 5.27A to G: (A to D) Placement of fragmentation cartilage graft and fascia strip. (E to G) Placement of a combined fascia and fragmented cartilage graft in the nose.

in its bed, it molds externally as if it were play dough. The placement of the combined graft is followed by a nasal splint: carefully place adhesive micropore tape first and then a plaster splint. Manually maneuver to fix the splint and shape the dorsum. The splint is removed after 1 week and replaced by a self-adhesive dressing tape (Micropore).

Clinical Cases

Case 19. ASD is a 24-year-old female patient with intermediate deviation of the nasal dorsum and hypertrophy of the nasal tip and alar cartilages (Figs. 5.28C and E). An aesthetic rhinoplasty was performed by placing fragmented cartilage graft covered with fascia to the radix and nasal dorsum, along with aesthetic correction of the nasal tip and nasal alar (Figs. 5.28A and B). Patient 1 year after with aesthetic nasal correction and improvement of nasal tip and wings (Figs. 5.28D and F).

Case 20. MVR is a 28-year-old patient with slightly depressed radix, intermediate nasal hump, droopy nasal tip, acute nasolabial angle, broad nasal pores, and receding chin (Figs. 5.29C to F). Treatment consisted of performing an increase to the radix with fascia and cartilage grafting, partial resection of the upper nasal septum, preseptal cartilage graft, cartilage graft to nasal tip, and chin augmentation implant. Additionally, a neck liposuction was performed (Figs. 5.29A and B).

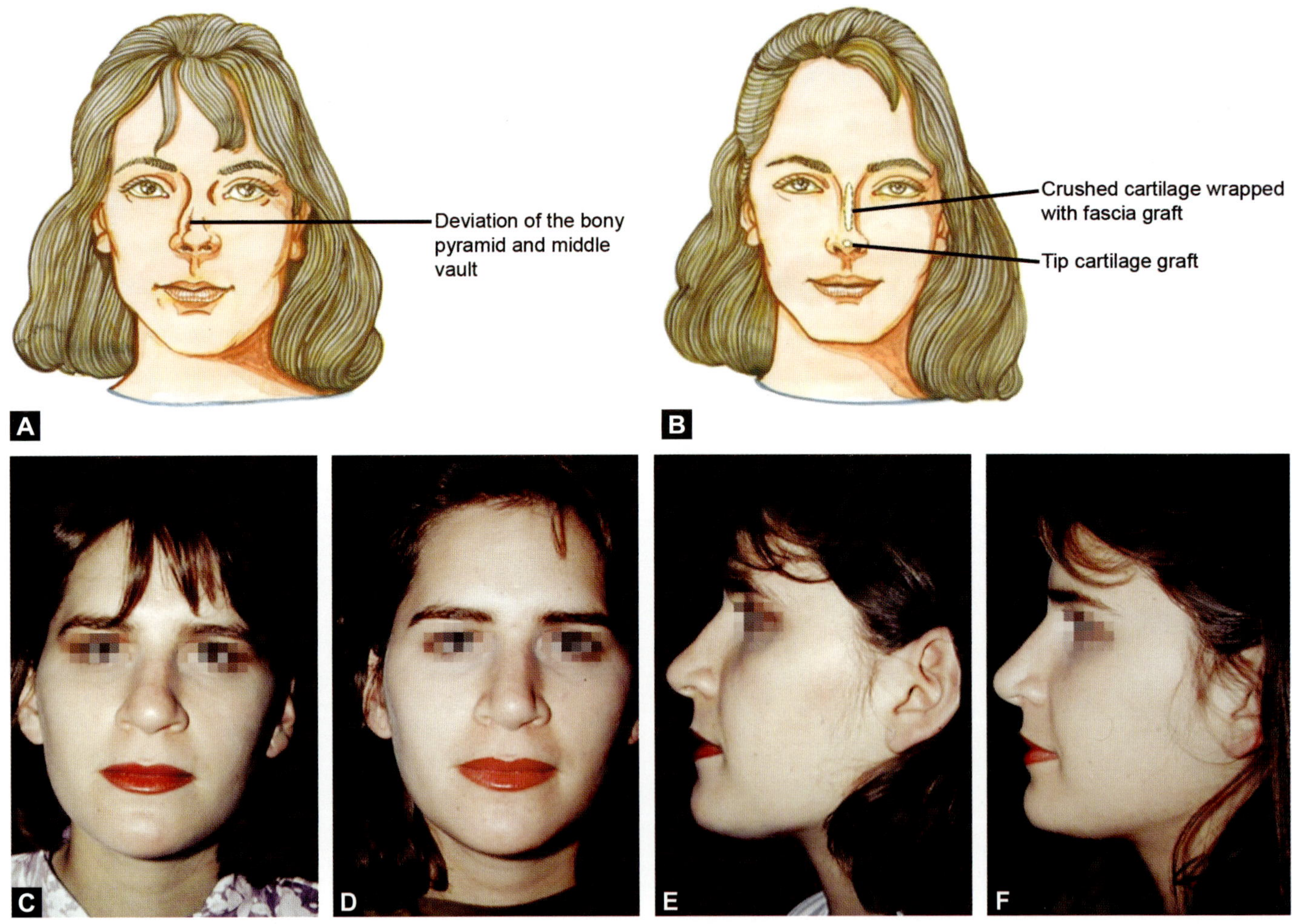

Figs. 5.28A to F: (A and B) Schematic of rhinoplasty placing combined fascia graft and fragmented cartilage in the dorsum and cartilage grafting in nasal tip. (C and E) Patient showing nasal deviation and hypertrophy of nose tip and wings. (D and F) Same patient 1 year after rhinoplasty.

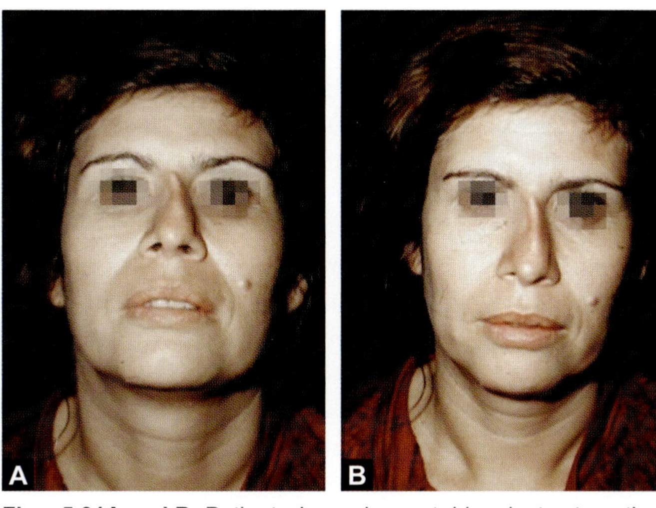

Figs. 5.31A and B: Patient who underwent rhinoplasty at another hospital showing a typical deformity developed when augmentation rhinoplasty is unsuccessful as a result of a deformed cartilage grafting produced by a very superficial cavity.

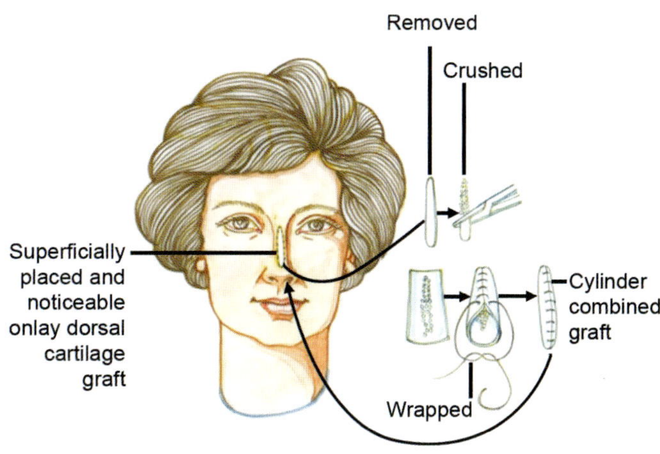

Fig. 5.32: Schematic secondary augmentation rhinoplasty.

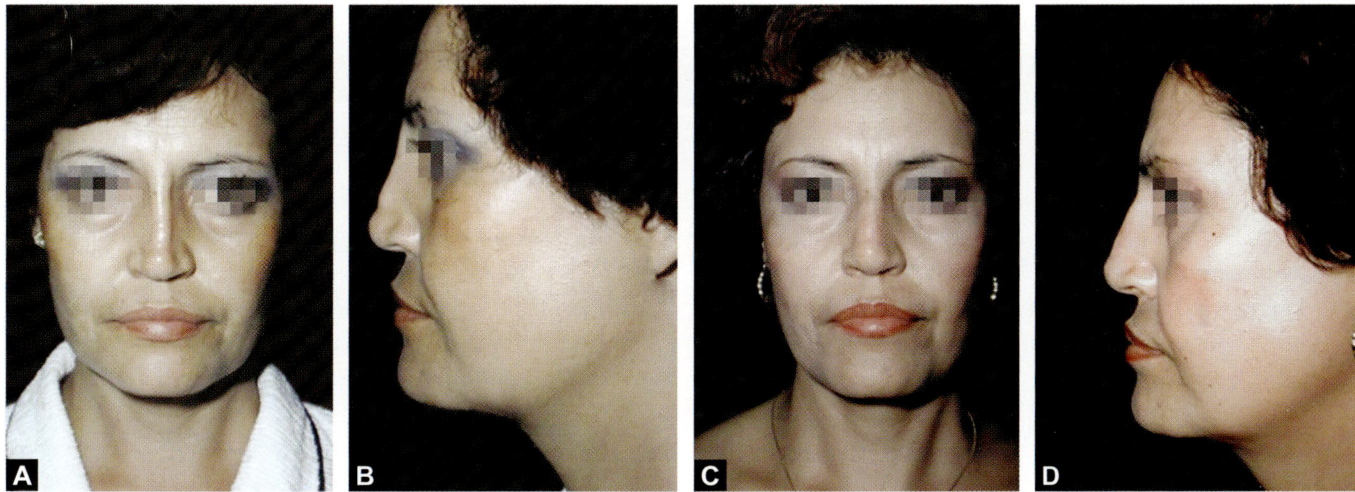

Figs. 5.33A to D: (A and B) Female patient after augmentation rhinoplasty for correction of nasal deformity. (C and D) Patient after secondary augmentation rhinoplasty with favorable aesthetic results.

The technique in correcting this deformity consists of the following: (1) The deformed graft is removed. After removal, it is fragmented and the pieces are placed in an adequately-sized fascia graft taken from the temporal region. (2) The fascia is sutured to form a combined cylinder-shaped graft and applied to a deep nasal dorsum cavity. (3) As in primary rhinoplasty, the combined graft is mounted. (4) The intranasal wound is closed (Fig. 5.32). (5) A nasal splint is placed; first a micropore splint and then a plaster splint. The nasal dorsum can manually be contoured when the before the plaster splint hardens.

CLINICAL CASE

Case 23. AJM is a 40-year-old female patient operated on at another institution where cartilage graft on the nasal dorsum was applied in a very superficial cavity. After surgery, the lumps were noticeable externally (Figs. 5.33A and B). The treatment consisted of performing the aforementioned procedure for secondary rhinoplasty. The result 1 year after was very satisfying. An aesthetic nasal dorsum can be seen with no irregularities (Figs. 5.33C and D).

PATIENTS WITH DEPRESSED DORSUM DUE TO EXCESSIVE RESECTION IN THE NOSE'S BACK IN PRIMARY AESTHETIC RHINOPLASTY

The 50s and 60s saw myriad cases of reduction rhinoplasty, as the procedure was extensively performed.

CLINICAL CASES

Case 24. AAI is a 22-year-old patient with over-resection of bone and cartilage who underwent primary rhinoplasty by another surgeon. On physical examination, there was radix and depressed nasal dorsum, supratip, valve collapse, exaggerated pig snout appearance, and acute nasolabial angle (Figs. 34C to E). Treatment included the application of multifragmented cartilage graft wrapped with fascia, valvuloplasty, and narrowing of the medial crura in the columella with cartilage suturing (Figs. 5.34A and B). Great improvements are visible 18 months after surgery (Figs. 5.34F to H). Picture of a satisfied patient 4 years later (Figs. 5.34I and J).

Case 25. LAF is a 40-year-old patient who underwent three previous rhinoplasties performed by general practitioners and not by plastic surgeons. On closer physical examination, there is a very depressed radix, a supratip, and a valvular collapse (Figs. 5.35A and B). Treatment consisted of two surgical procedures. The first surgery corrected the valvular collapse, which led to release of valvular retraction (Figs. 5.35C to G). Skin and auricular cartilage graftings were taken off and applied intranasally in the raw area formed as a consequence of the valvular collapse release, with skin out inside of the nose (Figs. 5.35H to K). The improvement achieved was positive. The second surgical procedure was performed 10 months following the previous one. The procedure involved placing a fascia-covered diced cartilage graft in the radix, correction of the supratip, removal of excess cartilage, application of spreader grafts, and cartilage grafting in nasal tip (Figs. 5.35L, N, O, and Q). Results 2 years after with corrected sequelae of previous rhinoplasties and aesthetic improvement of the nose (Figs. 5.35M, N, Q, and R).

Case 26. IVG is an 18-year-old patient with a bump on the nasal dorsum due to presence of a bone fragment. He had undergone primary rhinoplasty at another hospital (Figs. 5.36C and D). Scraping of the dorsum and application of a thinly fragmented cartilage graft wrapped in fascia was done (Figs. 5.36A and B). The surgical procedure achieved impressive results and high patient satisfaction (Figs. 5.36E and F).

Case 27. LAM is a 24-year-old patient presented with a mild irregularity of the nasal dorsum caused by inadvertent slash in the deep dermis and subcutaneous tissue when the primary rhinoplasty was done. In all likelihood nasal dorsum detachment was done with scissors (Figs. 5.37A to C). A slight rasping to the dorsum was done before applying a thin fascia fragmented cartilage graft. A favorable outcome after 1 year after surgery (Figs. 5.37D to F).

Simultaneous to the positive learning clinical experience of using fragmented cartilage graft in five volunteer

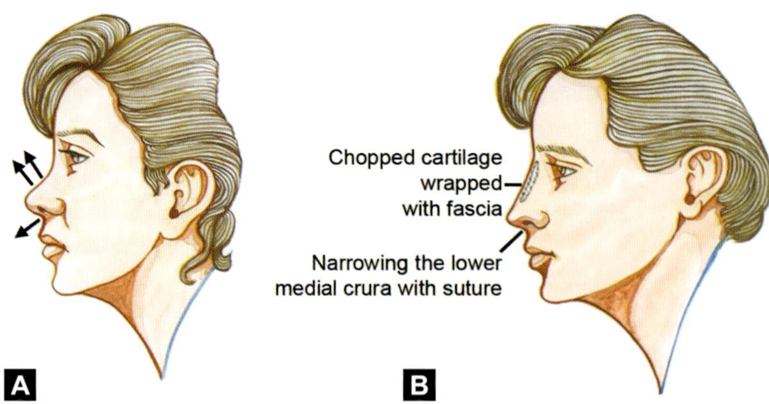

Figs. 5.34A and B: Basic treatment in secondary rhinoplasty includes the increase of the nasal dorsum, combined with fascia graft and fragmented cartilage, as well as other procedures.

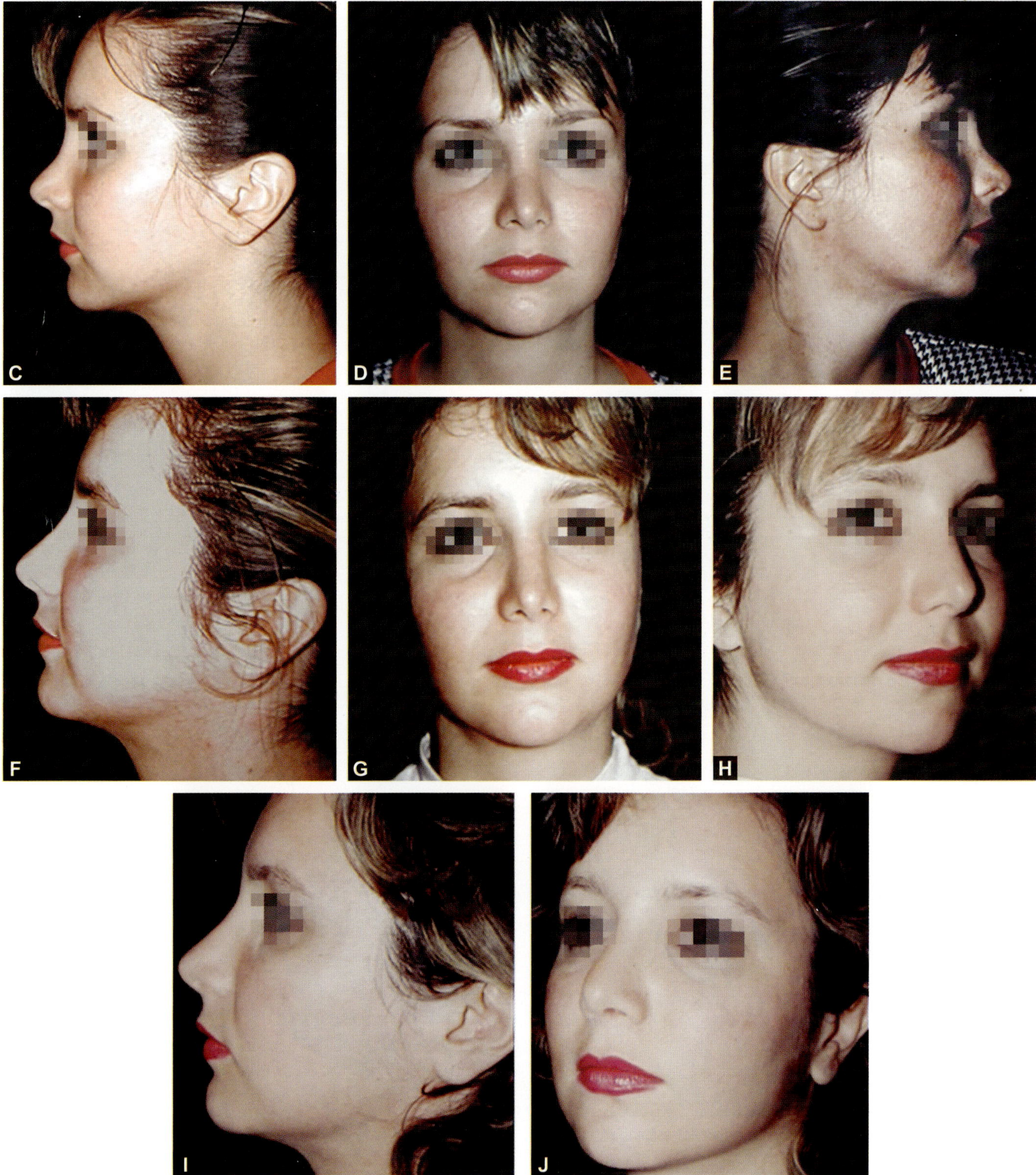

Figs. 5.34C to J: (C to E) Patient with radix and depressed nasal dorsum following primary rhinoplasty. (F to H) Patient after a year and a half following surgery. Excellent results. (I and J) Patient 4 years after secondary augmentation rhinoplasty.

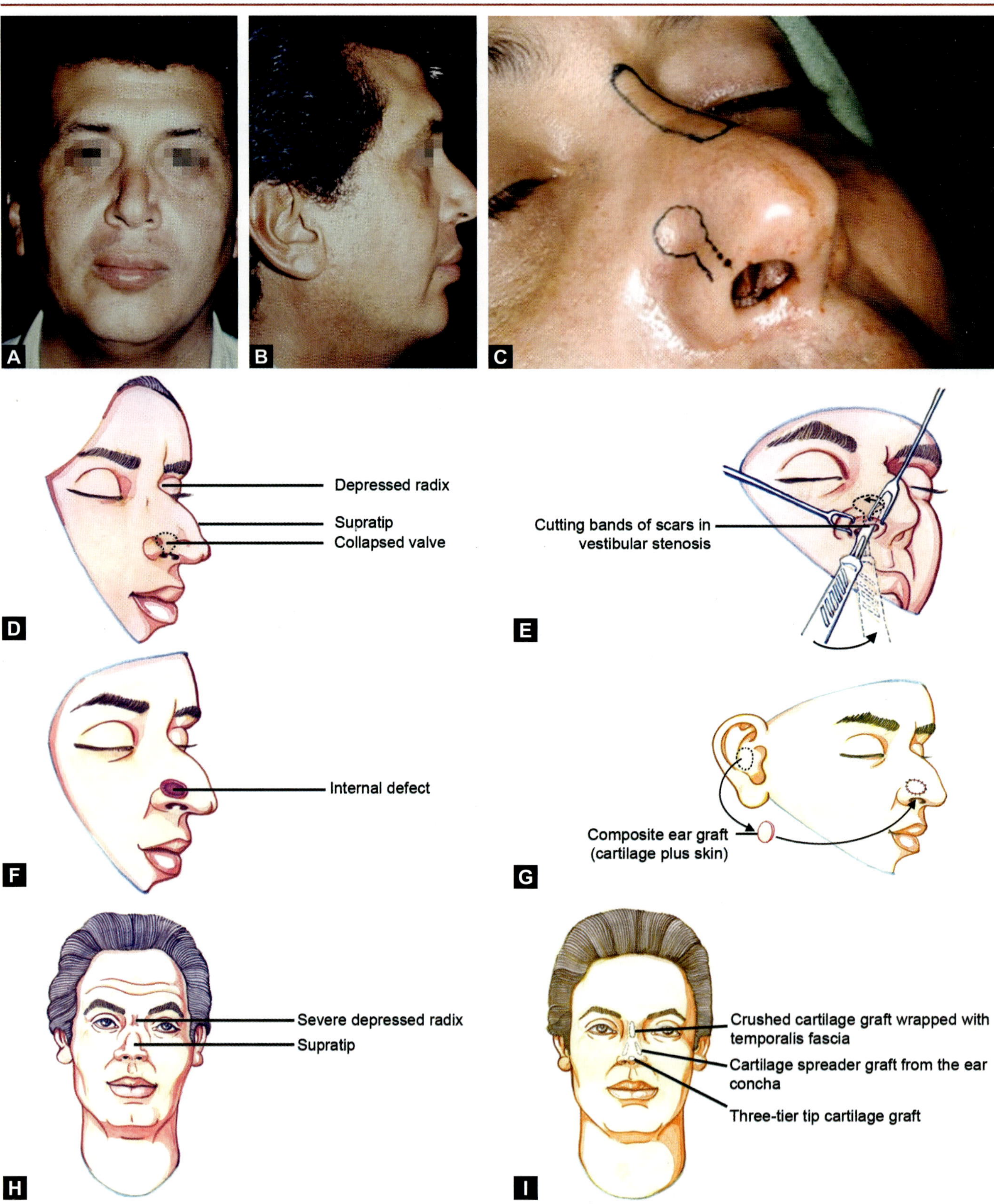

Figs. 5.35A to I

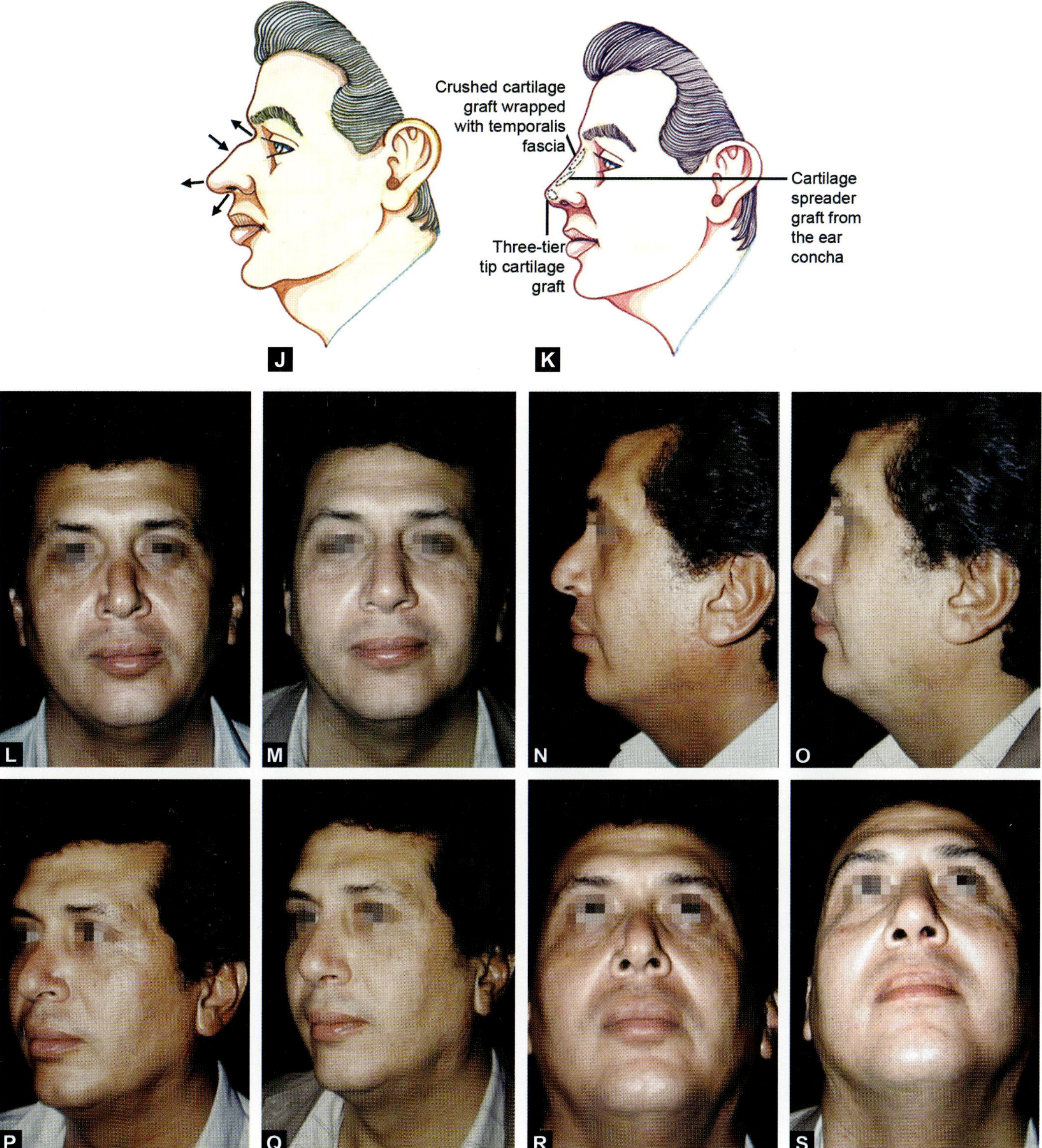

Figs. 5.35A to S: (A and B) Male patient with very deformed nose subjected to three previous rhinoplasties, in another hospital. (C to G) The first corrective surgery promoted liberation of valvular retraction by applying an intranasal skin cartilage. (H to K) In the second surgical procedure a fascia and cartilage graft was added to the radix, the supratip was corrected, cartilage spreader grafts were placed, as well as a cartilage graft to the nasal tip. (L to S) Patient before corrective rhinoplasty and 2 years following secondary correction.

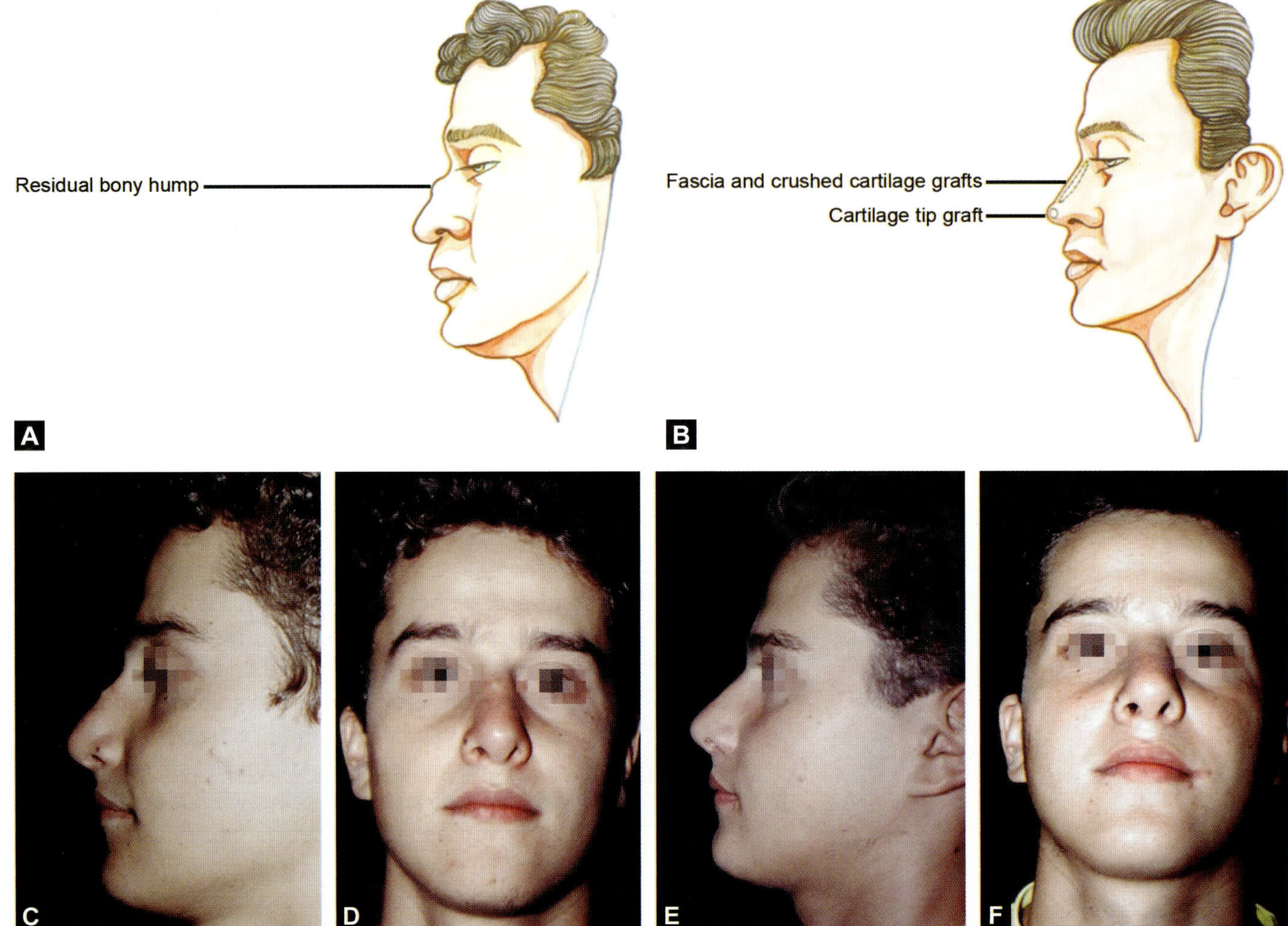

Figs. 5.36A to F: (A and B) Drawings of patient before and after correction using cartilage grafts with a fascial covering. (C and D) Patient with a mild deformity. (E and F). Cosmetic outcome following rhinoplasty.

patients at the Reconstructive Surgery Institute of Jalisco, fragmented cartilage grafts wrapped with fascia were applied subcutaneously to the back inner surface of the ear. Positive integration 6 months after, as histological report confirms (Figs. 5.38 and 5.39).

CONCLUSION

The use of fragmented or unfragmented cartilage graft wrapped with fascia is a procedure that yields good results. Fortunately, the two complications we have been confronted with, displacement, which is corrected by placing a plaster splint after shaping the grafted dorsum, and infection manifested as localized edema, erythema and presence of liquid, easily respond to treatment. The former is successfully treated through a small incision in the dorsum for liquid extraction; the latter by placing a micropore and plaster splint with constant pressure for 12 days, and by prescribing an antibiotic.

To avoid complications surgeons must comply with a meticulous surgical technique: careful cartilage and fascia grafts taking, careful preparation and making of nasal cavity where the combined graft will be mounted, and changing surgical instruments as necessary on suspected contamination.

The combined cartilage and fascia graft is an excellent alternative for augmentation rhinoplasty.

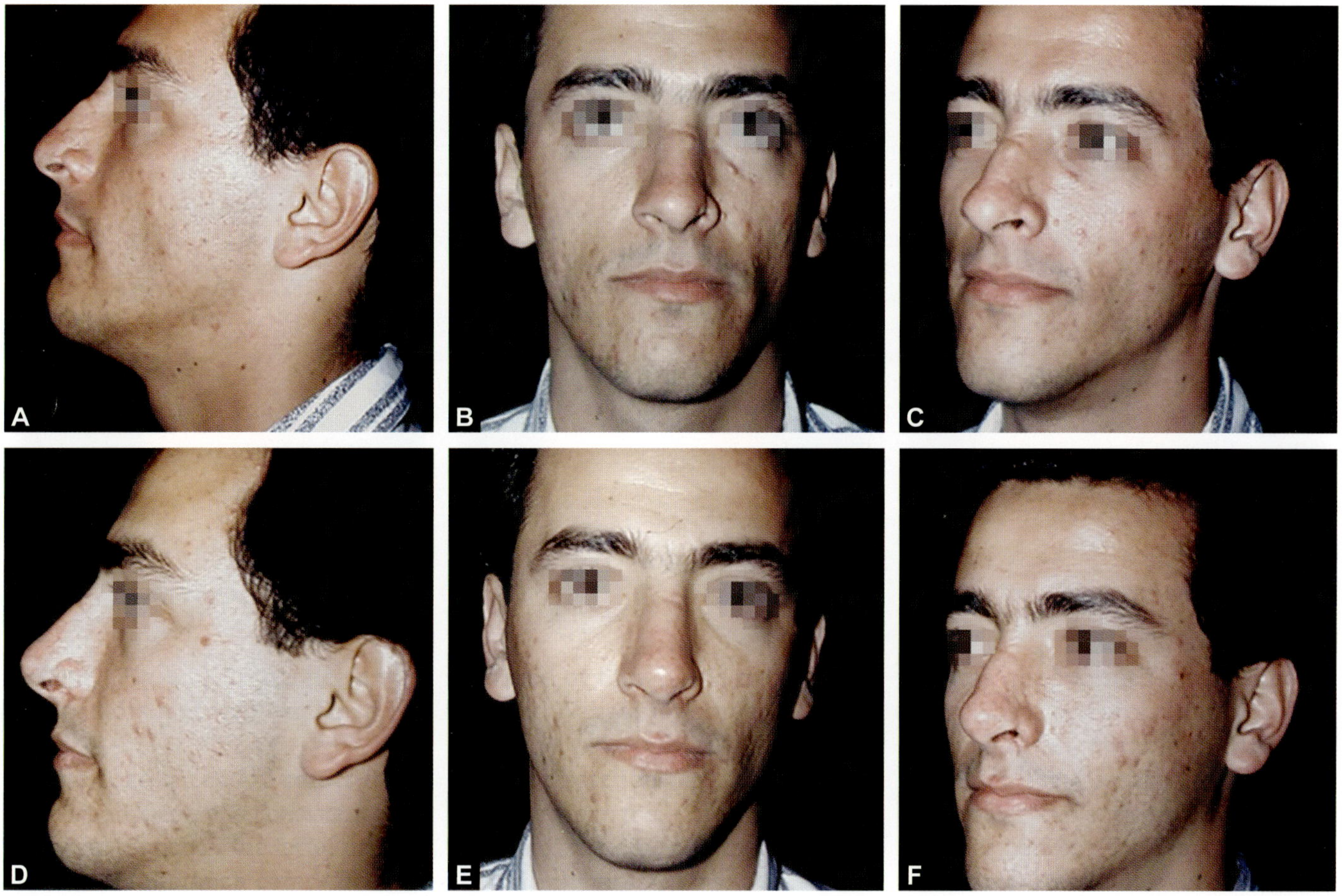

Figs. 5.37A to F: (A to C) Nasal dorsum depression after primary rhinoplasty. (D to F) The result achieved with fascia and crushed cartilage grafts.

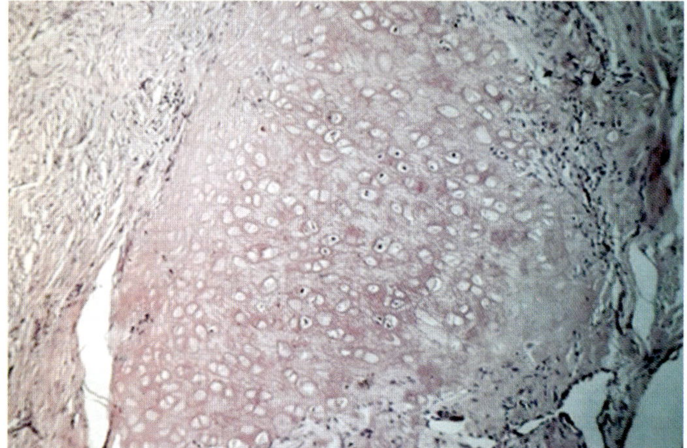

Fig. 5.38: Histological images of fascia and cartilage grafts applied to the retroauricular area. The excellent integration of this combined graft material can be seen 6 months after surgery.

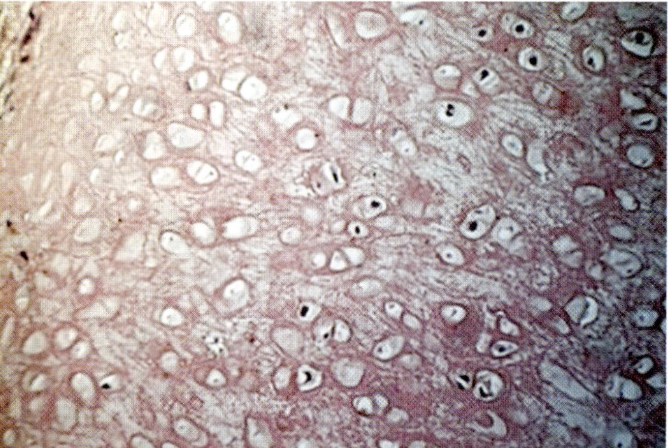

Fig. 5.39: Histological images of fascia and cartilage grafts applied to the retroauricular area. The excellent integration of this combined graft material can be seen 6 months after surgery.

REFERENCES

1. Stark RB, Frileck SP. Conchal cartilage grafts in augmentation Rhinoplasty and orbital floor fracture. Plast Reconstr Surg. 1969;43:6.
2. Ortiz-Monasterio F, Olmedo A, Oscoy LO. The use of cartilage grafts in primary aesthetic rhinoplasty. Plast Reconstr Surg. 1981;67:597.
3. Guerrerosantos J. Temporoparietal free fascia grafts in rhinoplasty. Plast Reconstr Surg. 1984;74:465-74.
4. Sheen JH. Conchal cartilage for dorsal grafts. Aesthetic Rhinoplasty, Vol. I. C.V. Mosby Company; St. Louis 1987. p. 428.
5. Ortiz-Monasterio F, Michelena J. The use of augmentation rhinoplasty: techniques for the correction of the non-caucasian nose. Clin Plast Surg. 1988;15:57-72.
6. Gunter JP. Augmentation rhinoplasty: dorsal onlay grafting using shaped autogenous septal cartilage. Plast Reconstr Surg. 1990;86:39-45.
7. Erol OO. The Turkish delight: a pliable graft for rhinoplasty. Plast Reconstr Surg. 2000;105:2229-41.
8. Guerrerosantos J, Trabanino C, Guerrerosantos F. Multifragmented cartilage wrapped with fascia in augmentation rhinoplasty. Plast Reconstr Surg. 2006;117:804-12.
9. Daniel RK. The role of diced cartilage grafts in rhinoplasty. Aesthet Surg J. 2006;26:209-13.
10. Daniel RK. Diced cartilage grafts in rhinoplasty surgery: current techniques and applications. Plast Reconstr Surg. 2008;122:1883-92.

6 Total Resection of the Alar Cartilages and Temporal Fascia Technique in Rhinoplasty

Salvador Rodríguez-Camps Devís

INTRODUCTION

This technique commenced in 1987 with a secondary rhinoplasty case with a highly unappealing nasal tip whose cartilages were completely broken (Figs. 6.1A and B). The author had to choose between eliminating the whole nasal dome and resetting it with a new cartilaginous structure or removing all the cartilage remains and covering with two-layered temporal fascia. The latter procedure was performed and follow-up years later showed the result to

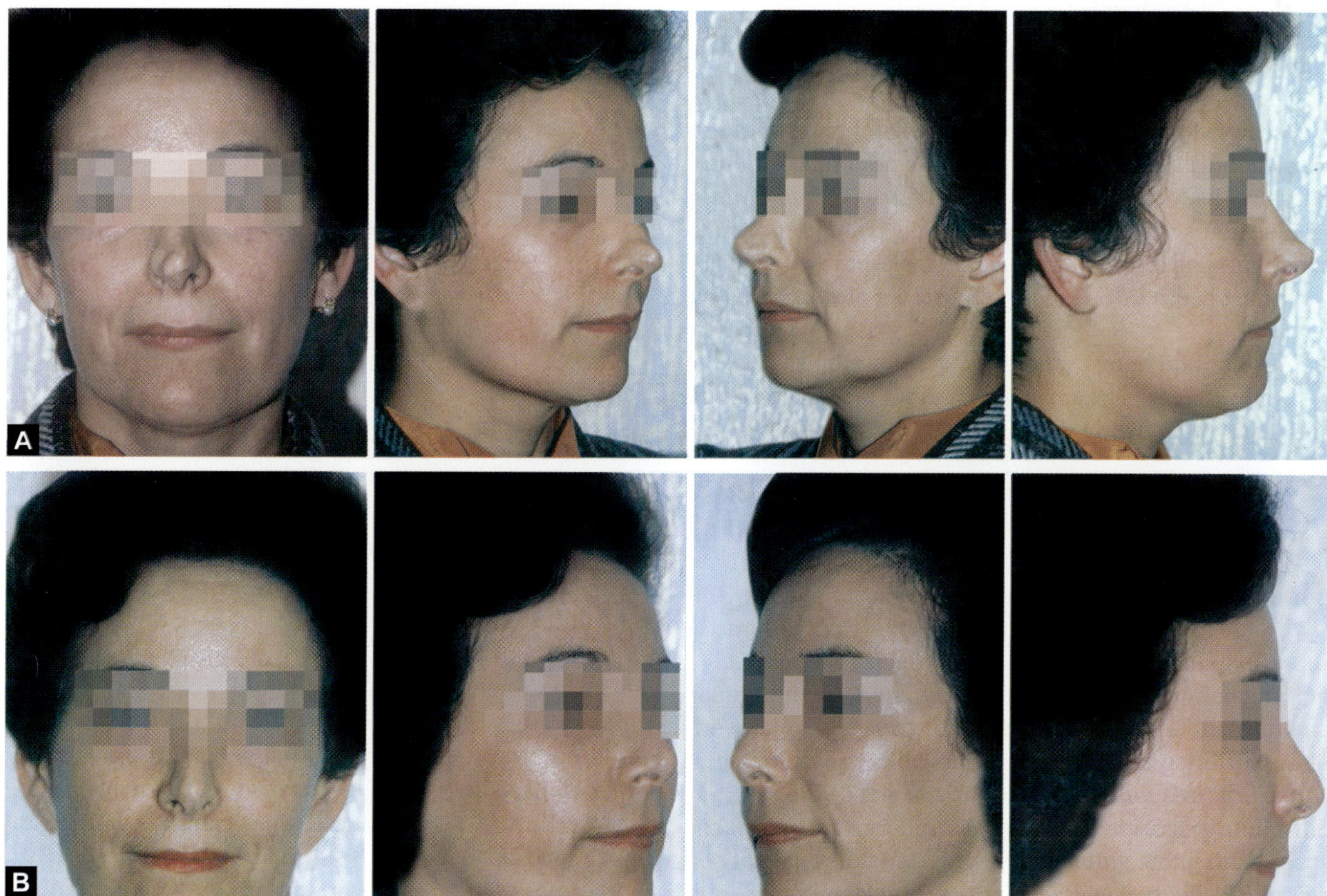

Figs. 6.1A and B: Author's first case in 1987. (A) Preoperative 38-year-old female who had been previously operated on twice at another clinic. The nasal tip is completely destroyed, with broken alar cartilages. (B) One year postoperative after type II resection-reconstruction.

remain stable. However, as all the plastic surgery treaties and publications warn us about the importance of conserving an alar cartilage band of no less than 3-5 mm on its caudal edge to avoid collapses, the author thought further cases should be performed. After performing more cases collapse did not occur. The indications were extended with particularly difficult primary rhinoplasty cases involving extremely domed, flat, and wide tips (Figs. 6.2 to 6.11).

Over the years the author continued improving and perfecting this process that went against what was "technically correct." The results were followed for as long as possible. After the operation, the results remained aesthetic and that the nasal base was checked to be equilateral and stable with a solid tripod and an equilateral stable base. To achieve this effect, some technical resources were introduced that helped convert to a long-pointed or flattened nose into what ensured good results with an equilateral base (Figs. 6.12 to 6.15). Then work was started with alar wedges, vestibular wedges, resecting or using a suture in the center of the crus medialis feet, partial reduction of the soft triangles, Converse suture, etc. to stabilize the tip. As the years passed, the indications continued to be extended and good results were obtained. However, the author was aware that what was being done was still "technically incorrect." The author decided to wait a little longer and acquire as much experience as possible to ensure that everything that was being done was not "incorrect by chance." The author wanted absolute security to be able to defend the technique when it emerged with all the consequences. The technique was presented at meetings[1-9] and published in medical journals.[10,11] There was acknowledgement that the results achieved have been excellent. Therefore, if the results are sound, the technique must be correct.

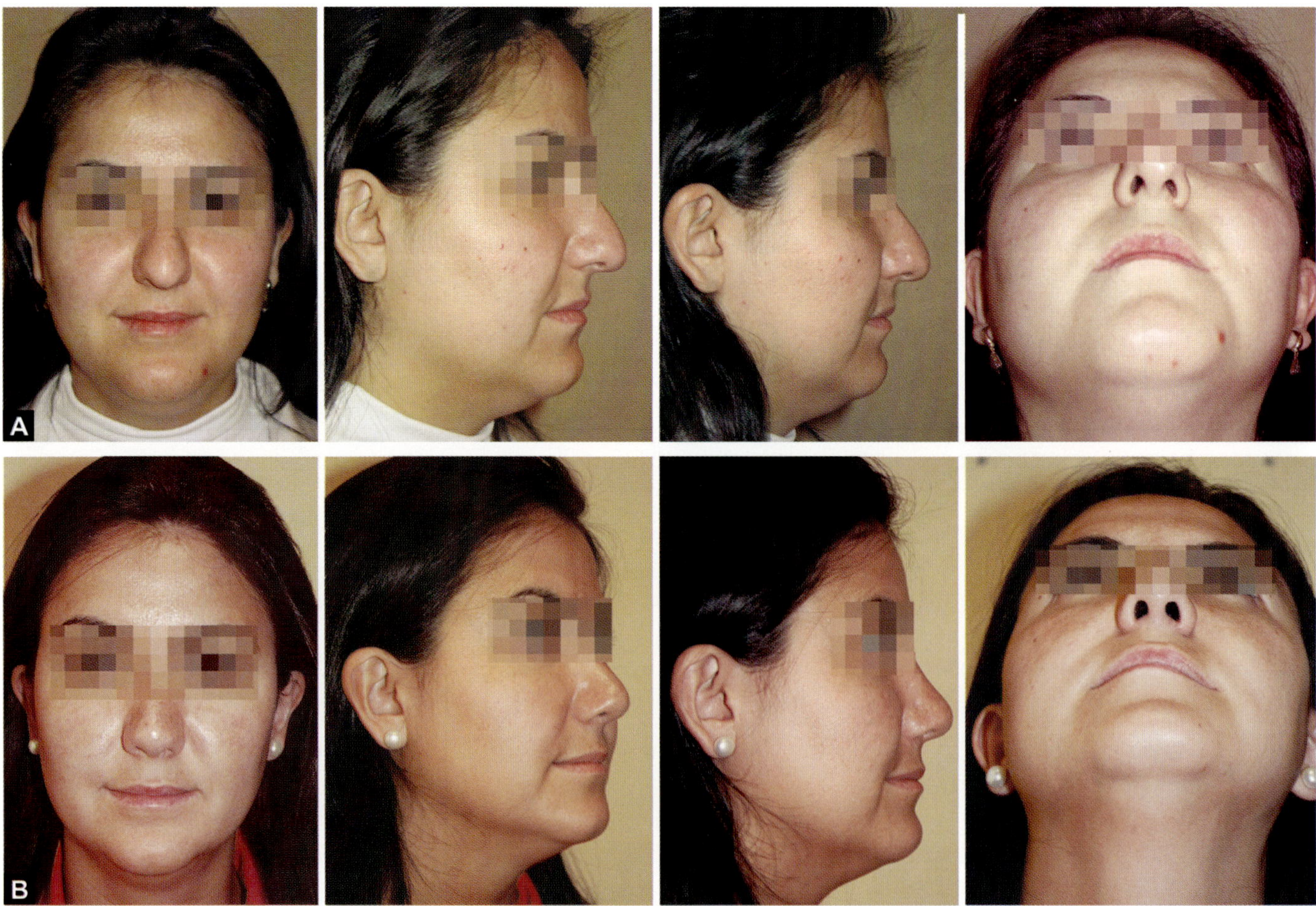

Figs. 6.2A and B: (A) Preoperative 26-year-old female with very thick skin. (B) One year postoperative after type II resection-reconstruction, but with a one-layered temporal fascial patch.

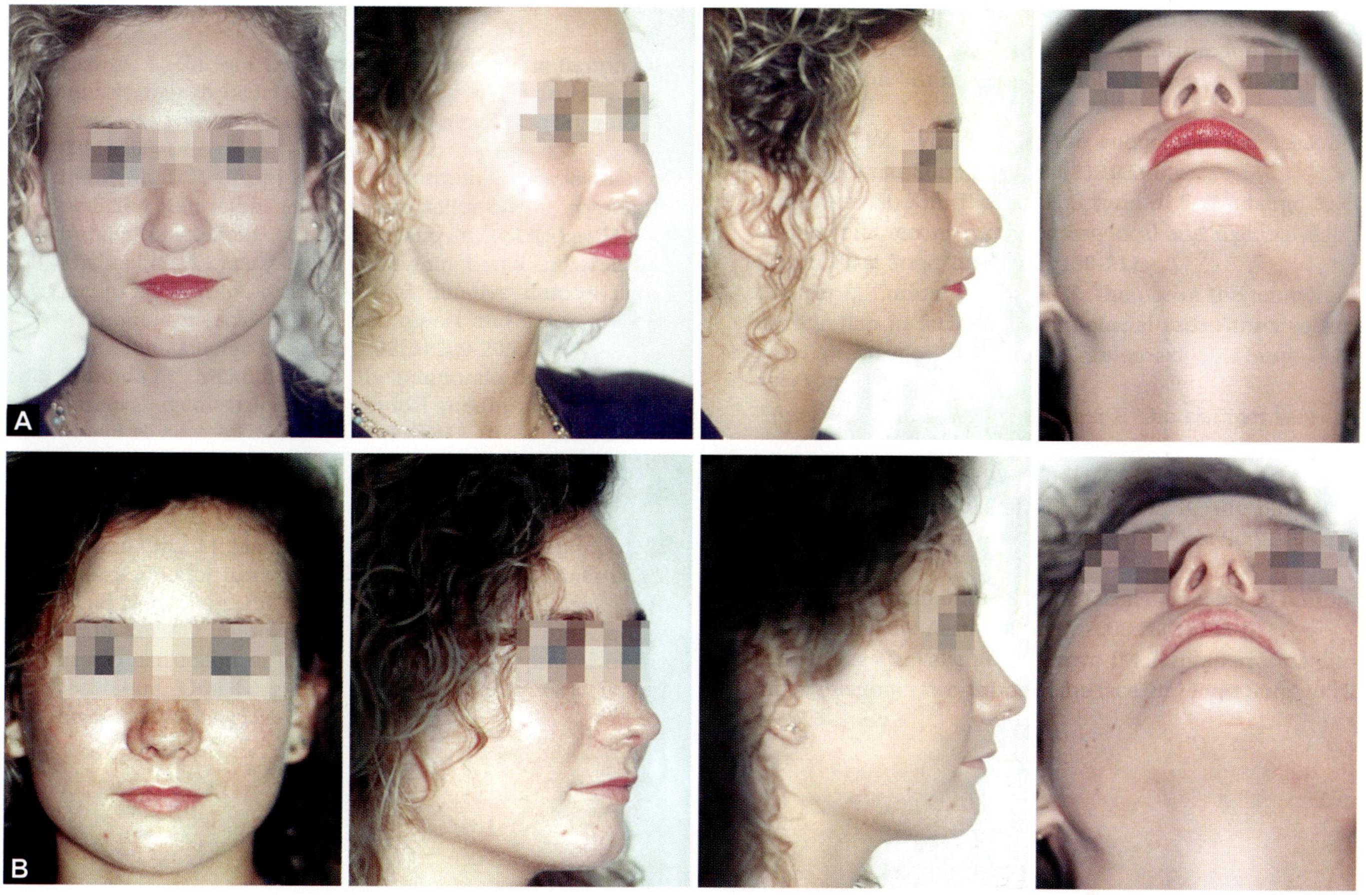

Figs. 6.3A and B: (A) Preoperative 21-year-old female with a wide and luxated nasal tip. (B) One year postoperative following type IV resection-reconstruction.

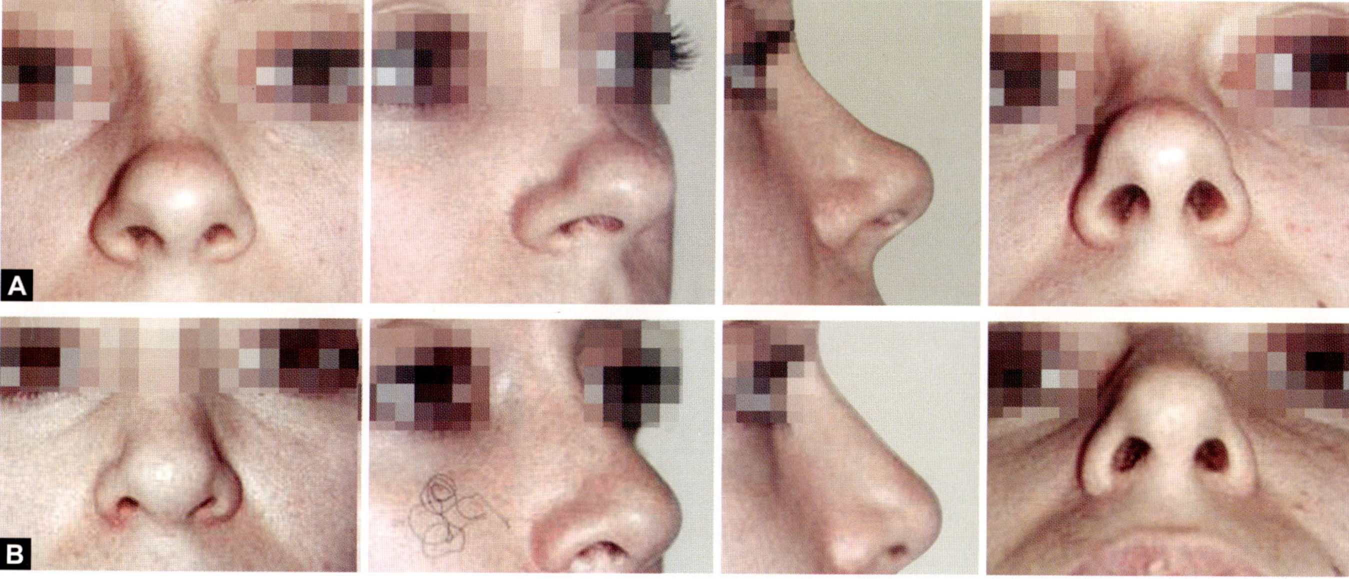

Figs. 6.4A and B: (A) Preoperative 26-year-old patient with a “clown tip.” (B) One year postoperative after type II resection-reconstruction.

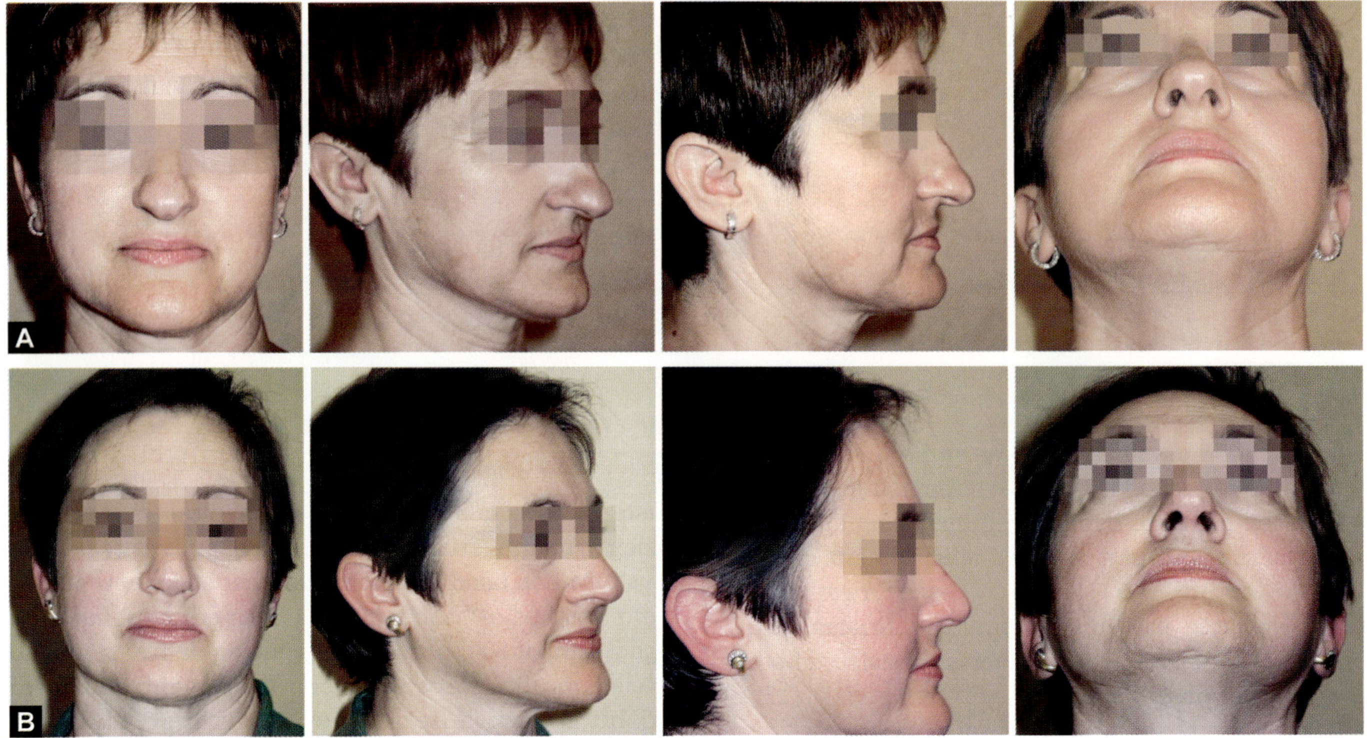

Figs. 6.5A and B: (A) Preoperative 52-year-old patient with large hypertrophied alar cartilages and excessively wide tip. (B) One year postoperative following type IV resection-reconstruction.

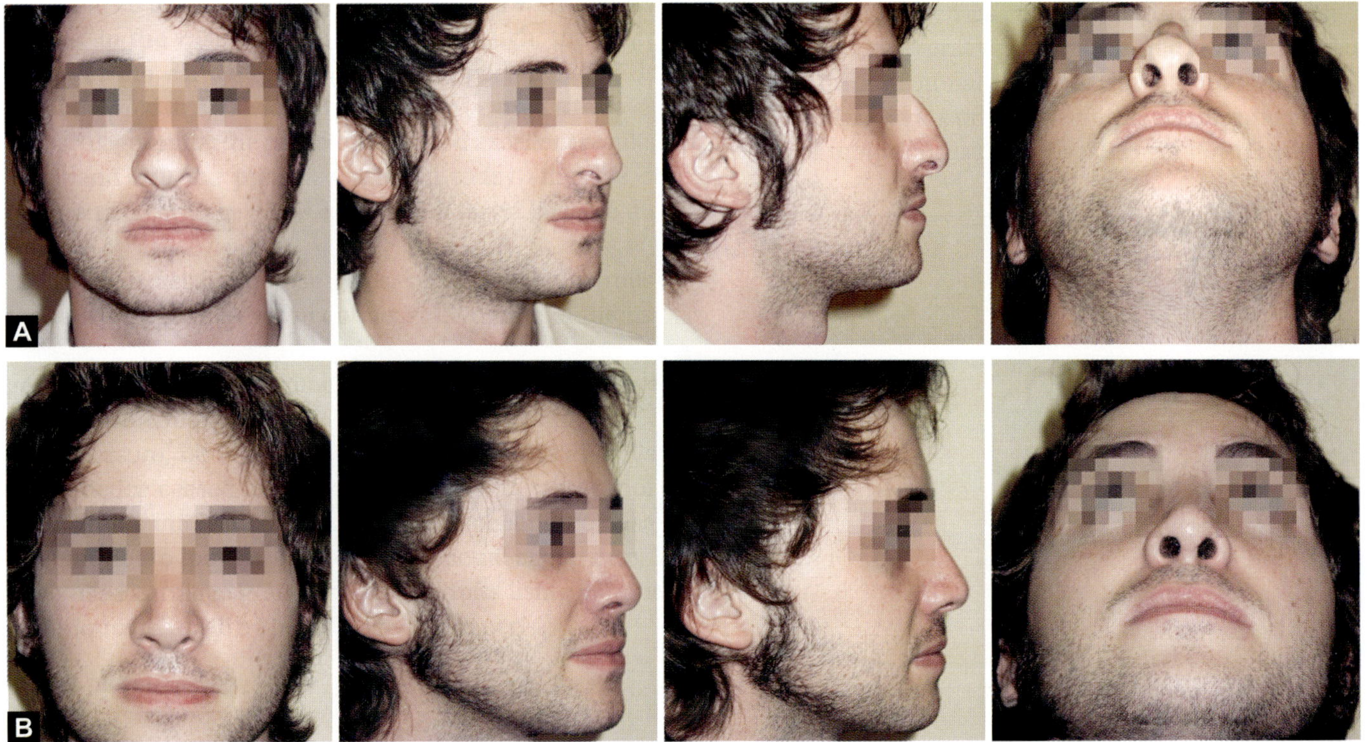

Figs. 6.6A and B: (A) Preoperative 25-year-old male with rounded and wide nasal tip. (B) One year postoperative following Type II resection-reconstruction.

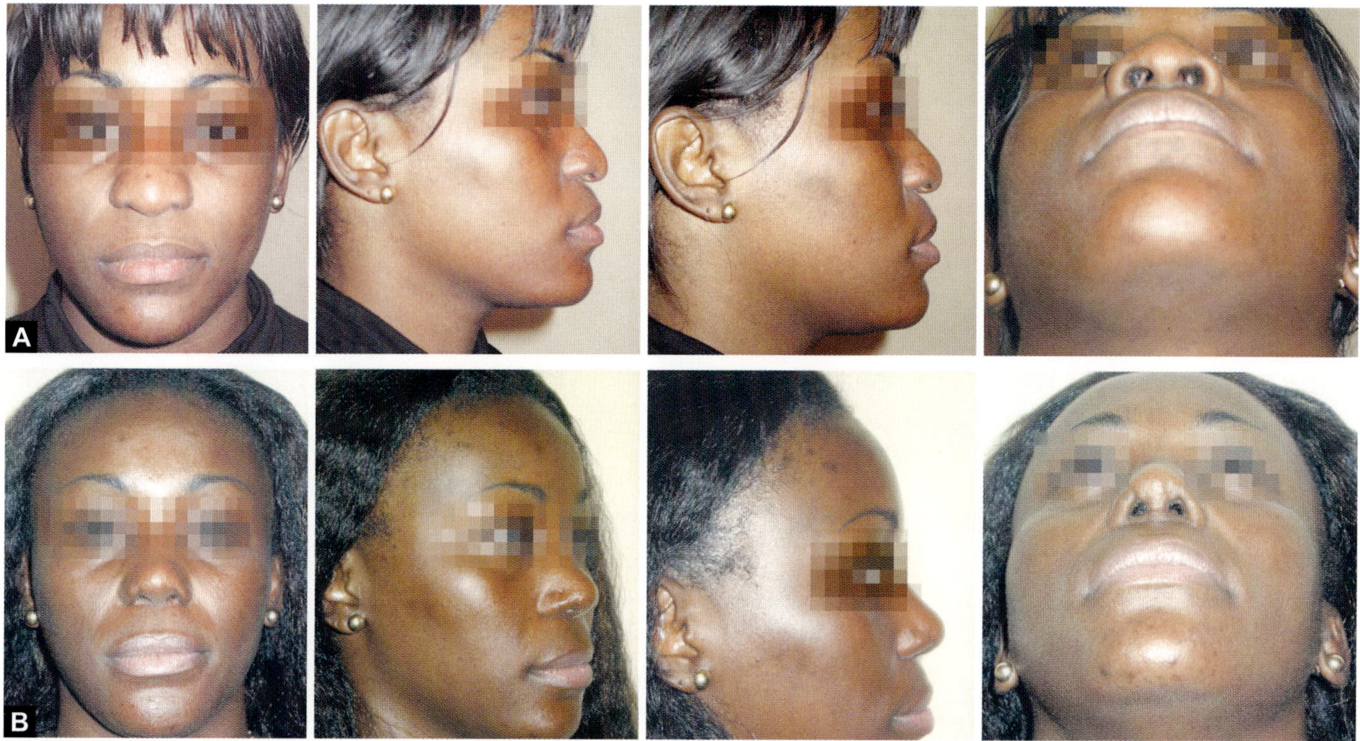

Figs. 6.7A and B: (A) Preoperative 35-year-old female with downward tip. (B) One year postoperative after type V resection-reconstruction

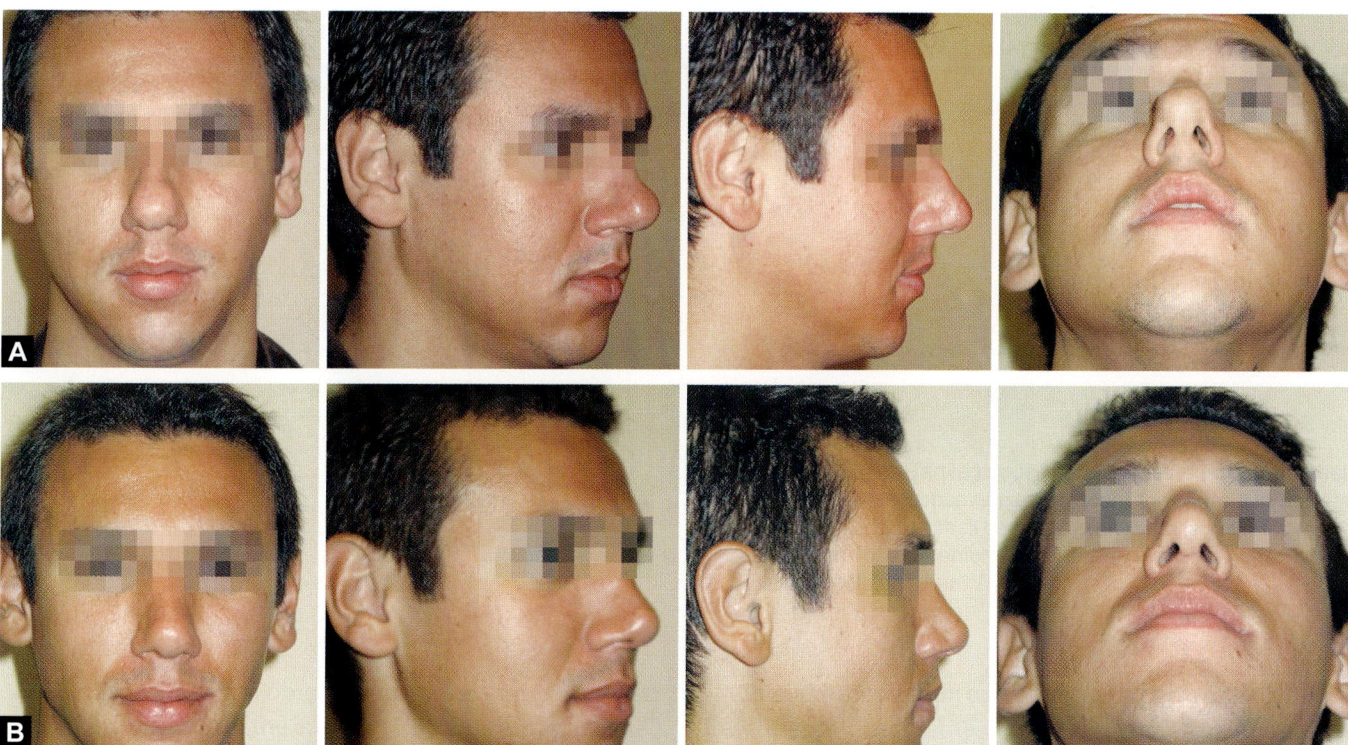

Figs. 6.8A and B: (A) Preoperative 28-year-old male with bulbous and hypertrophied tip. (B) One year after type III resection-reconstruction.

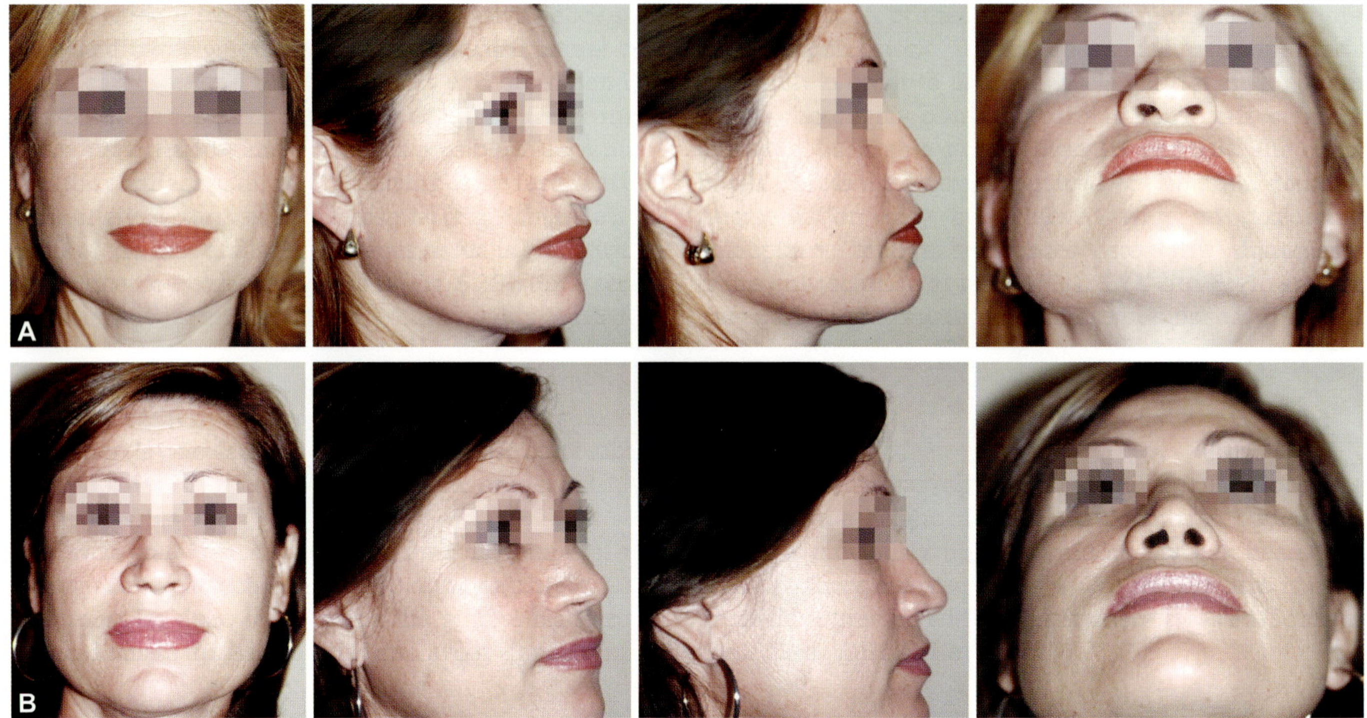

Figs. 6.9A and B: (A) Preoperative 48-year-old female with completely crushed and excessively wide nasal tip. (B) One year postoperative following primary rhinoplasty with type V resection-reconstruction.

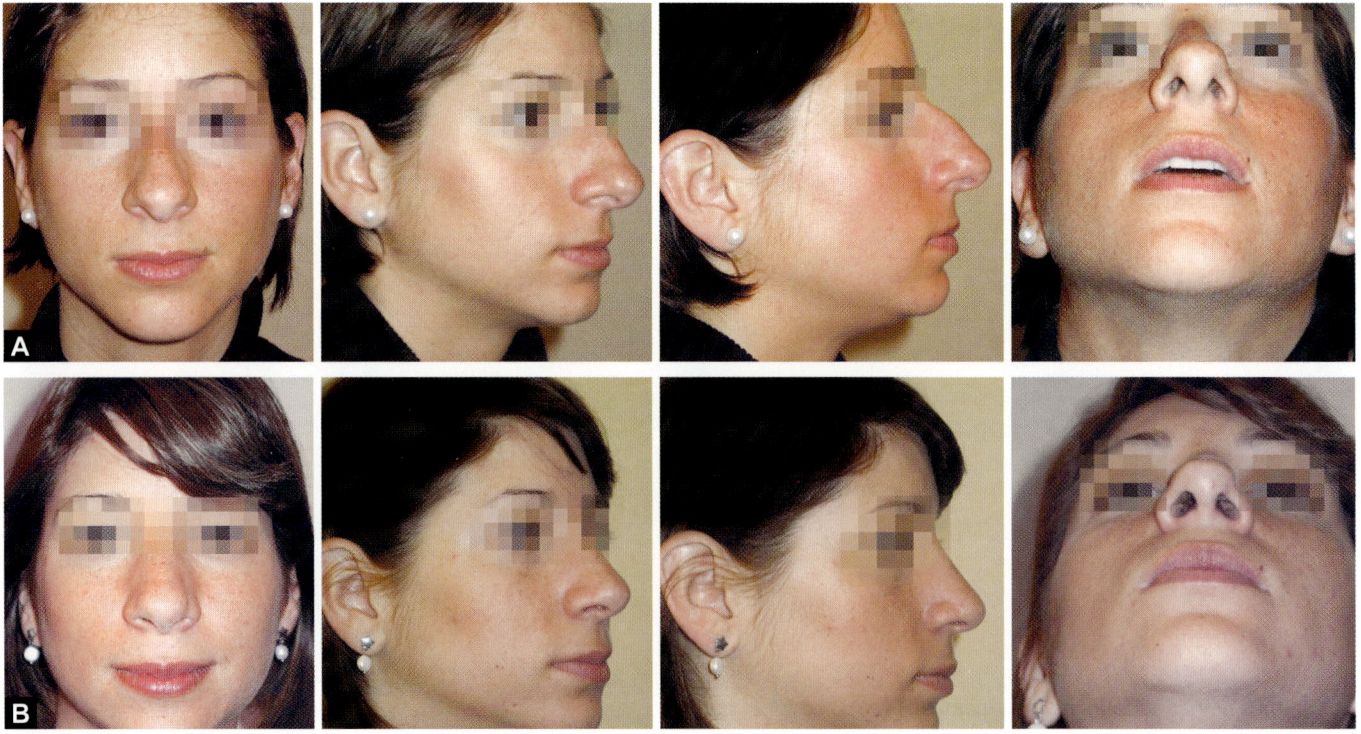

Figs. 6.10A and B: (A) Preoperative 26-year-old female with very thick and pronounced alar cartilages. (B) One year postoperative after type III resection-reconstruction.

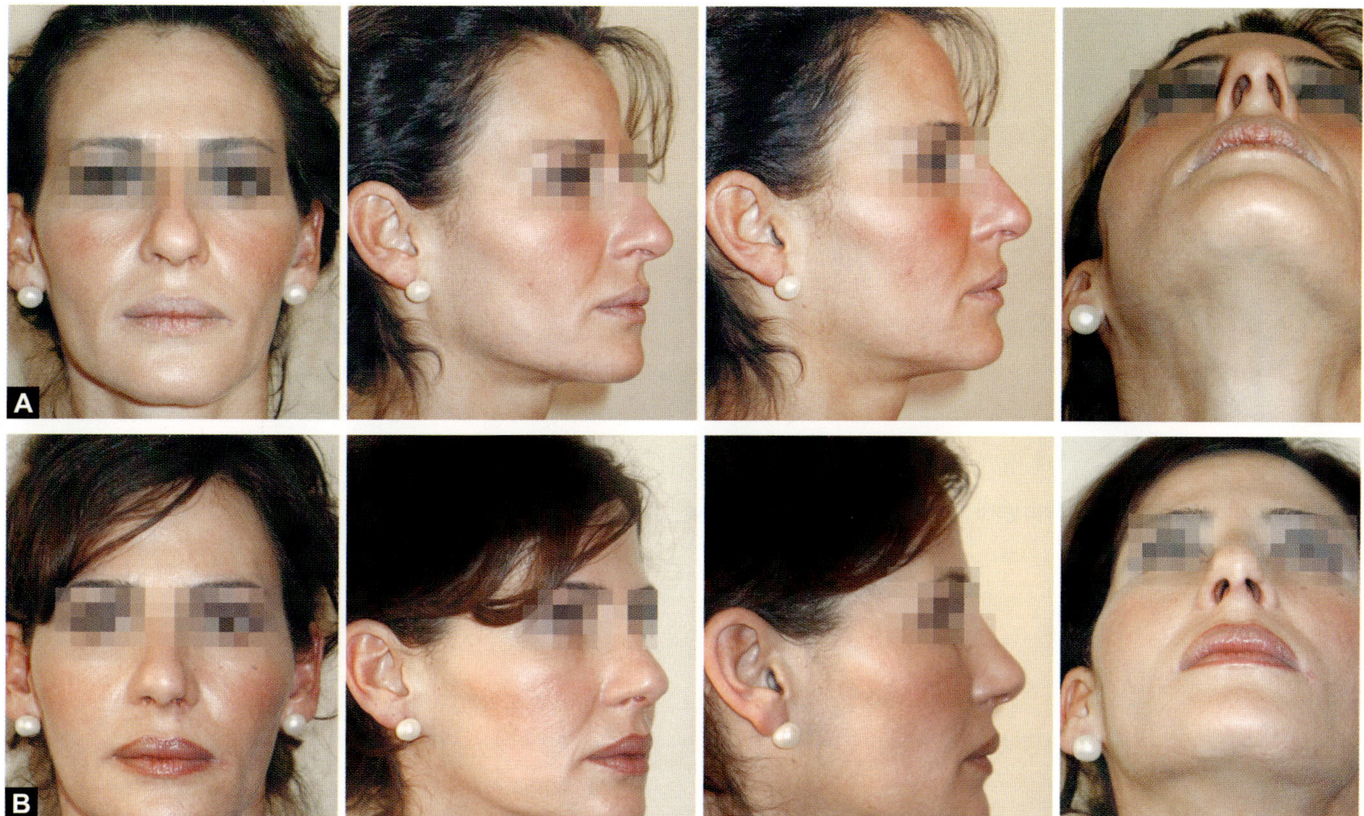

Figs. 6.11A and B: (A) Preoperative 35-year-old female with a bulbous tip. (B) One year postoperative following type IV resection-reconstruction.

TECHNIQUE

"Rhinoplasty is decidedly a very difficult operation although, technically, it seems deceptively easy" (Jack Sheen).

The author has operated on >500 patients with this technique and over 23 years (1987–2010) with highly satisfactory results. The technique, always Rethi (open rhinoplasty), is especially designed for secondary (Figs. 6.16 to 6.19) and traumatic (Fig. 6.20) rhinoplasty. Yet the author is increasingly employing it in primary rhinoplasty when the solution for a cartilaginous dome proves difficult with other techniques. The author has also gained experience in nasal reconstruction, mainly after cancer surgery on the nasal tip (Fig. 6.21).

The Resection

The main objective is an equilateral and stable nasal base (Fig. 6.22). To fulfill this objective, the author has classified resections into five types (although, in very special cases, it is convenient to make some little combinations between them):

Type I: Complete resection of alar cartilages, including domes and one trunk of the crus medialis. This is indicated for noses that are long-pointed, have a long columella, and for large and elongated nostrils. Here, we introduce some of our technical resources, such as alar wedges, and resecting the crus medialis feet (Fig. 6.23).

Type II: Complete resection of alar cartilages, including domes. This is indicated for noses with a slightly elongated nasal base (Fig. 6.24).

Type III: Total resection of alar cartilages, respecting domes. Applicable to noses whose nasal base is very close to the objective (equilateral nasal base) (Fig. 6.25).

Type IV: Total resection of alar cartilages, respecting domes, and leaving two small alar wedges whose latero-caudal length is no longer than 8 mm and is of an arrow-tip shape. Indicated for cases where the nasal base is equilateral (Fig. 6.26).

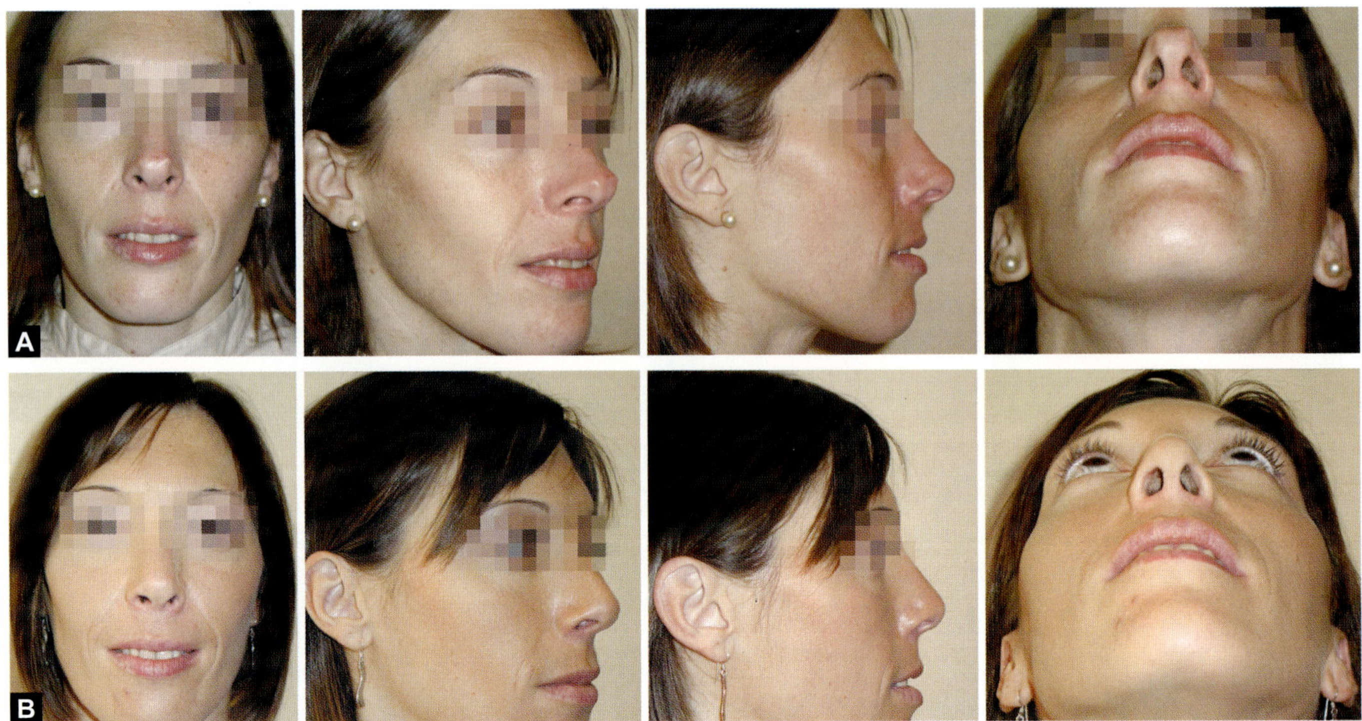

Figs. 6.12A and B: (A) Preoperative 32-year-old female with a bifid and sharp nasal cupola on both alar cartilages. (B) One-year postoperative after primary rhinoplasty with type III resection-reconstruction.

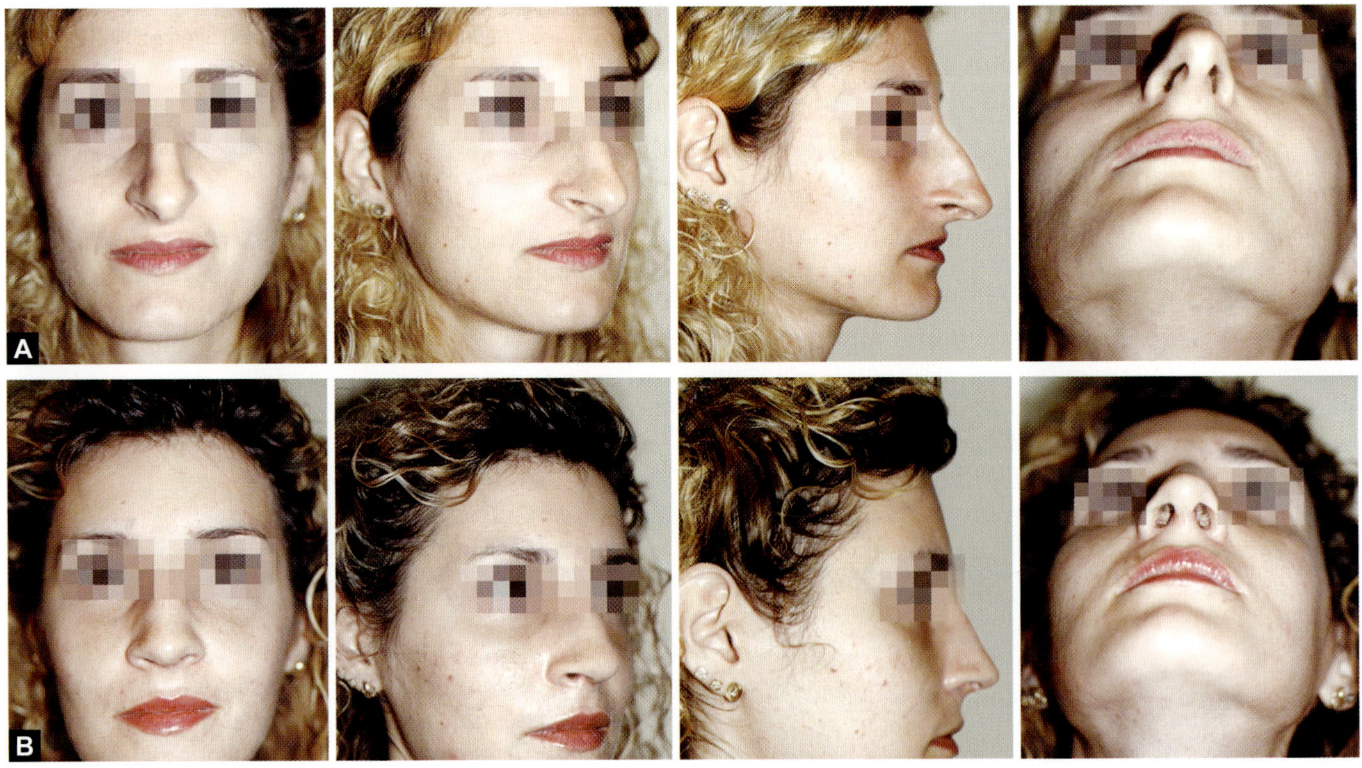

Figs. 6.13A and B: (A) Preoperative 27-year-old female with an excessively projecting nasal tip. (B) Two years postoperative after primary rhinoplasty with type I resection-reconstruction.

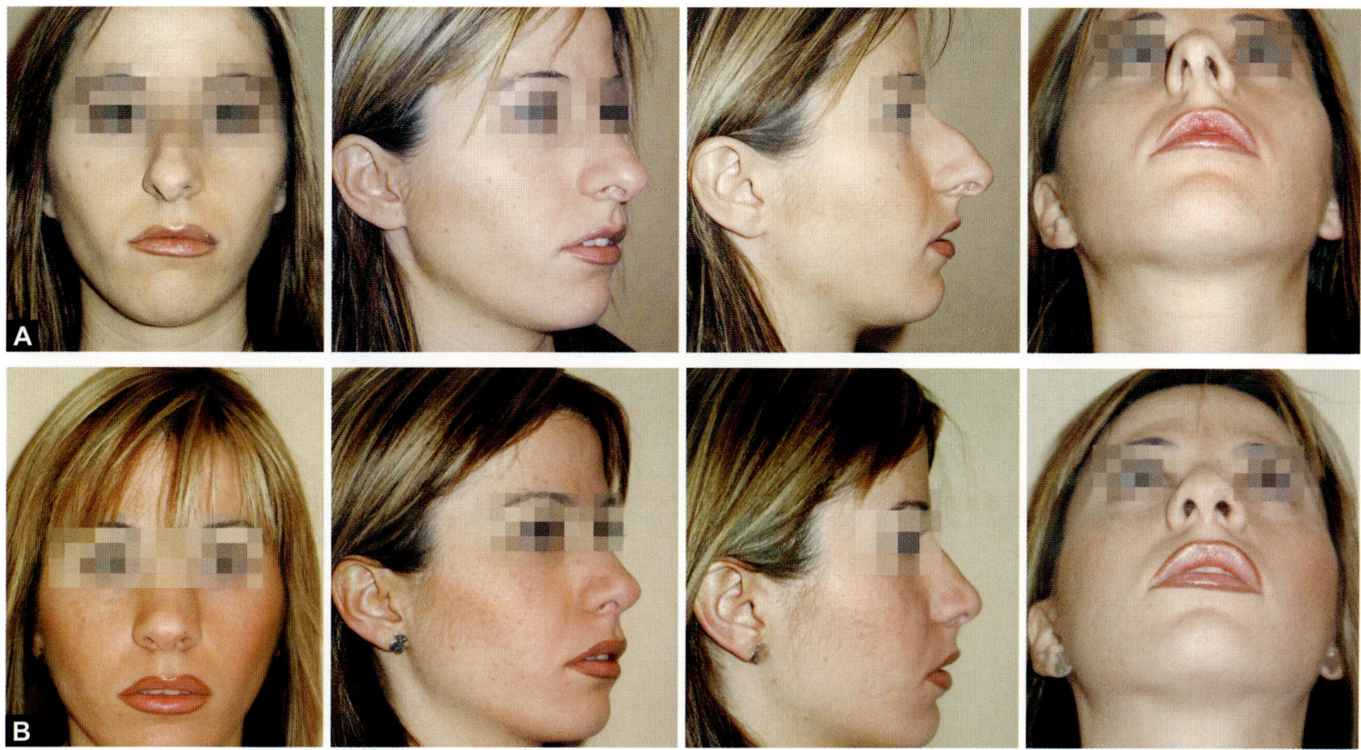

Figs. 6.14A and B: (A) Preoperative 22-year-old female with considerable rhinomegaly. (B) Two years postoperative after type I resection-reconstruction.

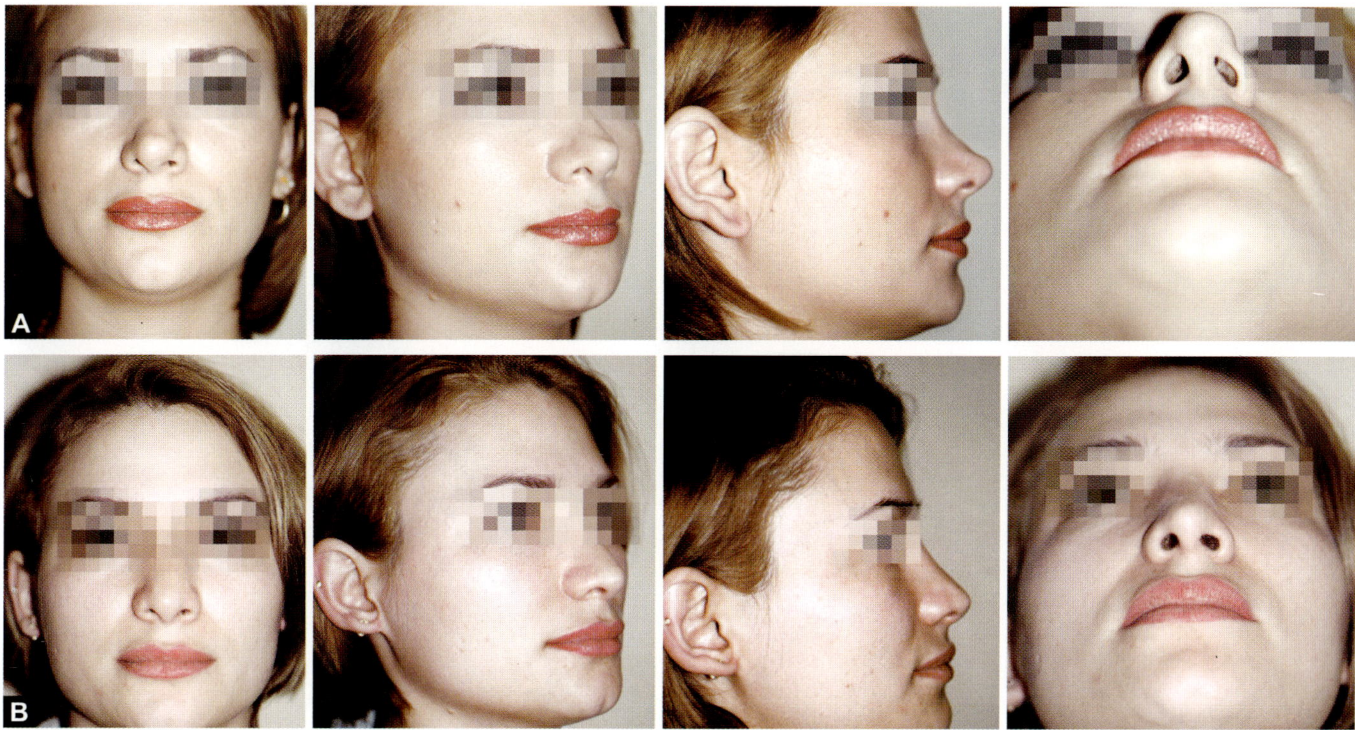

Figs. 6.15A and B: (A) Preoperative 32-year-old female with considerable asymmetry of the tip and cartilages with excess projection. (B) One year postoperative following type I resection-reconstruction.

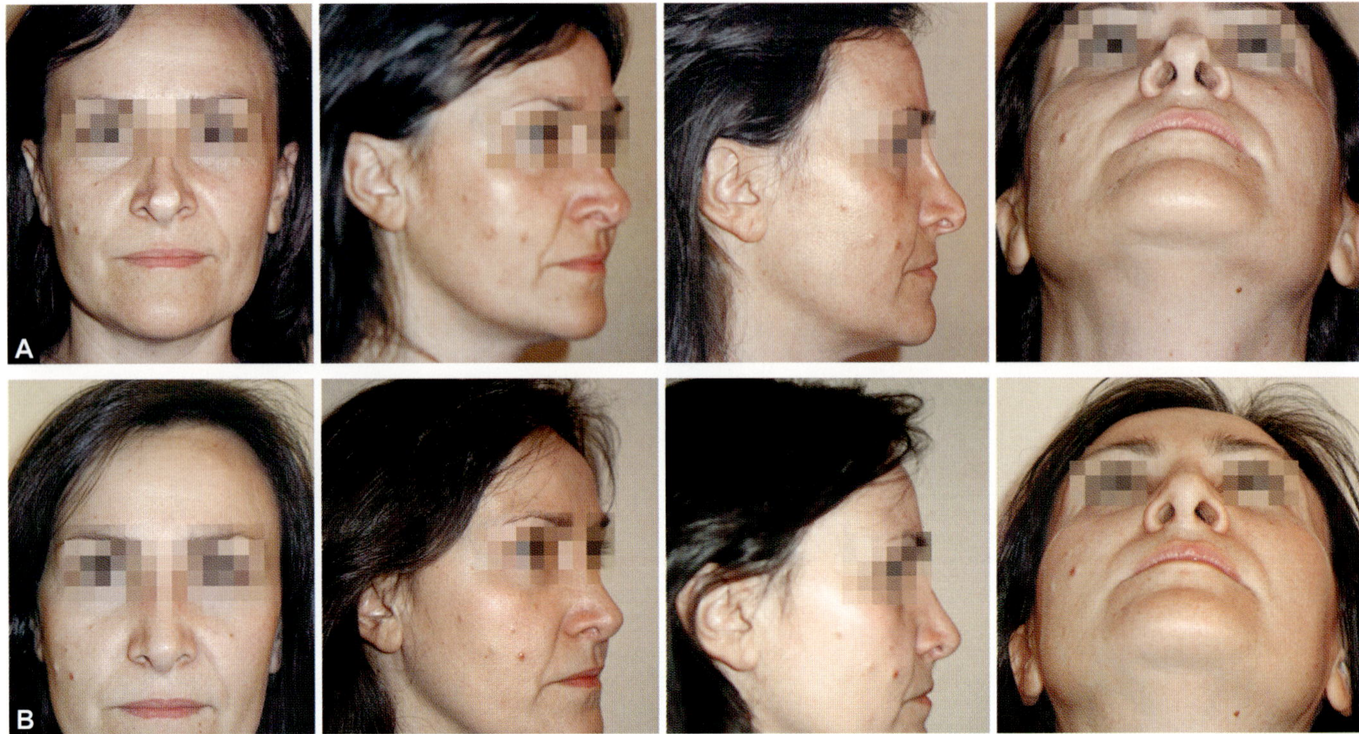

Figs. 6.16A and B: (A) Preoperative 36-year-old female previously operated on three times at other clinics. (B) One year postoperative after secondary rhinoplasty using type III resection-reconstruction.

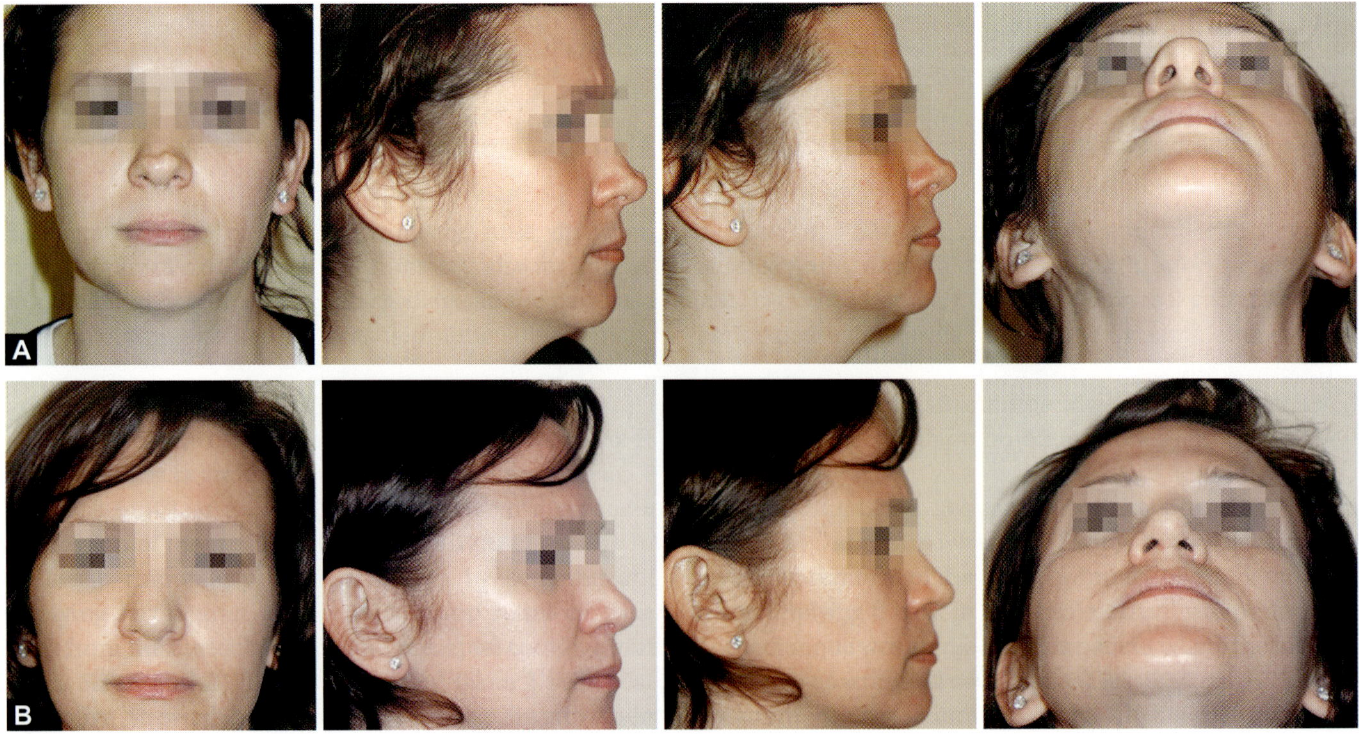

Figs. 6.17A and B: (A) Preoperative 24-year-old female with asymmetrical nasal tip and prominent cartilaginous remains. (B) Two years postoperative after secondary rhinoplasty using type II resection-reconstruction.

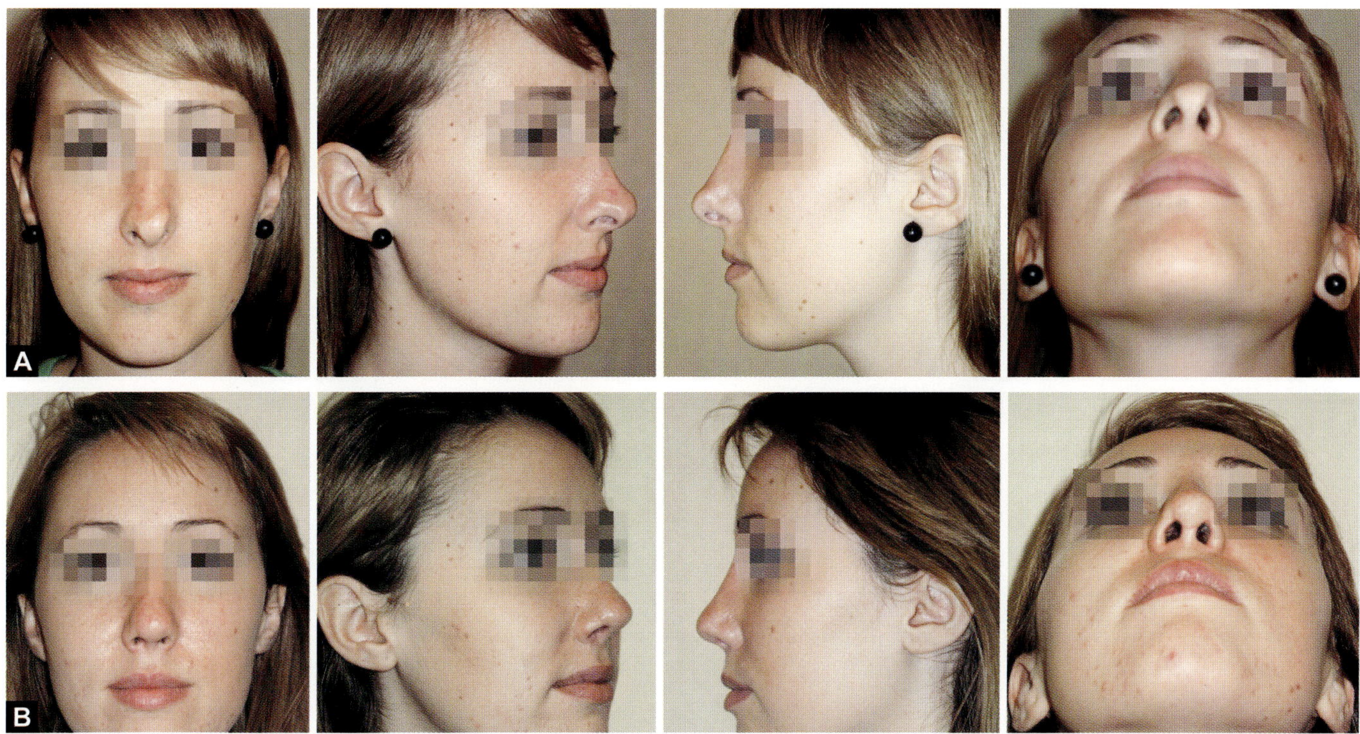

Figs. 6.18A and B: (A) Preoperative 27-year-old female whose tip and wings show high cartilaginous asymmetry. B) One year post-operative following secondary rhinoplasty using type III resection-reconstruction.

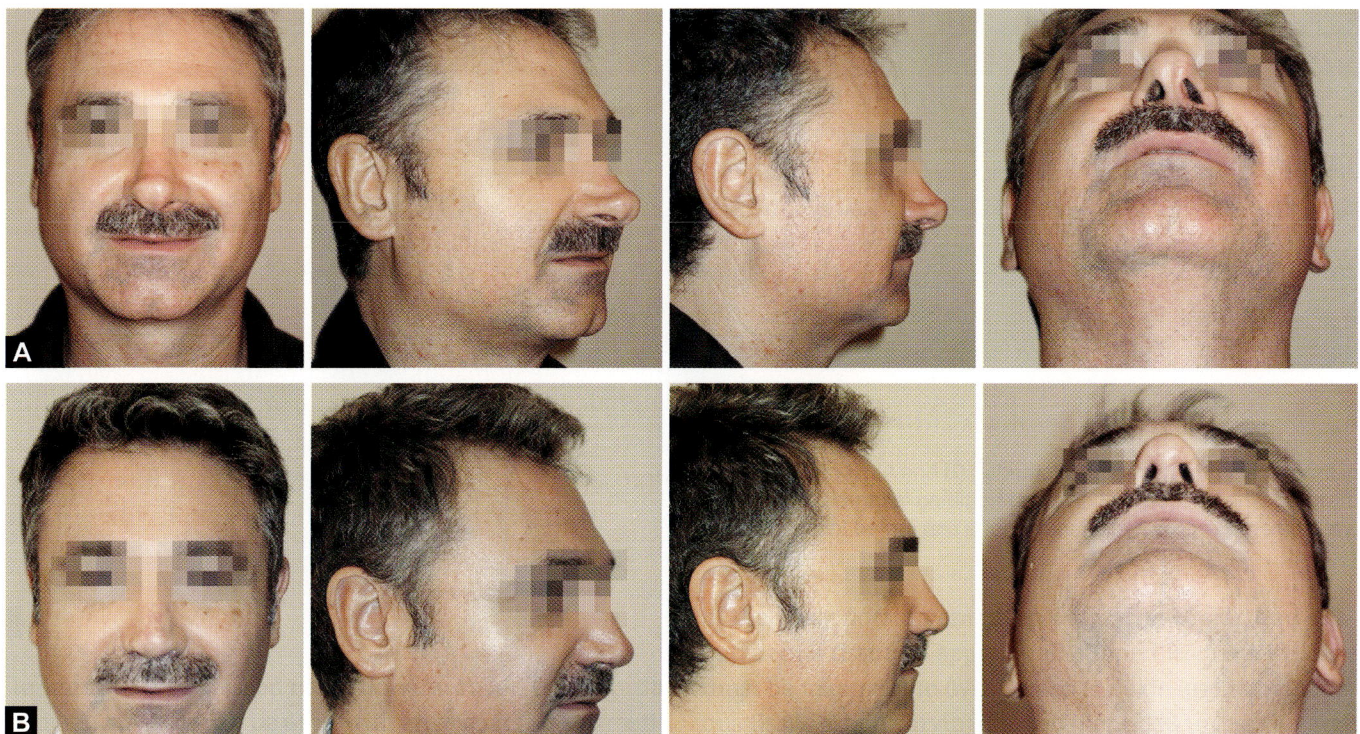

Figs. 6.19A and B: (A) Preoperative 52-year-old male previously operated on twice. The patient presents overprojecting and broken cartilaginous-structured remains. (B) One year postoperative after type I resection-reconstruction.

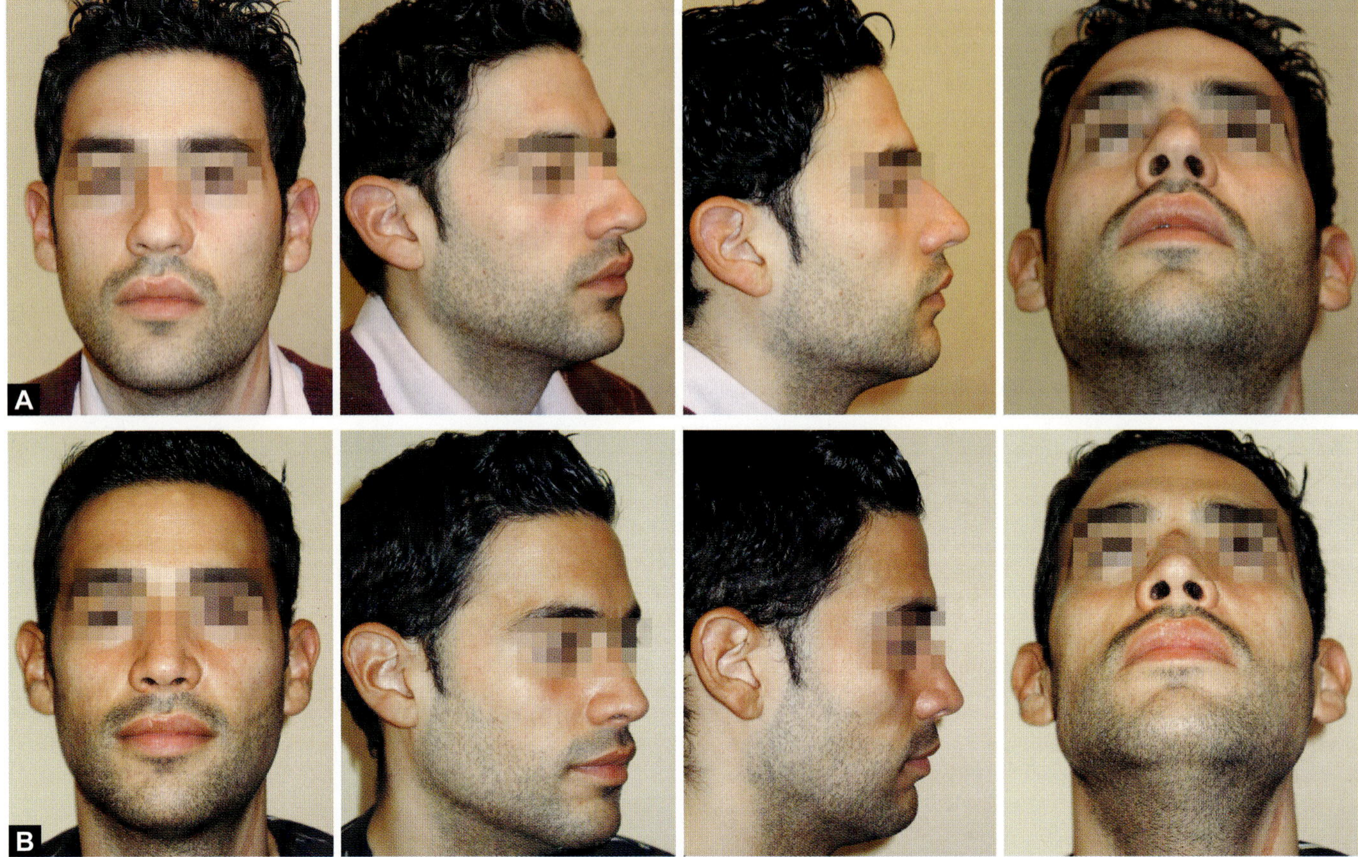

Figs. 6.20A and B: (A) Preoperative 28-year-old male previously operated for severe facial traumatism, whose bone-cartilaginous structure was completely fractured. (B) One year postoperative following type III resection-reconstruction.

Type V: Total resection of alar cartilages, respecting domes and approaching the Crus Medialis feet, and suturing domes as high as possible to accomplish projection. Then we remove vestibular wedges, place a converse stitch, smoothly reduce the soft triangles, release the columella of the base, and remove a trunk of the septum depressor muscle. Generally, it is only here where we introduce a septum tutor intercrus to prolong and strengthen the columella projecting the nasal tip. This is indicated for flat and negroid noses with a short columella, separated nasal wings, and broad nostrils (Fig. 6.27).

Reconstruction

Two apposition sutures with 5-0 nylon are placed with the knots concealed on top of the crus medialis to keep them firmly together. There are times when this is not necessary if the approach is complete.

The Temporal Fascia

The use of temporal fascia was introduced by Guerrerosantos in 1984[12] (Fig. 6.28) to increase the dorsal unit of the nose and to fill the nasofrontal angle. The author uses it to achieve a firm covering and a beautiful, smooth protection in terms of both sight and touch by joining it as a single plane to the fibroadipose covering to the skin (Fig. 6.29). Temporal fascia is only excluded in those nasal tips with a thick skin, with abundant sebaceous glands and a dense fibroadipose covering. Conversely in Caucasian females with delicate skin, its placing is essential to avoid a pointed nasal tip.

Depending on requirements and the resection type, one- or two-layered temporal fascia is placed (Fig. 6.29), and sometimes muscle fibers are included to provide bulk (Fig. 6.30). The seal extension will also depend on the thickness of the wings' skin. In this way, the anatomy of

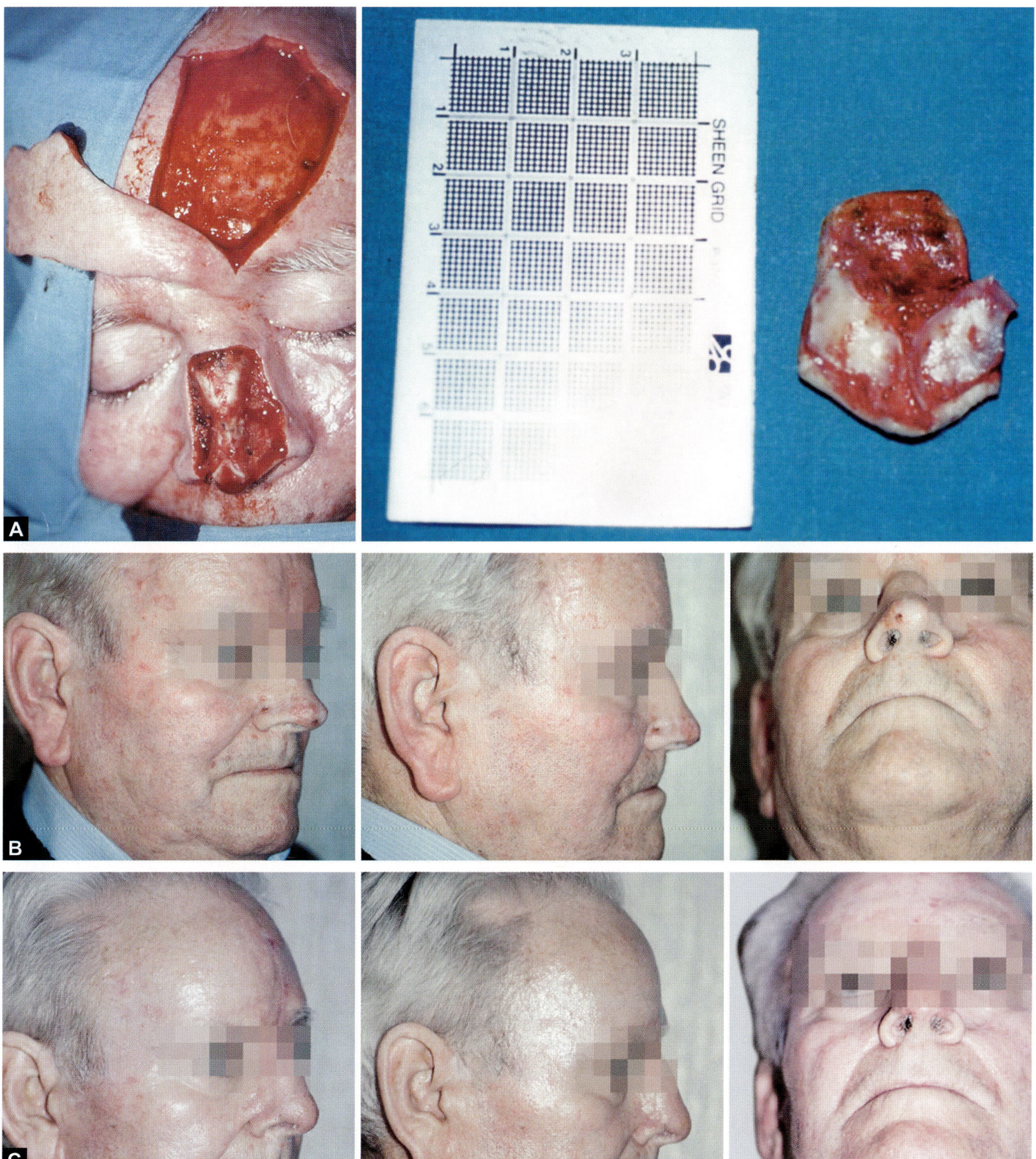

Figs. 6.21A to C: (A) Resected tissues include the alar cartilages of the tip. (B) Preoperative 77-year-old male. (C) Two years postoperative after reconstructive rhinoplasty by resecting the nasal tip due to recidivist cancer without repositioning the cartilaginous structure.

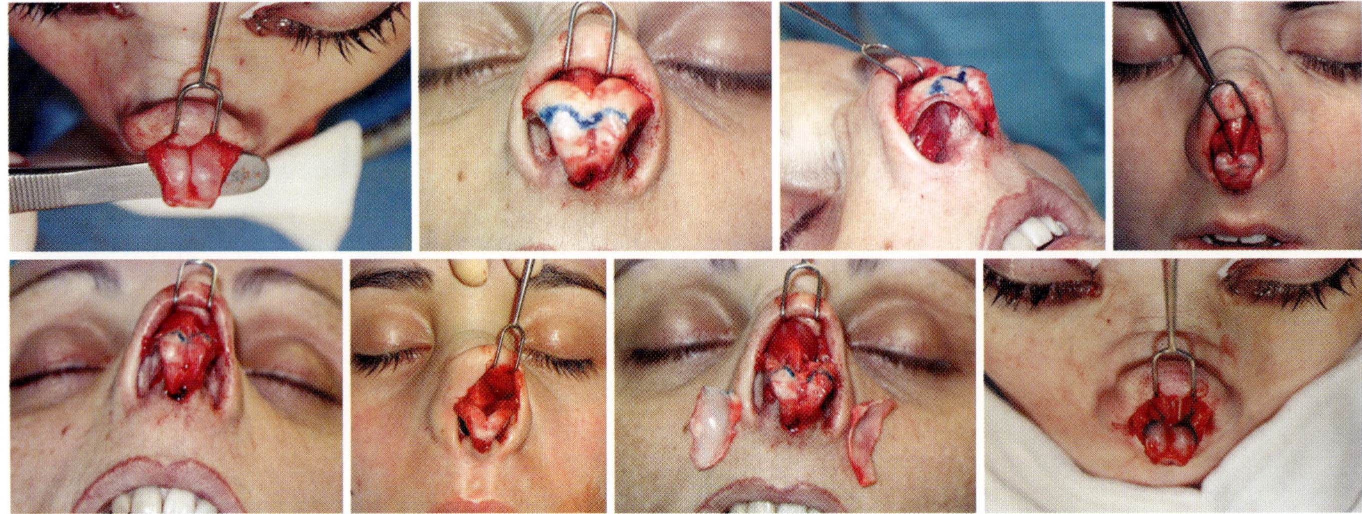

Fig. 6.22: Marking and resection details of the alar cartilages.

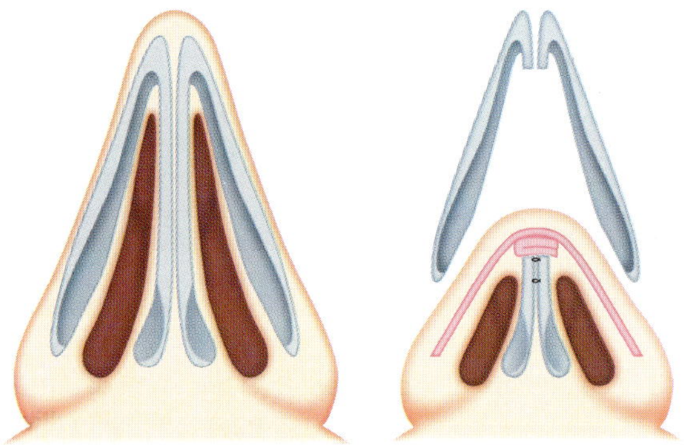

Fig. 6.23: Type I: Total resection of the alar cartilages, including domes and a trunk of the crus medialis. Covering with a temporal fascia patch and layer.

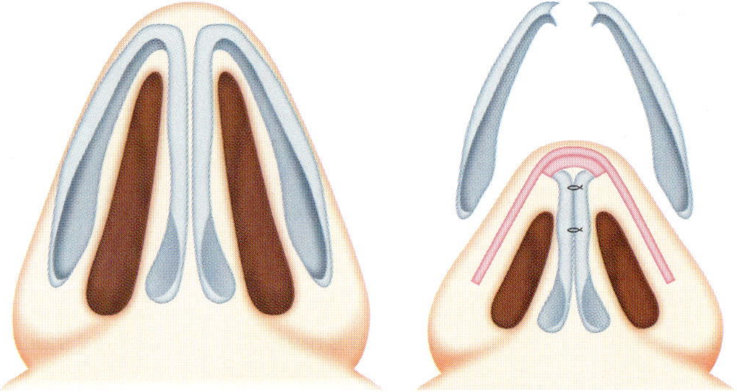

Fig. 6.24: Type II: Total resection of the alar cartilages, including domes. Covering with a temporal fascia patch and layer.

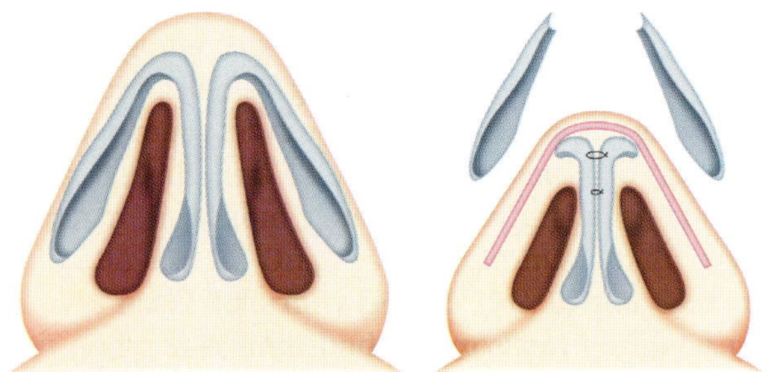

Fig. 6.25: Type III: Total resection of the alar cartilages by respecting the domes, and using a temporal fascia layer.

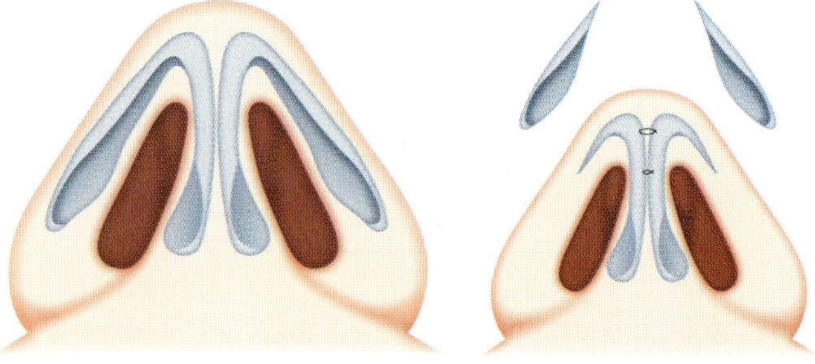

Fig. 6.26: Type IV: Subtotal resection of the alar cartilages by respecting the domes and a small tip-shaped band measuring some 8 mm. No temporal fascia.

the new nasal tip and the wings will outwardly to inwardly comprise the following single-body layers:

- Superficial skin
- Fibroadipose covering
- External fibrous lamina
- Temporal fascia
- Internal fibrous lamina
- Internal vestibular skin

The Technical Resources

To achieve an equilateral nasal base, and according to the former shape of the nasal base, we use a series of technical details that enable a firm, consistent base that resists alar collapse during inspiration: reduction of soft triangles, resecting a trunk of the septum depressor muscle, converse stitch, releasing the columella, alar wedges, resection or approach of the Crus Medialis Feet, tutor intercrus, vestibular wedges, septoplasty (Killian), luxation or cauterization of the nasal turbinates, and filling the nasal-labial angle with resected remains.

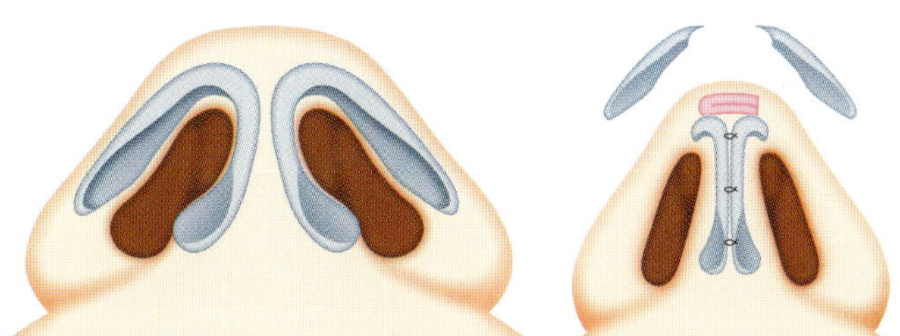

Fig. 6.27: Type V: Total resection of the alar cartilages by respecting the domes with a two-layered temporal fascia patch.

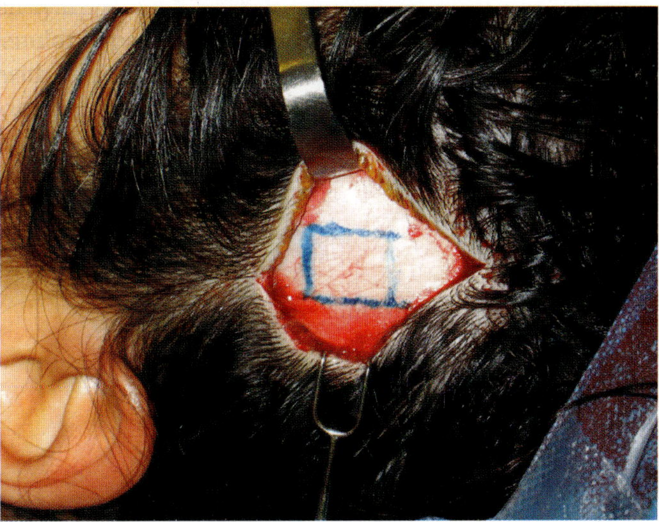

Fig. 6.28: Temporal fascia. An incision of no >3 cm is all that is needed to obtain all the fascia required.

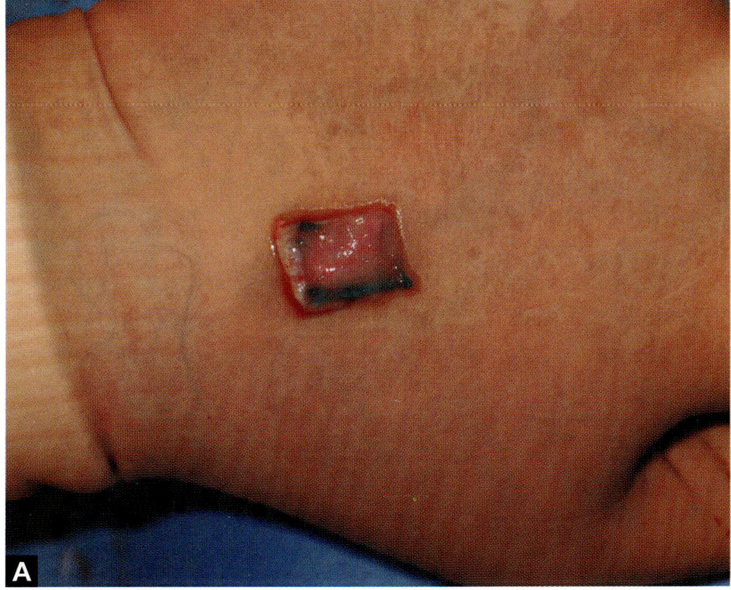

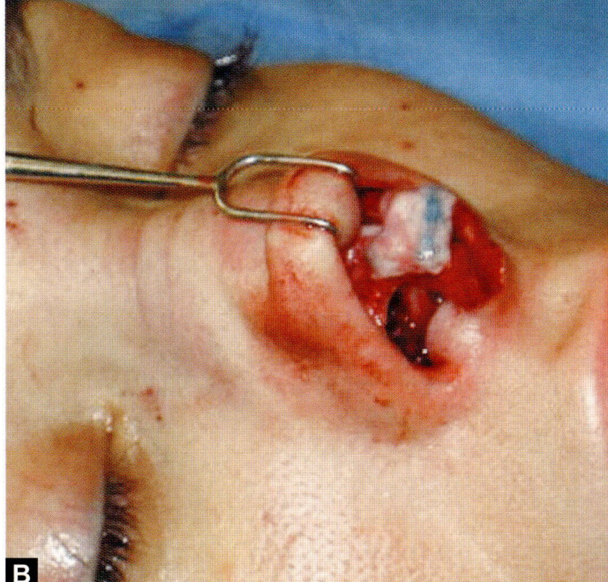

Figs. 6.29A and B: (A) Details of a temporal fascia patch ready to be placed on the crus medialis. (B) Patch in place.

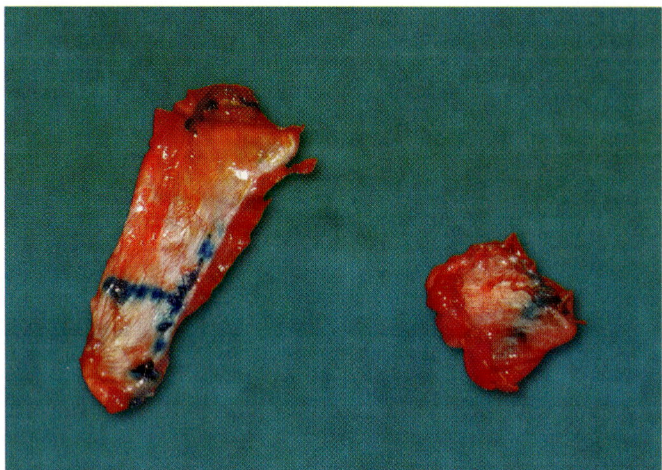

Fig. 6.30: It is sometimes advisable to take the fascia with some muscular fibers to increase crus medialis protection and to improve the covering.

The Postoperative Period

With this technique, the postoperative period does not differ much from that of other techniques (if anything, recuperation is shorter). However, the author has to maintain the vestibular plugging pushing the domes for 4–5 days. A plaster splint remains in place for 7 days, and a double layer of Steri-Strip is used for 7 additional days.

RESULTS

The results obtained since 1987 to date in 2010 range from very good to excellent judging from the patients' degree of satisfaction. Other nasal tip reconstruction techniques performed with complex cartilaginous structures did not provide the best results because a "surgical tip" emerged when the edema disappeared, with traces of barely admissible tips and edges.

Personally, the author reached the conclusion some time ago of not using cartilaginous grafts in the nasal tip, provided this is feasible, for ultimate problems of displacement, reabsorption, distortion, and an unappealing presentation in terms of sight and touch. The nasal tip is reconstructed using the cartilages that are available and if they do not serve this purpose, they are resected directly. Very rarely has the author resorted to cartilaginous grafts since this technique was adopted.

Regarding complications, there is nothing particular to highlight in either aesthetic or functional terms. There have been no problems with the ever-feared alar collapse, which is most certainly due to other factors such as an excessive resection of the triangular cartilages, a vestibular valve lesion without correcting a significant deviation of the septum during surgery, or hypertrophic turbinates which could contribute to or even cause nasal respiratory failure with a uni- or a bilateral collapse.

DISCUSSION

The author wishes to express his maximum respect and admiration to all the Rhinoplasty Masters from whom he has learnt.

From the very beginning, the author realized that this technique was controversial, and that our Rhinoplasty Masters did not advise an excessive resection of alar cartilages, but preferred to maintain a cartilage band of a width of no less than 3–5 mm in the laterocaudal sense to avoid alar collapse. However, the author has verified and demonstrated that this may be avoided by following the steps of the technique and by maintaining its main objective: an equilateral, solid nasal base with a firm, yet soft nasal tip in terms of sight and touch, with no cartilaginous remains in view.

Nonetheless, all this involves experience in rhinoplasty and a totally accurate technique. It proves a most useful technique, but to be used only in extremely difficult nasal tip cases.

CONCLUSION

This technique has matured sufficiently over time in casuistry and has posed no problems when well indicated, diagnosed, and performed.

In the end, the nasal tip becomes as firm and consistent, or more, than prior to surgery. Its five anatomical layers retract in a uniform fashion without distortions. To the touch, it is solid yet smooth and, aesthetically, it offers a beautiful result. Only a biopsy would enable us to verify the state of the stratification, but it is complicated proposing this to a patient who is satisfied with his or her nose, and the author is well aware of the possible negative consequences of extracting a cylinder of tissue with the more than likely alteration to the vector system and to shape. It would be rather like requesting a "structural sampling" in a cathedral vault to learn the characteristics or state of its materials. Thus, our colleagues should trust in the technique thanks to its results.

Rhinoplasty is undoubtedly the most difficult plastic surgery operation and, within it, nasal tip cases are extremely difficult. Nonetheless, the operation is the most appealing and fascinating of our specialty, but great care must be taken while performing it.

The author literally cites: "The complete and permanent removal of what Mother Nature has designed requires the broadest experience, competence and an aesthetic feel by a Master Craftsman in a procedure that permits a minor error, or absolutely none. I therefore completely agree with the author that this procedure cannot be generally applied to all nasal tip operations, and that it is not suitable for enthusiastic beginners in surgery who lack both experience and aesthetic criteria"... "It is likely that the author has found temporal fascia an ideal substitute after totally resecting alar cartilages." (Dr Neeta Patel, in her commentary on this technique in the *Aesthetic Plastic Surgery Journal*, January 2009).

"We are well aware that the nasal tip is one of the most difficult parts of rhinoplasty, and that all of us have the technique that provides the best results available; but we also know that some rhinoplasty cases are very difficult to solve. Dr. Rodríguez-Camps' technique of totally removing alar cartilages and then introducing temporal fascia is novel and interesting"... "Needless to say, the results obtained by Dr Rodríguez-Camps are excellent and we are enthusiastic about using this nasal aesthetic technique." (Dr Guerrerosantos in his commentary on the technique in *Cirugía Plástica Iberolatinoamericana*, January-February-March 2010).

The author concludes that when it seemed that everything had been described and that the results depended only on the author's hands, something new and fresh appears: "The Total Resection of the Alar Cartilages and Temporal Fascia Technique."

REFERENCES

1. Rodriguez-Camps S. Miscellaneous rhinoplasty: primary and secondary. XXXIV Spanish National Plastic, Reconstructive and Aesthetic Surgery Society (SECPRE) Congress, Marbella, Spain, April 1999.
2. Rodriguez-Camps S. Rhinoplasty: primary, secondary and reconstructive. II Plastic, Reconstructive and Aesthetic Surgery Society Meeting of the Valencian Community (SCPRECV), Alicante, Spain, February 2000.
3. Rodriguez-Camps S. Aesthetic nasal reconstruction. XXXVII Spanish National Plastic, Reconstructive and Aesthetic Surgery Society (SECPRE) Congress, Oviedo, Spain, June 2002.
4. Rodriguez-Camps S. Secondary rhinoplasty: our procedure. Total resection of the alar cartilages and domes with a temporal fascia stamp on the tip. XLI Spanish Plastic, Reconstructive and Aesthetic Surgery Society (SECPRE) Congress, Paper, Pamplona, Spain, May 2006.
5. Rodriguez-Camps S. Nasal reconstruction. VII Plastic, Reconstructive and Aesthetic Surgery Society Meeting of the Valencian Community (SCPRECV) Meeting, Alzira, Valencia, Spain, October 2006.
6. Rodriguez-Camps S. Reconstructive rhinoplasty. Teaching Course on Plastic, Aesthetic and Reconstructive Surgery, School of Medicine, University of Barcelona, Spain, November 2006.
7. Rodriguez-Camps S. Rhinoplasty. The difficult nasal tip: Total resection of the alar cartilages. XIX Congress of the International Society of Aesthetic Plastic Surgery, (ISAPS), Panelist, Melbourne, Australia, February 2008.
8. Rodriguez-Camps S: New technique to treat a very difficult nasal tip. Total resection of the alar cartilages and temporal fascia covering. XLV Spanish Plastic, Reconstructive and Aesthetic Surgery Society (SECPRE) Congress, Gerona, Spain, May 2010.
9. Rodriguez-Camps S. Demonstrating the Total Resection of the Alar Cartilages and Temporal Fascia Technique on a Corpse as Part of the VI Theoretical-Practical Course on Anatomical Dissection Organized by the Spanish Association of Aesthetic Plastic Surgery (AECEP). I Course on Rhinoplasty and Facial Implants, Department of Human Anatomy and Embryology II, School of Medicine at the Complutense University of Madrid, Madrid, Spain, July 2010;105-217.
10. Rodriguez-Camps S. Rhinoplasty. The difficult nasal tip: total resection of the alar cartilages. Aesthetic Plast Surg. 2009;33(1):72-83.
11. Rodriguez-Camps S. Un paso adelante en rinoplastia: Técnica de resección total de los cartílagos alares y fascia temporal. Span Assoc Aesthetic Plast Surg J. 2010;12: 13-24.
12. Guerrerosantos J. Temporoparietal free fascia grafts in rhinoplasty. Plast Reconstr Surg. 1984;74(4):465-74.

FURTHER READING

1. Burget G, Menick F. Aesthetic Reconstruction of the Nose, 1st edition. St Louis, MO: Mosby; 1993.
2. Converse J. Reconstructive Plastic Surgery, 2nd edition. Philadelphia, PA: WB Saunders Co; 1977. pp. 1040-281.
3. Ezquerra Carrera F, Sainz-Arregui J, Berrazueta Fernández M J. La rinoplastia "No basica primaria." Cir Plast Iberlatinamer. 2001;27(1):45-54.
4. Gubisch W, Eichhorn-Sens J. Overresection of the lower lateral cartilages: a common conceptual mistake with functional and aesthetic consequences. Aesthet Plast Surg. 2009;33(1):6-13.

5. Gunter JP, Rohrich RJ, Adams WP Jr. Dallas rhinoplasty. In: Gunter JP, Rohrich RJ, Adams WP Jr (Eds). Nasal Surgery by the Masters, 2nd edition. St Louis, MO: Quality Medical Publishing, Inc; 2007. pp. 303-590.
6. Juri J, Juri C, Grilli D, Zeaiter MC, et al. Correction of the secondary nasal tip. Ann Plast Surg. 1986;16(4):322-32.
8. Meyer R. Secondary and functional rhinoplasty. The Difficult Nose, 1st edition. Orlando, FL: Grune & Stratton, Inc; 1988.
9. Peck G Techniques in Aesthetic Rhinoplasty, 1st edition. New York: Gower Medical Publishing Ltd; 1984.
10. Rodriguez-Camps S. Augmentative rhinoplasty with an auricular gibbus. Aesthet Plast Surg. 1998;22(3)196-205.
11. Rodriguez-Camps S. Nose Reconstruction with medial forehead flap after Mohs surgery. Int Video J Plast Aesthet Surg. 1995;2(3).
12. Rodriguez-Camps S. Reconstrucción nasal tras cirugía micrográfica de mohs. Cir Plast Iberolatinoamer. 1995;21 (3):215-23.
14. Rodriguez-Camps S. Una nueva técnica para el tratamiento de la punta nasal difícil. Experiencia personal de 22 años (1987-2009). Cir Plást Ibero-latinoam. J Cir Plast Iberolatinoam. 2010;36(1):3-12.
15. Rodriguez-Camps S Nasal reconstruction after epithelioma. Aesthet Plast Surg. 2001;25(4):273-7.
16. Sheen J. Aesthetic Rhinoplasty, 2nd edition. St Louis, MO: The C.V. Mosby Company; 1978.
17. Soria JH, Pintos JC, Conde, CG, Losardo RJ. Sobrepunta Nasal como Expresión de una Comunicación Septal. Cir Plast Iberolatinoam. 2009;35(4):243-8.
18. Tardy ME Jr. Surgical Anatomy of the Nose, 1st edition. New York: Raven Press, Ltd; 1990.

7 Correction of Auricular Deformities after Failed Otoplasty

Alexander Berghaus

ANALYSIS OF DEFORMITIES AFTER OTOPLASTY

Unwanted results after failed otoplasty include minor, but sometimes also severe deformities difficult to correct. Such deformities range from minor forms of under- or overcorrection, asymmetry and distorted proportions to the formation of aesthetically very annoying edges or even to partial or subtotal loss of the auricle.[1]

For revision surgery of such deformities, knowledge of the different otoplasty techniques is substantial to understand the cause of the actual deformity. The surgeon should therefore be familiar with the basic concepts and variations of the cutting technique of converse, the scoring technique of Stenströem, and the suture technique of Mustardé, which are not explained here with reference to the corresponding literature.[2-4] All otoplasty techniques using cartilage incisions, resections, or aggressive scoring bear an increased risk of causing severe deformities.[5-8] A systematic analysis of deformities after otoplasty includes the unwanted results summarized in Table 7.1.

Standardized photographs of the auricles (frontal, posterior, and lateral view) are taken to objectify the actual deformities. Additionally, the dimensions of the auricle are measured, especially height, breadth, and projection. The distance of the helical rim to the skull is determined in three measuring points (cranial, central, and caudal) using the method of Wodak,[9] normal values are within the range of approximately 18 mm. Thus, both auricles can be mutually compared. Only in total loss of the auricle a position check with a template as used in microtia reconstruction is necessary, achieving symmetry to the contralateral healthy side with the help of facial landmarks (corner of the eye, eyebrow, nasal bridge).

The corrective surgical procedure naturally depends on the cause and extent of the actual deformity.

Table 7.1: Deformities after otoplasty

Undercorrection	Unilateral Bilateral
Overcorrection	Unilateral Bilateral
Distorted proportions	"Telephone handle deformity" (relative overcorrection of the middle third) Protruding upper third Protruding lobule
Formation of edges	Without cartilage loss With thinned cartilage With cartilage loss
Deformities with skin defects	Mainly postauricular region
Deformities with loss of cartilage and skin	Partial loss of the auricle Total loss of the auricle

UNDERCORRECTION

If one or both auricles are still protruding after otoplasty, this is due to insufficient correction of an incomplete folding of the antihelix and/or insufficient flattening of a large conchal cavum.

Undercorrection only in the upper third of the auricle is mainly connected to an insufficient folding of the antihelix during primary otoplasty. An elegant method in revision cases is the "incisionless" technique of Fritsch.[10] If the surgeon is not familiar with this technique, the recommended alternative for revision surgery is the method of Mustardé.[3]

The most reliable and predictable method for correcting an insufficient approximation of the auricle to the skull in cases of a large conchal cavum is the Furnas technique.[11] After resection of soft tissue between the conchal cavum and the mastoid, sutures between the perichondrium of the cavum and the periosteum of the mastoid are set for flattening of the cavum and for approximating the auricle to the skull. The extent of these secondary corrections can be controlled by comparing both sides using the method of Wodak,[9] as in primary otoplasty. The more laterodorsally the approximating sutures are positioned, the stronger is the resulting effect.

A protruding lobule can be annoying in distinctive cases or when there is asymmetry to the contralateral side. It can be corrected using the restraining suture described by Siegert and Weerda. Similar to the positioning of Mustardé sutures, the soft tissue of the lobule is approximated to the stable cartilage of the conchal cavum.[12,13] The needle should be guided with some distance to the anterior skin of the lobule to avoid a "navel formation" on the lobule when tightening the suture.

OVERCORRECTION

Overcorrections after otoplasty, with distances of the helical rim to the skull of 15 mm or less, are usually more difficult to correct than undercorrections.

If the overcorrection is the result of previous otoplasty with suture techniques, the sutures can usually be released at least in the early stage up to 1 year after the operation, followed by revision otoplasty with suture techniques (this time with less approximation of the auricle to the skull).

However, if overcorrection is the result of previous otoplasty with cutting or scoring techniques, the following steps can be necessary (Fig. 7.1):

1. Reopening of the postauricular incision
2. Complete releasing of the dorsal cartilage skeleton
3. Identification of the previously performed incisions and releasing of the cartilage from the frontal skin coverage in these areas
4. Subsequent repair of the incision defects in the cartilage by adapting the edges accurately in their previous position by a series of stable single sutures.

Subsequently, the auricle will often retake its original, protruding position. Then it is necessary to perform otoplasty once again on the repaired cartilage skeleton within the same session. To avoid additional weakening of the injured cartilage, only pure suture techniques should be

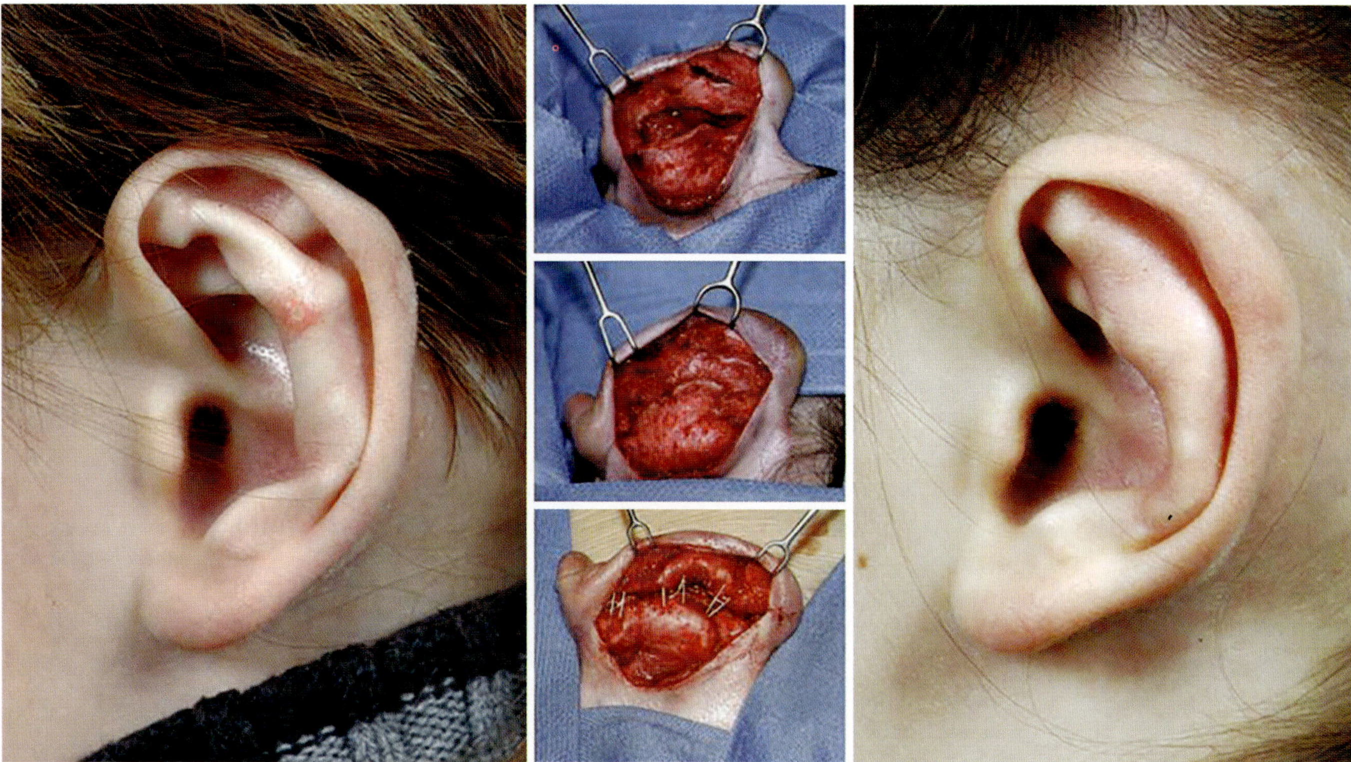

Fig. 7.1: Deformity after otoplasty. Left: Creases and extreme antihelical folding after otoplasty. Central top: Several radical cartilage incisions and additional use of sutures were found as the cause for the deformity. Central middle and bottom: Readaptation of the cartilage skeleton freed of scar tissue followed by revision otoplasty using suture techniques. Right: Two years postoperatively.
Source: Reprinted with permission from Berghaus A, Braun T, Hempel JM. Revision otoplasty: how to manage the disastrous result. Arch Facial Plast Surg. 2012;14(3):205-10. Copyrighted ©, 2012, American Medical Association.

used in this context. Sutures passing the cartilage have to be positioned and tightened very carefully, with meticulous control of the distance between the helical rim and the skull, since cartilage weakened by previous incisions is more easily folded despite the applied "repairing sutures."

If overcorrection is connected with excessive approximation of the cavum to the skull, revision surgery must seek to enlarge the distance between the mastoid and the conchal cavum again. This is achieved by lifting the auricle from the mastoid and interposition of volume-giving materials. Rib cartilage is basically an appropriate material, although only a relatively small interposition is needed, which is cut to a sickle- or half-moon-shape with a maximal breadth of 5–10 mm. Harvesting of rib cartilage for such a small interposition means a possibly inadequate effort and an additional thoracic scar. Therefore, the author prefers an implant of porous polyethylene. This material has an excellent biocompatibility, can be cut to the desired form, penetrated by a needle, and thus easily fixed with sutures.[14] An extrusion is extremely rare when the implant is covered by enough healthy tissue. The author has not seen extrusion of porous polyethylene implants in eleven cases with this indication.[1] An additional protection against extrusion can be achieved by coverage of the implant in the postauricular sulcus with a broadly pedicle flap of muscle, fascia, and connective tissue.

DISTORTED PROPORTIONS

The most frequent deformity with distorted proportions after otoplasty is the so-called telephone handle deformity. The middle third is approximated too close to the skull, while the upper and lower third (i.e. the lobule) are protruding too much. For correction, a combination of the different operative procedures for the individual deformities as described above have to be applied; the middle third has to be elevated, while the upper and lower third have to be approximated to the skull.

FORMATION OF EDGES

Incisions of the cartilage during otoplasty can lead to the formation of extremely annoying, clearly visible edges or bends. These changes become more severe and conspicuous over time due to scar contraction and skin atrophy. Sometimes the auricle has a "saw tooth"- or "rat bite"-like contour, so that the operated auricle actually looks uglier and more conspicuous than the previously protruding ear (Fig. 7.2). With increasing deformity, patients tend to cover their ears with long hairs. Over time, the patients' desire for operative revision is continuously growing, especially when there are matters of partnership involved. We have seen patients with such deformities rebuffed by several specialized surgeons with the statement that no corrections of such deformities are possible; fortunately, this does not hold true. Simply lifting the ventral skin over the deformity and covering the edges with fascia, however, will not be successful in the long run. The fascia will atrophy, and the crease will reappear.

The most advantageous cases are when cartilage was only incised, but not resected. The subsequent formation of edges, regardless if connected with over- or undercorrection, can be corrected by the technique describe above: releasing of the cut cartilage skeleton using a dorsal approach, releasing of the frontal skin around the cartilage incisions, reattachment of the edges into their original position, and repair of the cartilage by a series of long-term resorbable single sutures, e.g. 5–0 or 6–0 Maxon (United States Surgical Corporation, Norwalk, CT, USA). If repair of the original cartilage configuration leads to a protruding auricle again, revision otoplasty using suture techniques is necessary and possible in the same session (Fig. 7.3).

More difficult are the cases when not only cartilage incisions but also superficial scoring with Stenströem's technique[4] has been previously applied. The cartilage is more or less weakened, so that in cases of overcorrection, suturing the incision edges together does not always reproduce the original form. For sufficient restoring and stabilization of the original form, implants of porous polyethylene,[14] cut exactly to the appropriate size and shape, are fixed to the cartilage from dorsally. For this indication, very delicate and individually fitted implant pieces are needed. Commercially available implants of porous polyethylene for auricular reconstruction (Medpor "Ear Base" and "Helical Rim," Stryker Corporation, Newnan, GA, USA) are suitable primary materials.

Also when not only cartilage incisions but even resections leading to defects of the cartilage framework were performed during the previous operation, adequately cut implants of porous polyethylene can be used for partial reconstruction of the destroyed auricular framework. Such implants do not necessarily have to be covered with an additional layer of fascia between the foreign material and the skin to prevent extrusion if the ventral skin coverage is healthy and stable. The author has used such implants repeatedly, also in combination with additional implants to increase the distance between the cavum and the skull

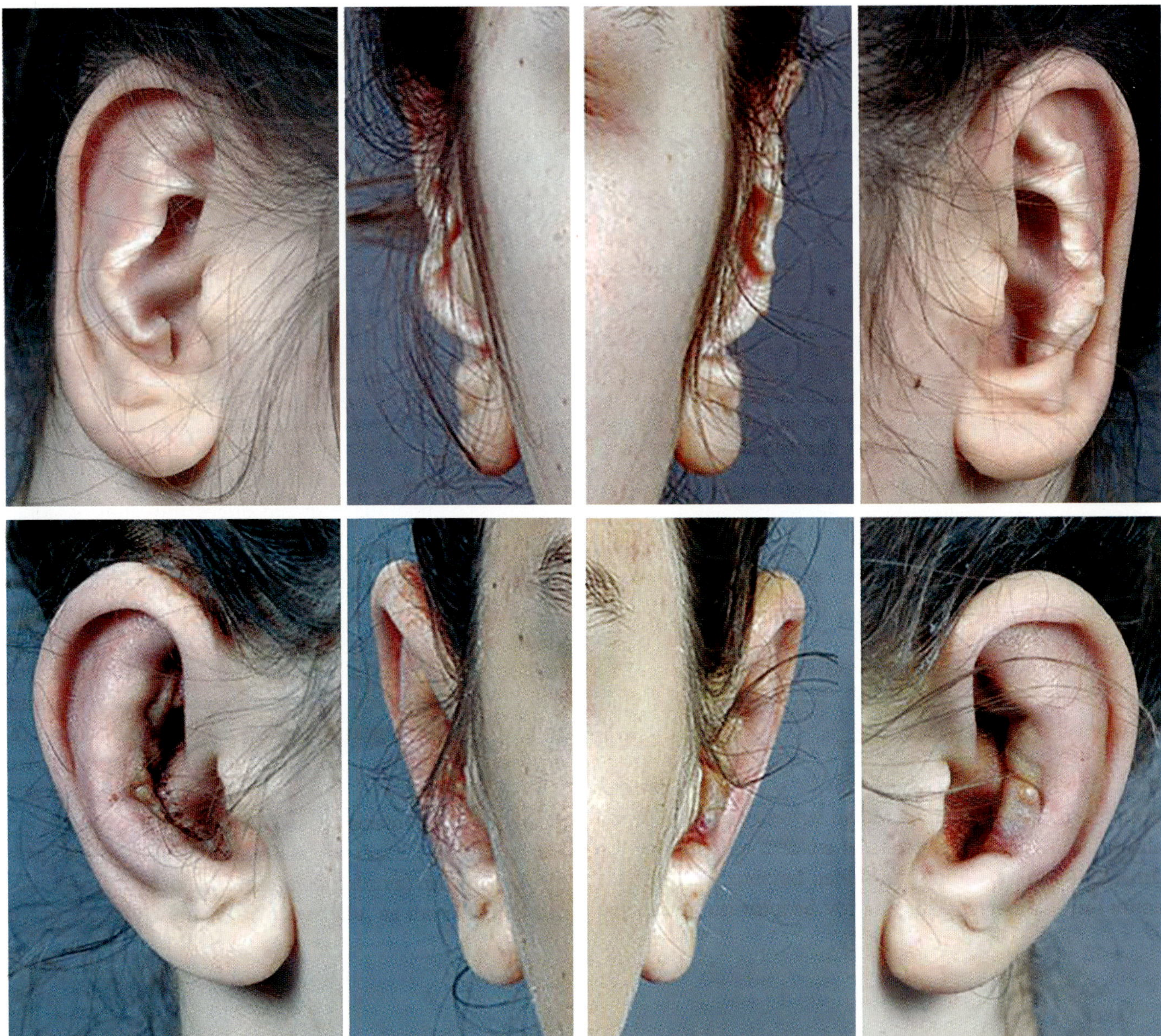

Fig. 7.2: Deformity after otoplasty. Top: Extreme garland-like edges and creases in the cavum conchae and antihelix as well as a too small concha-mastoid angle after overcorrection of protruding ears by applying cartilage incisions and sutures. Bottom: Two days postoperatively after smoothing and readaptation of the cartilage skeleton followed by revision otoplasty using suture techniques. Copyrighted ©, 2012, American Medical Association.

(see above) without seeing any spontaneous skin perforations[1] (Fig. 7.4). However, for a better prevention of lesion in the postauricular sulcus by temples or hearing aids, implants can be covered dorsally with broadly pedicled flaps of connective tissue and fascia of the mastoid region before closure of the postauricular skin.

Alternatively, smaller cartilage fragments missing in the framework can be replaced by transplants from the conchal cavum fixed by sutures. Should the patient need a septoplasty at the same time, it suggests itself to use transplants of nasal septal cartilage, which is also a material very suited for auricular repair with limited extent.

DEFORMITIES WITH SKIN DEFECTS

It is known for more than a century that postauricular skin resections are not suitable for achieving harmonic results in otoplasty, in contrast to corrections carried out on the

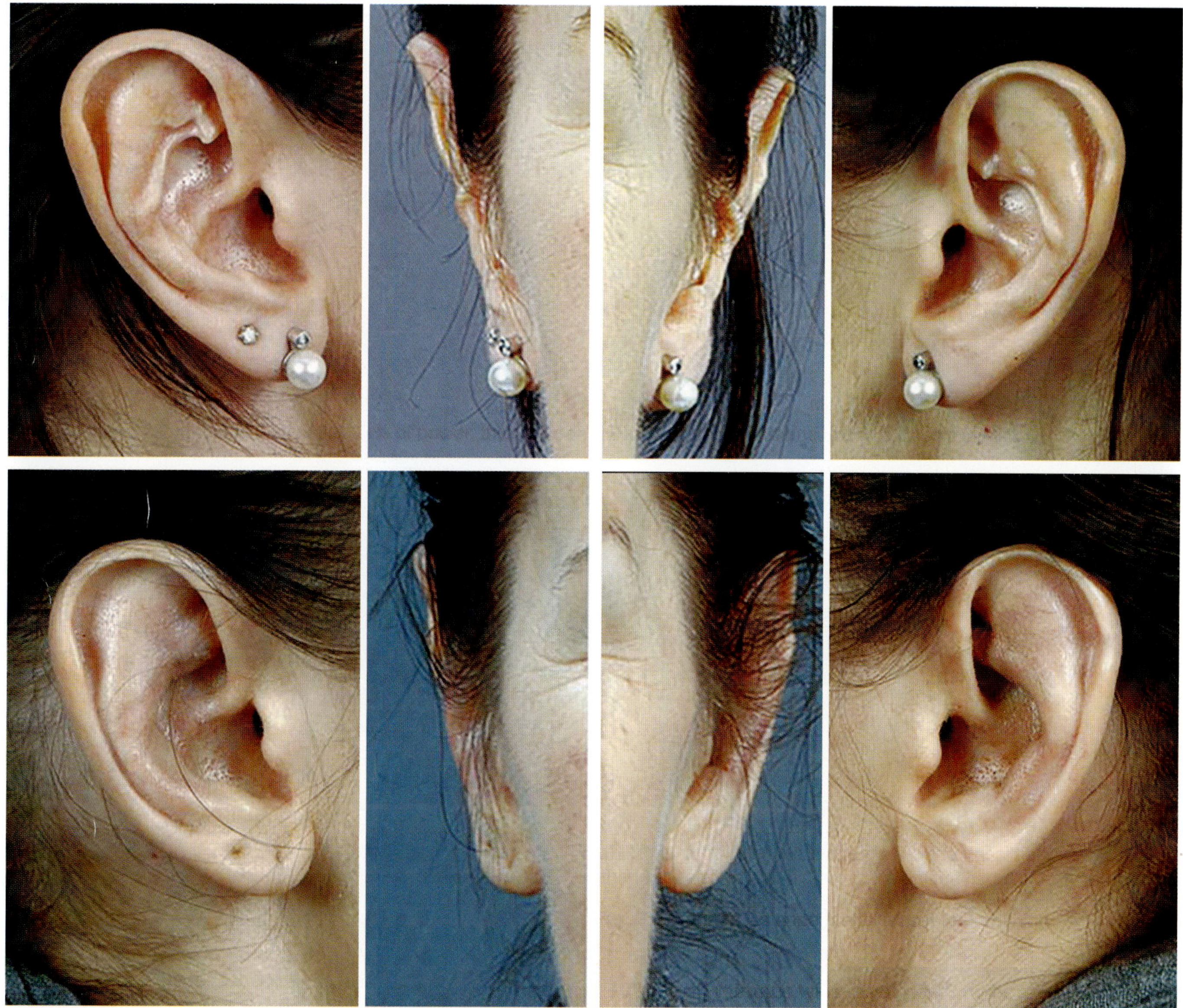

Fig. 7.3: Deformity after otoplasty. Top: Creases in the antihelix as well as a too-small concha-mastoid angle after overcorrection of protruding ears by applying cartilage incisions. Bottom: Four weeks postoperatively after smoothing and readaptation of the cartilage skeleton followed by revision otoplasty using suture techniques. *Source*: Reprinted with permission from Berghaus A, Braun T, Hempel JM. Revision otoplasty: how to manage the disastrous result. Arch Facial Plast Surg. 2012;14(3):205-10. Copyrighted ©, 2012, American Medical Association.

cartilaginous framework.[15,16] Nonetheless, also nowadays many surgeons routinely resect a more or less broad strip of postauricular skin when performing otoplasty. The author has abandoned this step of otoplasty for 15 years without seeing any disadvantages. Skin resections in the postauricular sulcus increase the risk of keloid formation due to increased tension of the sutures, a complication dreaded especially in the auricular region. In contrast, none of the many ears operated by the author has shown formation of keloids in the scar, and the results of otoplasty were completely satisfying also without any skin resections, e.g. also no annoying skin excess was noted.[17,18]

Moreover, loss of the postauricular fold can hamper patients wearing glasses or hearing aids and is also an additional problem in revision otoplasty. In order to replace missing skin behind the auricle during revision otoplasty, which is sometimes substantial in cases of overcorrection, skin grafts or local flaps are needed. As in auricular reconstruction, thinned full-thickness skin grafts are needed, since split-skin grafts may look promising at

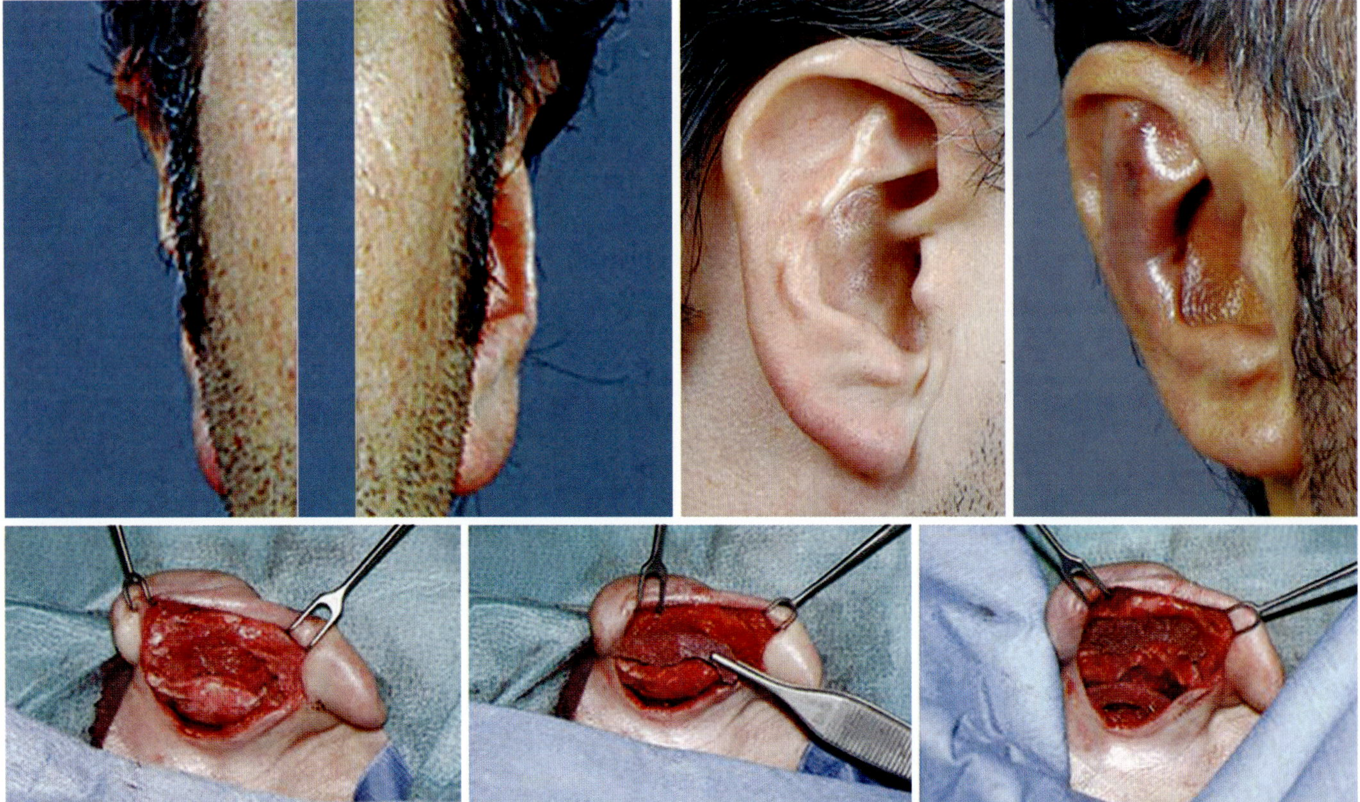

Fig. 7.4: Deformity after otoplasty. Top left three: Overcorrection of both ears, with an additional postoperative deformity on the right side. Top right: Five days postoperatively. Bottom left: Intraoperatively, it was revealed that a cartilage bar 1-cm wide was removed in the prior otoplasty, making readaptation of the cartilage skeleton impossible. Bottom middle: Insertion of the first porous polyethylene for bridging of the skeleton defect. Bottom right: Insertion of a second porous polyethylene implant for raising the concha-mastoid angle. *Source*: Reprinted with permission from Berghaus A, Braun T, Hempel JM. Revision otoplasty: how to manage the disastrous result. Arch Facial Plast Surg. 2012;14(3):205-10. Copyrighted ©, 2012, American Medical Association.

first, but tend to contract considerably over time, so that the preoperative state is finally reached again. We prefer to harvest thin full-thickness skin grafts from the groin in the "bikini zone."[19] Other possible harvesting areas are the supraclavicular area or the medial upper arm. To allow sufficient engraftment, skin grafts in the postauricular region should be strongly attached to the surface for 8–10 days using prolate pads knotted firmly by sutures for maximal compression.

An elegant alternative is the use of translational skin flaps cut in different configurations behind the auricle to improve the skin coverage of the postauricular sulcus. Two basic considerations when planning such flaps are that no hair-bearing skin should be moved to the sulcus and incisions and thus scar formation should not reach the neck region below the lobule to avoid aesthetic impairment due to visible scars. The author has had excellent experience with modified Z-plasties or cranially and caudally formed antidromic rotation flaps.

In cases with a previously harvested full-thickness skin graft from the groin with a scar existing in this area, it can be advisable to excise the more or less broad scar from the groin, thin the scarred skin and use it as a graft for the postauricular sulcus. Using firmly attached pads, also this kind of skin heals well to the underground in the author's experience. The scarred texture of this graft is not annoying in the inconspicuous postauricular region, and an additional advantage is the concomitantly narrowed groin scar.

DEFORMITIES WITH LOSS OF CARTILAGE AND SKIN

Defects with larger missing parts of the cartilaginous framework and also of the skin coverage are rarely solely due to aggressive otoplasty techniques. However, when severe bacterial infections occur after otoplasty, partial or even total loss of the auricle can be the result. Revision surgery must then seek to replace larger parts of the cartilaginous framework and of the skin coverage. In such cases only techniques of auricular reconstruction as used for the rehabilitation of microtia can be successful. For many years, the author prefers auricular reconstruction with a porous polyethylene framework covered by a temporal-parietal fascia flap vascularized by the superficial temporal artery. Skin coverage is completed, as far as possible, by full-thickness skin grafts from the retroauricular region of the healthy contralateral ear and from the groin in the "bikini zone." The details of this technique are elaborately explained in the literature.[20–23]

CONCLUSION

Otoplasty techniques using aggressive incisions or resection bear a substantial risk for later deformities even more annoying than the previous protruding ear. While minor over- or undercorrections can be revised with relatively simple means, major deformities can imply such problems for a revision that even experienced surgeons experience. Fortunately, for all kinds of deformities, even subtotal loss of the auricle, surgical techniques for repair are known to allow the patients showing their ears in the public again without feelings of shame. Since relatively aggressive techniques are still used frequently, and thus patients continue to seek help for the resulting consequences, the dedicated facial surgeon studying the options available for correction will be rewarded.

To avoid the risk of severe deformities through otoplasty, the author strongly recommends not to use incision or resection methods, in favor of pure suturing techniques with nonabsorbable material, and to abstain from postauricular skin resection. Following these principles lead to very good results with otoplasty.[18]

ACKNOWLEDGMENTS

The author would like to thank Dr Thomas Braun, Department of ORL-HNS at Ludwig Maximilian University, Munich, Germany, for assistance with translation and editing of the manuscript.

REFERENCES

1. Berghaus A, Braun T, Hempel JM. Revision otoplasty: how to manage the disastrous result. Arch Facial Plast Surg. 2012;14(3):205-10.
2. Converse JM, Nigro A, Wilson FA, et al. A technique for surgical correction of lop ears. Plast Reconstr Surg. 1995;15(5): 411-8.
3. Mustarde JC. The correction of prominent ears using simple mattress sutures. Br J Plast Surg. 1963;16:170-8.
4. Stenströem SJ. A "natural" technique for correction of congenitally prominent ears. Plast Reconstr Surg. 1963;32: 509-18.
5. Adamson PA, Mcgraw BL, Tropper GJ. Otoplasty: critical review of clinical results. Laryngoscope. 1991;101(8):883-8.
6. Kelley P, Hollier L, Stal S. Otoplasty: evaluation, technique, and review. J Craniofac Surg. 2003;14(5):643-53.
7. Mandal A, Bahia H, Ahmad T, Stewart KJ. Comparison of cartilage scoring and cartilage sparing otoplasty—A study of 203 cases. J Plast Reconstr Aesthet Surg. 2006;59(11): 1170-6.
8. Szychta P, Orfaniotis G, Stewart KJ. Revision otoplasty: an algorithm. Plast Reconstr Surg. 2012;130(4):907-16.
9. Wodak E. Über die Stellung und Form der menschlichen Ohrmuschel. Arch Klin Exp Ohren Nasen Kehlkopfheilkd. 1967;188(2):331-5.
10. Fritsch MH. Incisionless otoplasty. Laryngoscope. 1995;105 (5 Pt 3Suppl70):1-11.
11. Furnas DW. Correction of prominent ears by conchamastoid sutures. Plast Reconstr Surg. 1968;42(3):189-93.
12. Siegert R. Correction of the lobule. Facial Plast Surg. 2004; 20(4):293-8.
13. Weerda H. Surgery of the Auricle. Stuttgart: Thieme; 2007.
14. Berghaus A. Porous polyethylene in reconstructive head and neck surgery. Arch Otolaryngol. 1985;111(3):154-60.
15. Braun T, Hempel JM, Berghaus A. Otoplasty: focusing on patient benefit and health-related quality of life. In: Shiffman MA (Ed). Advanced Cosmetic Otoplasty: Art, Science and New Clinical Techniques. Berlin: Springer; 2013. pp. 569-73.
16. Gersuny R. Über einige kosmetische Operationen. Wien Med Wochenschr. 1903;48(7):2253-7.
17. Berghaus A, Braun T. Otoplasty today: maximal benefit with state-of-the-art surgery. Prime. 2012;2(3):46-54.
18. Braun T, Hainzinger T, Stelter K, et al. Health-related quality of life, patient benefit, and clinical outcome after otoplasty using suture techniques in 62 children and adults. Plast Reconstr Surg. 2010;126(6):2115-24.
19. Braun T, Patscheider M, Berghaus A, et al. Scars after total ear reconstruction with porous polyethylene: the patients' perspective. Eur J Plast Surg. 2013;36(7):413-6.
20. Berghaus A. Porecon implant and fan flap: a concept for reconstruction of the auricle. Facial Plast Surg. 1988;5(5): 451-7.
21. Braun T, Gratza S, Becker S, et al. Auricular reconstruction with porous polyethylene frameworks: outcome and patient benefit in 65 children and adults. Plast Reconstr Surg. 2010;126(4):1201-12.
22. Hempel J, Gratza S, Berghaus A, et al. Patient benefit from ear reconstruction with porous polyethylene in severe cases of hemifacial microsomia. Eur J Plast Surg. 2013;36(4): 219-24.
23. Reinisch JF, Lewin S. Ear reconstruction using a porous polyethylene framework and temporoparietal fascia flap. Facial Plast Surg. 2009;25(3):181-9.

8 Focal Nerve Lesions with a Monopolar Radiofrequency Device for Cosmetic Enhancement

Diane I Duncan, Doug McBurney, Brian Kinney

INTRODUCTION

The possibility of attaining long-lasting relaxation of dynamic lines without the need for repeated botulinum toxin injections is an attractive idea to many patients. The need for multiple visits to the physician for injections is annoying for many. Patients who get these injections complain of the discomfort, lack of immediate results, difficulty finding time for the appointment, and the cost of repetitive treatment.

Another complaint is that the effect is not complete. As more and more practitioners offer botulinum toxin injections, the skill level of the injectors and the quality of the botulinum toxin injected becomes more and more variable. The option of a long-term solution for reduction of glabellar frown lines, crow's feet, and transverse forehead lines has initially been well received among patients who have undergone monopolar RF nerve ablation in these areas.

THE DEVICE

The "Symphony RF" device (distributed by Thermigen, Inc, Southlake, TX, USA) is a Class II 20 W monopolar, electrothermal generator cleared by the FDA for sale under 510K # K033981 dated February 25, 2004. The device is cleared for the indication of creation of lesions in nervous tissue by pinpoint application of heat. The device is similar to the single channel RF nerve ablation devices used by physicians in chronic pain practices.

The device's 5 cm cannula has an RF tip with a small area of action (isotherm) of a few millimeters. The 22-gauge tip is about 1 mm in diameter. When the internal maximum temperature of the tip reaches 65°C, an active area (isotherm) extends out about 3 mm and reaches temperatures of 50°C at the outer margin. This precision of heating allows safe treatment of small regions with accuracy that was previously unavailable.

When heated to 85°C, theoretical considerations and clinical observations suggest a comparably small annulus of heating at the tip. This is an important point, as nerves in the treatment region are often superficial. Treatment safety is a top concern. An important innovation in the tip is the presence of a microthermistor providing essentially real-time temperature monitoring along with electrical impedance monitoring. The concomitant use of a FLIR camera monitors the external skin temperature. This allows maintenance of a targeted temperature during treatment in order to prevent skin burns. Typically, temperatures are targeted at 85°C for nerve ablation, 70°C for adipolysis, and 50°C–60°C for connective tissue contouring and tightening. The automatic gain control (AGC) circuit in the device varies the power delivery to maintain effective tissue heating, much like a cruise control device on a car during temperature-controlled applications.

The device emits pulsed or continuous radiofrequency (RF) energy in the 480 Hz range. In the stimulation mode, pulsatile voltage amplitude is set at low levels (3–8 mA) in the "stim" mode to map nerves. In the RF lesion mode, amplitude is much higher and power output is controlled by the AGC circuit and peaks at 20 W to achieve the preset temperatures in a variety of applications.

SAFETY

Studies by DiBernardo[1] suggest that skin temperatures about 45°C sustained for >1–2 minutes are associated with burns of the overlying skin. These are often second degree, but occasionally can be third degree burns. Lack of precision in monitoring skin temperature has led to many complications in transcutaneous RF devices, in spite of simultaneous administration of a cryogen spray. Temperature monitoring in that setting is highly challenging and localization of temperature zones is not available.

A recent safety innovation is the addition of surface skin temperature monitoring in real time on a tablet computer via wireless connection to a forward-looking infrared camera (FLIR) camera. This improvement is a standard feature with the Thermigen device. Initial monitoring by visual inspection or palpation for a feeling of heat was predictably imprecise. A standard infrared one-pixel temperature probe (commonly used temperature "guns") provided poor accuracy at one specific location. The addition of a 19,200 pixel real-time, mapping temperature camera (FLIR) has brought safety to tissue heating. A color-coded, mapped real-time video of tissue temperatures allows for maximum heating with a controlled impact on the skin. The surgeon can easily view the internal tissue temperature and the maximum skin temperature simultaneously as the treatment progresses.

HISTORY

Radiofrequency nerve ablation, in practice for over 30 years, has seen a dramatic increase in use over the past 15 years.[2] A common use is treatment of chronic low back pain by ablation of the medial branch nerves supplying the facet joints. Testing prior to treatment with a lidocaine nerve block increases the likelihood of achieving significant pain relief.[3] The single channel RF ablation device has been succeeded by multichannel devices that can create a number of lesions at once.

Other uses for RF ablation included treatment of cardiac conduction defect and ablation of both primary and metastatic tumors. Other types of chronic pain and arthritis pain can be improved with RF ablation techniques.[4] Ultrasound-guided RF ablation for the treatment of varicose veins has a high success rate.[5] Treatment of Barrett's esophagus, cautery of bleeding uterine fibroids, and uvuloplasty are other applications of RF ablation.

An advantage of the high frequency alternating current is that it does not directly stimulate muscle contraction nor nerve signaling. In many cases, the procedure can be easily performed under local anesthesia. Care must be taken to avoid using so much local anesthetic that the nerve in question will not respond to stimulation.

Historical duration of nerve lesion duration is 6–18 months. The nerves do regenerate, so creation of more lesions and lesions that are close together does prolong the effect. Usually done under X-ray or ultrasound guidance, nerve ablation in chronic pain patients is most commonly performed by anesthesiologists or interventional radiologists. Cardiologist with electrophysiology expertise practice RF ablation for nerve conduction problems, with gastroenterologists and general surgeons use RF ablation while performing endoscopic procedures.

Rhizotomy (the creation of nerve lesions) is usually performed with a RF-emitting probe set at 85°C to 90°C. The probe is located at a nerve location responding to internal stimulation. The administration of a small amount of local anesthetic prior to lesion creation greatly helps the patient to be more comfortable. The duration of the continuous RF pulse is usually 80–90s. When treating a chronic pain patient, more than one lesion is needed in order to generate the best result and duration of effect.

HISTORY OF COSMETIC NERVE ABLATION

The first application of RF neuroablation of motor nerves for the reduction of glabellar furrows was described by Hernandez-Zendejas and Guerrero-Santos[6] in 1994 using a bipolar RF device. Clinical results in 21 patients showed that nerves could be located via electrical stimulation, and that RF could be applied accurately to reduce motor nerve function, and thus reduce the appearance of "frown lines." In 1999, Utley and Goode[7] published results of RF application via a bipolar device to achieve results similar to Hernandez-Zendejas and Guerrero-Santos. Knize[8] dissected ten fresh cadaver heads in order to better understand the effect of stimulation of the temporal and zygomatic branches of the facial nerve on brow mechanics. He identified the depressor supercilii as a separate muscle. He performed a nerve block study to support the need for treatment of the angular branch of the facial nerve.

In 2004, after almost a decade of off-label use by early pioneers, botulinum toxin type A (Botox Cosmetic, Allergan Inc, Irvine, CA, USA) was approved for the reduction of glabellar furrows by the FDA.[9] Botox proved to be a simple and safe treatment and was widely accepted by patients and physicians. The introduction for cosmetic purposes has been a true revolution in treatment of facial wrinkles from the glabella, to the crow's feet, around the mouth and elsewhere. Adoption by the medical profession and the public has been enthusiastic and overwhelming—millions of injections are performed yearly. Its acceptance has increased to the point of the product essentially becoming a verb in common parlance. To "botox" is to inject a botulinum toxin for cosmetic purposes.

The relative ease of use, safety, low cost, and attractive business model for injection of botulinum toxin type A is believed to have limited commercial and clinical interest in pursuing nerve ablation as a treatment option. However, a major limitation is the duration, generally about 4 months, gradually increasing slightly after several years of use. A recent study by Flynn[10] compared the duration of botulinum toxin relaxation of glabellar frown lines by gender. He reported a 3- to 5-month duration in women and a 4- to 6-month duration in men. Most patients completely relapsed at 6 months. Flynn noted in a head-to-head trial that Botox patients had a 23% relapse rate at 16 weeks, while Dysport patients noted a 40% relapse rate at the same interval. Recent reports suggest a chance of antibody formation and resistance to the effects of toxin injection in a small percentage of patients.[11]

The "GFX" device was FDA cleared for application of RF lesions to nerve tissue in 2008, and separate publications in 1999 by Newman[12] and Nahm WK et al.,[13] respectively, began to investigate the efficacy of such treatments using a single needle bipolar RF needle.

Investigators used a peripheral nerve stimulator to map nerve pathways prior to insertion of the percutaneous nerve stimulator/RF needle. This improvement would better guide the treating physician in nerve location. RF nerve ablation was proving effective as an alternative to botulinum toxin type A injection, but the pain associated with the procedure, limited data regarding longevity of effect, and the inability to accurately monitor skin surface temperature led to limited clinical and commercial appeal. Because patients were expected to be "tough" and endure nerve ablation without local anesthetic, which would diminish the ability to map the nerve, few said they would repeat the treatment or recommend it to others.

In 2009, Hantash BM et al.[14] published results obtained using the bipolar GFX device for nerve ablation for cosmetic purposes. A newer monopolar device study was performed by Kim,[15] who published findings using a monopolar device that applied RF in a temperature controlled manner. Results were similar to previous investigations, showing effective reduction in muscle action. Temperature control (meaning real time monitoring and maintenance of a specific temperature for a specific time) mitigated concerns regarding the precise delivery of RF. Nerve ablation could be reliably achieved. These findings encouraged engineers, physicians, and device manufacturers and led to further investigation of the modality for cosmetic purposes.

In 2012, the Symphony RF device (Thermigen Inc, Southlake, TX, USA) was introduced. The process used similar technology as applied by Kim el al.,[15] but had two significant advances. The first was injection of anesthetic precisely to the area of ablation (first performed in 2012 by Carruth via syringe directly introduced into the RF cannula, and later in 2013 by Carruth via a specially designed injector port). Local anesthesia was originally achieved by 2% lidocaine administration; it was modified by increasing the concentration to 4% by Kinney (on the guidance of Chao). The second was real time monitoring of surface skin temperature, achieved using a FLIR camera, first used by Kinney in 2012. Temperature data were streamed live to the screen of a tablet computer, and could be monitored alongside displays of internal temperature and impedance. Patient comfort and muscle response could also be reliably assessed during treatment; finally giving the physician more complete control of the entire procedure. A third innovation was the addition of cutaneous mapping of all the branches of the facial nerve prior to percutaneous insertion of the probe. Precision in probe placement and heating leads to both safety and efficacy of the outcome.

The Symphony RF device effectively addressed the issues believed to have prevented wide clinical and commercial acceptance of RF nerve ablation for cosmetic purposes. Pain issues were addressed by precise external and internal mapping of the nerve, and pinpoint delivery of anesthetic immediately prior to energy application. Concerns regarding safety and control of the precise amount of heat applied were addressed by the new ability to monitor both internal and external temperature using an internal thermistor in the probe, and high resolution and accurate FLIR monitoring for the skin. Longevity of effect has been established to be 18 months to 5 years (Rivlin, personal conversation).

In 2013, Key[16] submitted findings regarding the off label use of the Symphony RF device for soft-tissue contraction at the annual meeting of the American Society of Lasers in Medicine and Surgery (ASLMS). Also presented at the 2013 ASLMS were Duncan's[17] findings regarding off label use of the Symphony RF device for heat-mediated tissue tightening in the lower face, neck and breast. In 2013 as well, Kinney[18] presented at the Hot Topics forum of the American Society for Aesthetic Plastic Surgery on nerve ablation.

ANATOMY

A new interest in defining the musculature and innervation of the medial brow unit has improved our understanding of the "difficult" glabella. The anatomy of the depressor supercilii, first described by Knize was further outlined by Janis in a two-part elucidation of the bony landmarks and variations in supraorbital branching patterns.[19,20] Cook[21] also described this muscle in detail after dissecting eighteen cadaver muscles. He noted that the origin of the depressor was the frontal process of the maxilla, about 1 cm above the medial canthal tendon. Insertion into the dermis occurred 13–14 mm above the medial canthal tendon. Two heads are most common.

Bartolin and Lalo[22] gave a detailed description of the corrugator supercilii in a review article published in 2008. Knize's[8] extensive dissection of the entire complex confirms the need to look at the medial brow as a cooperative and complex unit. Isolated treatment of a single component rarely results in a satisfactory outcome.

POTENTIAL USE FOR BROW LIFTING

The traditional coronal brow lift technique has been in use since 1910.[23] Due in part to the global trend for minimally invasive procedures, more conservative approaches to brow lifting were a hot topic during the past decade. Temporal or lateral brow approaches[24] were used for isolated lateral brow lift and upward suspension of the frontalis. However, this approach did not allow correction of the medial brow and corrugator region. The endoscopic brow lifting technique pioneered by Saltz[25] and others[26,27] overcame that limitation. Knize's[28] technique using a limited incision achieved good results without the need to buy endoscopic equipment. Both techniques greatly reduced the problems of numbness and alopecia that were associated with the traditional coronal approach. However, fixation of the brow continued to be a problem. Honig et al.[29] performed a study in which half of his patients underwent fixation of the lateral brow with a single suture, while the other half had suspension with the Endotine device. His conclusion was that neither technique provided prolonged lateral brow elevation, but the Endotine had better longevity of medial brow correction. Pascal et al.[30] used the Endotine ribbon device in addition to the standard endotine fixation device to enhance the long-term outcome of brow lifting. Application of percutaneous RF energy for cosmetic purposes continues to be investigated, and utilized in a variety of treatment protocols. This therapeutic approach may hold as yet unrealized potential for cosmetic application.

Early use of the Thermigen device for expanded indications has yielded promising results. Indications for treatment include prominent glabellar frown lines, and an off label use for soft-tissue tightening in small regions such as the neck and lower jawline. Patients with dynamic lines in the periorbital regions have requested treatment of crow's feet, transverse forehead lines, and possible improvement of disappointing results of a previous brow lift. Similar treatment parameters were used for these indications, with the exception of treatment for transverse lines. The pilot treatment protocol for this indication combines lesion creation in the medial frontal branch of the facial nerve. Due to suboptimal response observed on the table, treatment of the dermal insertion of the nerve was performed as well at 1.5-cm intervals using an 80°C temperature and a 60-second duration, due to the superficial location of the probe.

TECHNIQUE: TREATMENT PROTOCOLS ON LABEL

Nerve Ablation Brow

Warning: do not treat your Botox patient until full relapse at 3–4 months has occurred:

1. Cutaneous mapping of the facial nerve branches with an external nerve stimulator to the temporal branch of the facial nerve. This runs along the top of the brow; sometimes within the brow. Mapping is begun 1–2 cm lateral to the tail of the brow. Location of each active site is marked with a permanent marker. The second branch to be mapped with the external nerve stimulator is the angular branch. Mapping usually begins at the lateral base of the nose above the ala. This branch can continue up to the medial canthal tendon. Locations of nerve activity should be marked about 0.5–1 cm apart. The more closely together the lesions are located the better success with outcome.
2. Prepare the skin with sterile prep solution. Povidone-iodine, Hibiclens, or pHisoderm can be used.
3. Inject 0.1 mL of 1% lidocaine/1:100,000 epinephrine about 2 cm lateral to first nerve lesion to be treated, usually 1–3 mm superior to the lateral most portion of the brow. Be careful not to inject within the distribution of the nerve; you may knock out the response to stimulation.
4. Make stab wound with 18-gauge needle for cannula access.

5. Insert the 22-gauge probe advance under the first cutaneous mark.
6. Set the device to "motor stim." Stimulate the nerve at the minimum amplitude necessary to detect motion in the corrugator muscles, usually 3–4 mA. This may be gradually turned up if needed. When checking for external stimulation after several lesions is created, a higher amplitude may be needed.
7. Inject 0.1 mL of 4% lidocaine and wait 1 minute for full anesthetic effect. If you treat too soon, the patient will experience significant discomfort. If 4% lidocaine is not available, 0.15 mL of 2% lidocaine can be substituted.
8. Switch device front panel setting to RF lesion on controller.
9. Set temperature to 85°C and timer for 1 minute.
10. Monitor skin with FLIR camera to keep temperatures below 42°.
11. Check for loss of muscle action in lateral portion of muscle by asking patient to frown.
12. Advance to next lesion, usually about 0.5–1 cm medially.
13. Repeat steps 7–11 for each lesion.
14. Check muscle action medially as each lesion is treated. Voluntary motion is more reliable than the external stimulator.

Nerve Ablation Angular

1. Cutaneous mapping of the facial nerve branch in the angular position starts about 1 cm inferior eyelid skin and medial to the vertical mid-line of the pupil.
2. Mark 2–3 lesions as the nerve courses superiorly and medially toward the medial canthus. More lesions may need to be created in order to get full effect:
3. Steps 4–11 are similar as above.
4. Check for loss of muscle action in the medial portion of muscle.
5. Complete procedure when muscle no longer responds voluntarily, or on electrical stimulation.

Postoperative treatment consists of compression garment at night as necessary and over the counter analgesics. Mild-to-moderate edema is expected for 1–3 days with minimal to no pain after treatment.

CASE STUDIES

Glabellar Frown (Figs. 8.1A and B)

This 41-year-old female with strong glabellar frown with frontalis recruitment while animating. Two months after treating with Symphony RF nerve ablation creating 8–10 lesions in the temporal branch leading to the corrugator muscle. Four to five lesions were created along the angular nerve.

It is very important to persist in treating patients. The procedure is not complete until the patient cannot longer voluntarily animate and the muscle cannot be mechanically stimulated. With four to five lesions along the brow, about a 50% reduction in corrugator activity can be achieved. With a lot of attention to detail, a more thorough correction can be created. This may take eight lesions or more. If the medial frontalis is mapped out and treated, further correction of strong glabellar frowns can be achieved.

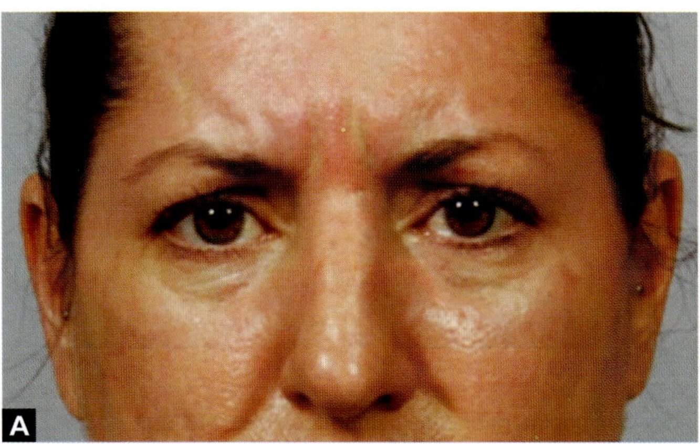

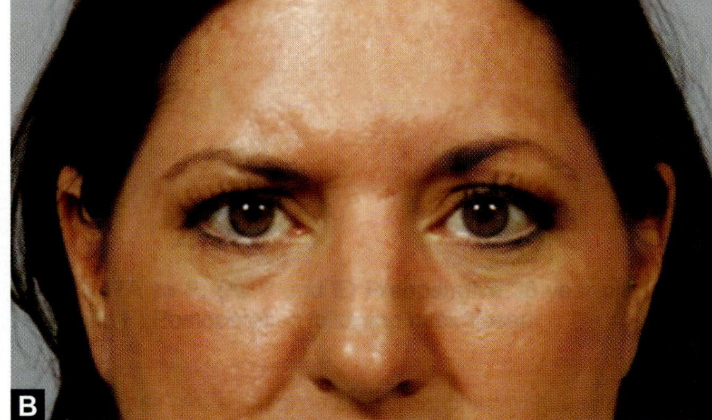

Figs. 8.1A and B: (A) Preoperative 41-year-old female with strong glabellar frown with frontalis recruitment. Photograph was taken while animating. (B) Two months postoperative after treating with Symphony RF nerve ablation.

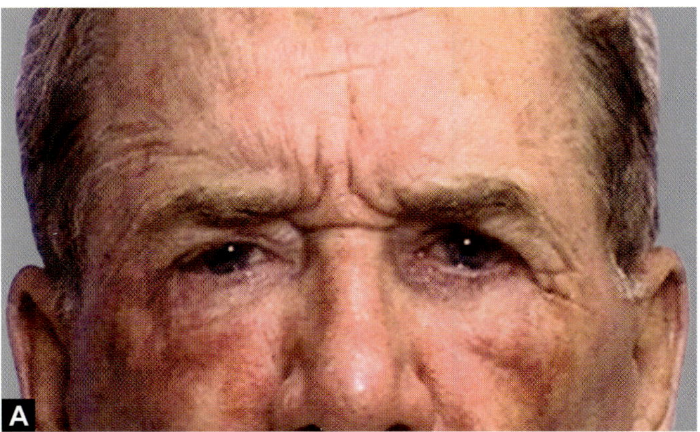

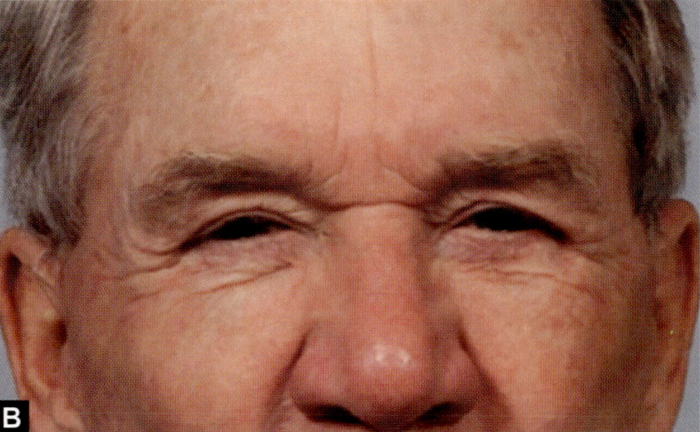

Figs. 8.2A and B: (A) Preoperative 66-year-old male had been getting Botox injections for many years. He was tired of the repeated trips, and was eager to try a more long-lasting solution. (B) Two-month post-treatment shows the improvement.

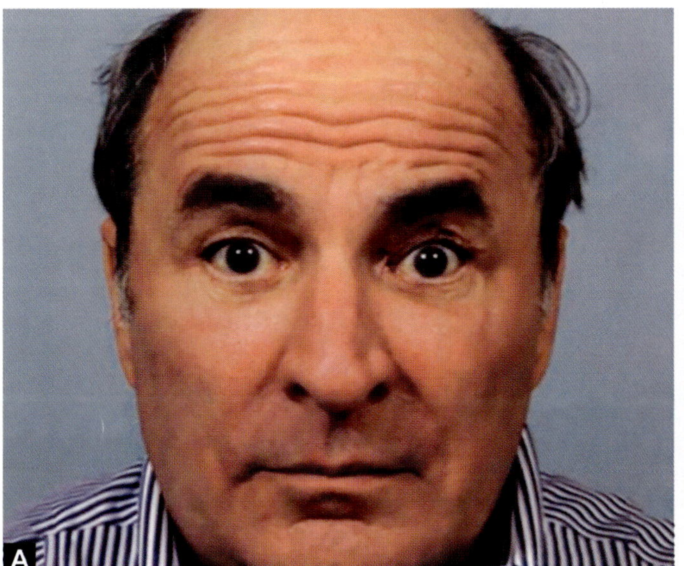

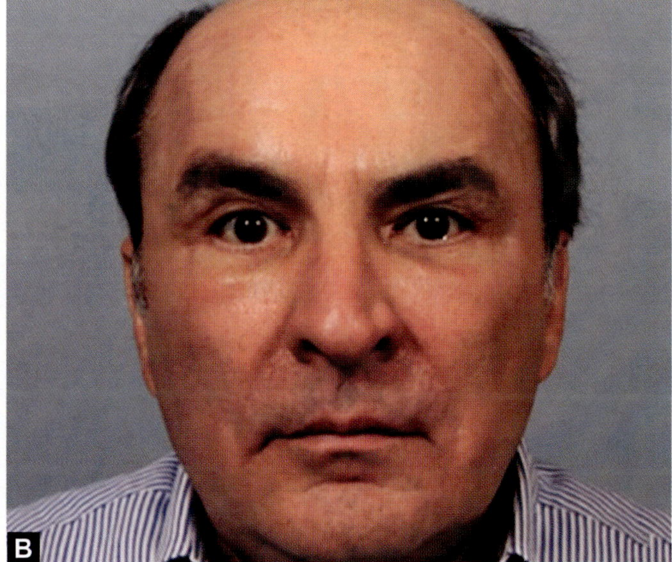

Figs. 8.3A and B: (A) Preoperative 65-year-old male had very strong transverse forehead lines. Glabellar frown lines and strong crow's feet were also present. (B) Postoperative animation 3 weeks post-treatment.

Male with Glabellar Frown and Brow Ptosis (Figs. 8.2A and B)

This 66-year-old male had been getting Botox injections for many years. He was tired of the repeated trips, and was eager to try a more long-lasting solution. The standard protocol was followed in performing his nerve ablation. This patient was treated until voluntary motion was no longer present in both the angular and temporal regions. There is some frontalis recruitment in his frown with animation. Therefore, the medial frontal branch was also treated with RF lesions. He had sixteen lesions per side, including treatment of the medial frontal, temporal, lateral orbicularis, and angular branches. Two months post-treatment shows the improvement.

Transverse Forehead Lines (Figs. 8.3A and B)

This 65-year-old male had very strong transverse forehead lines. Glabellar frown lines and strong crow's feet were also present. He desired a significant difference, but would not agree to a traditional brow lift approach. Three weeks post-treatment following three treatment areas that were

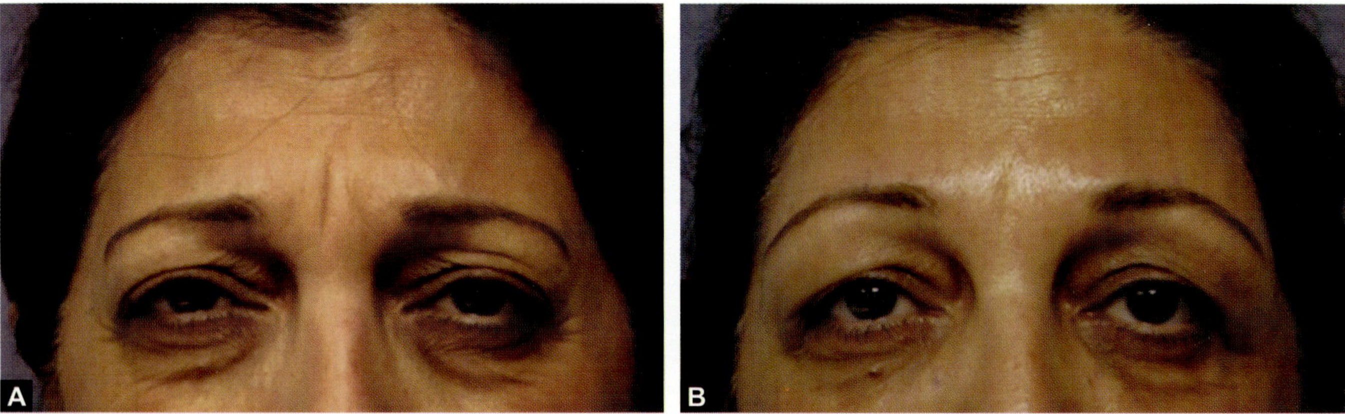

Figs. 8.4A and B: (A) Preoperative 45-year-old female with prominent glabellar frown. (B) Postoperative, while animating, shows definite improvement of the glabellar frown.

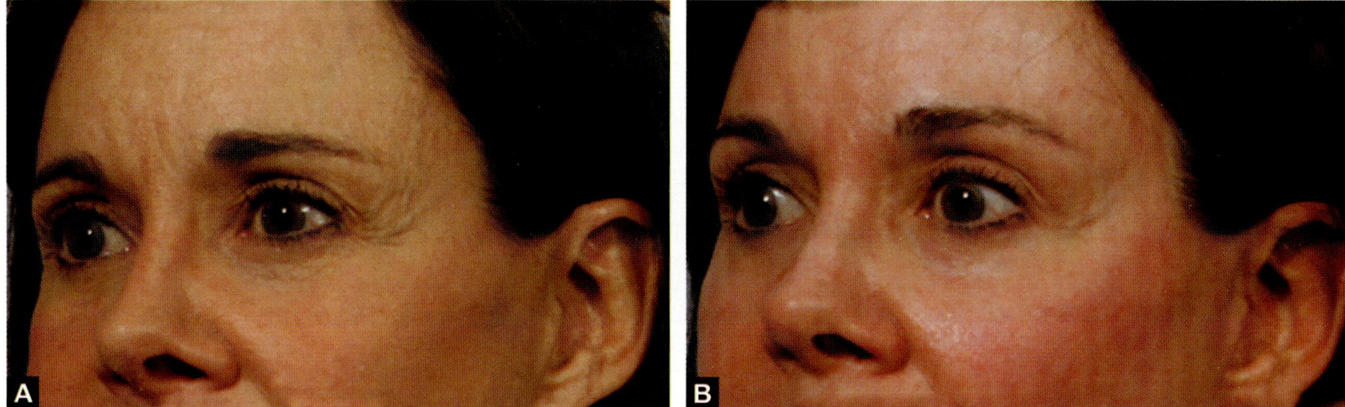

Figs. 8.5A and B: (A) Preoperative 52-year-old female had facial rejuvenation procedures in another state. She noted that she had some residual drooping of the lateral brow which she would like improved. (B) Six weeks postoperative post-treatment with Erbium laser resurfacing and RF nerve ablation. Note improvement in her glabellar frown, her brow position, and crow's feet.

addressed: transverse lines, glabellar frown, and crow's feet. The transverse lines were treated by creating lesions along the medial frontal branch bilaterally. In addition, focal heating of the muscular insertion points was performed for 45 seconds at 80°. These were placed 1.5-cm apart. Animation shows improvement.

Female with Glabellar Frown (Figs. 8.4A and B)

This 45-year-old female had a prominent glabellar frown. The path of the corrugator branch was delineated with the external nerve stimulator. Three lesions were created using the Thermigen RF ablation device on each side. The lesions were produced with settings of 85°and duration of 90 seconds each. One day post-treatment there is the mild edema in the upper lids. While animating there is definite improvement of the glabellar frown.

Female with Glabellar Frown, Crow's Feet, and Failed Previous Brow Lift (Figs. 8.5A and B)

This 52-year-old female had facial rejuvenation procedures in another state. She noted that she had some residual drooping of the lateral brow that she would like improved. Her glabellar frown made her appear worried. She was also hoping for some improvement of her crow's feet. Six weeks post-treatment with Erbium laser resurfacing and RF nerve ablation, this patient has improvement in her glabellar frown, her brow position, and crow's feet.

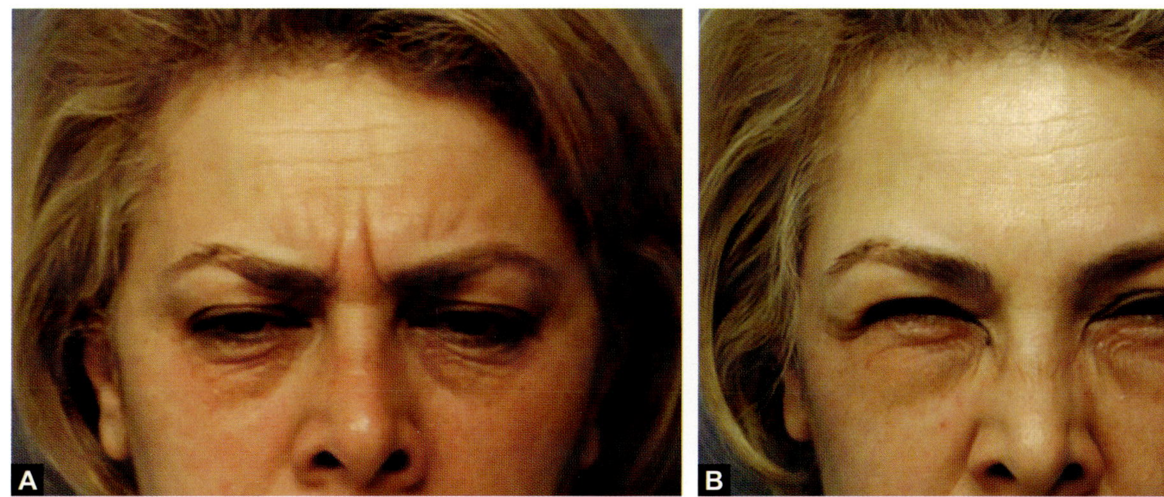

Figs. 8.6A and B: (A) Preoperative 42-year-old female had a strong glabellar frown. (B) Two weeks after treatment with RF nerve ablation to the corrugator branch.

Female with Glabellar Frown (Figs. 8.6A and B)

This 42-year-old female had a strong glabellar frown. Two weeks after treatment with RF nerve ablation to the corrugator branch shows improvement. Three lesions were created just above each brow after external and internal stimulation was used to map out the nerves.

CONCLUSION

Radiofrequency nerve ablation has new and expanded uses for cosmetic indications. With the addition of a local anesthetic injection prior to nerve lesion formation, patient comfort is greatly improved over the original GFX procedure. The safety feature of an indwelling thermistor and a high-resolution temperature camera for skin monitoring has greatly reduced the risk of burns. The quality of outcome is operator dependent. While the procedure is straightforward and very reproducible, persistence in treatment can make the difference between a modest improvement and a dramatic outcome. Practitioners with prototype devices report 5-year results with attention to detail during treatment and a possible touch-up after several years.

REFERENCES

1. DiBernardo BE, Reyes J, Chen B. Evaluation of tissue thermal effects from 1064/1320-nm laser-assisted lipolysis and its clinical implications. J Cosmet Laser Ther. 2009;11(2):62-69.
2. Radiofrequency ablation—Wikipedia, the free encyclopedia. http://www.en.wikipedia.org/wiki/Radiofrequency_ablation. [Accessed May 1, 2013].
3. Health and nutrition facts for you—UW Health. http://www.uwhealth.org/healthfacts. [Accessed May 1, 2013].
4. Chen JQ, Xie H, Deng HY, et al. Endovenous laser ablation of great saphenous vein with ultrasound-guided perivenous tumescence: early and midterm results. Chin Med J (Engl). 2013;126(3):421-5.
5. Radiofrequency ablation for arthritis pain—Webb MD. http://www.webmd.com/radiofrequency_nerve_ablation. [Accessed April 17, 2013].
6. Hernandez-Zendejas G, Guerrero-Santos J. Percutaneous selective radio-frequency neuroablation in plastic surgery. Aesthetic Plast Surg. 1994;18(1):41-48.
7. Utley DS, Goode RL. Radiofrequency ablation of the nerve to the corrugator muscle for elimination of glabellar furrowing. Arch Facial Plast Surg. 1999;1(1):46-48.
8. Knize DM. Muscles that act on glabellar skin: a closer look. Plast Reconstr Surg. 2000;105(1):350-61.
9. Botox history and development—Allergan. http://www.allergan.com/assets/botox-history-and-development.pdf. [Accessed May 20, 2013].
10. Flynn TC. Botulinum toxin: examining duration of effect in facial aesthetic applications. Am J Clin Dermatol. 2010;11(3):183-99.
11. Flynn TC. Advances in the use of botulinum neurotoxins in facial esthetics. J Cosmet Dermatol. 2012;11(1):42-50.
12. Newman JP. Radiofrequency energy for denervation of selected facial muscles: clinical experiences at six months. Internet J Plast Surg. 2009;5(2):4-8.
13. Nahm WK, Su TT, Rotunda AM, Moy RL, et al. Objective changes in brow position, superior palpebral crease, peak angle of the eyebrow, and jowl surface area after volumetric radiofrequency treatments to half of the face. Dermatol Surg. 2004;30(6):922-8.

14. Hantash BM, Renton B, Berkowitz RL, Stridde BC, Newman J, et al. Pilot clinical study of a novel minimally invasive bipolar microneedle radiofrequency device. Lasers Surg Med. 2009;41(2):87-95.
15. Kim JH, Jeong JW, Son D, et al. Percutaneous selective radiofrequency nerve ablation for glabellar frown lines. Aesthet Surg J. 2011;31(7):747-55.
16. Key D. Improving the clinical response of skin tightening by "targeted temperature" subdermal RF probe heating using a method of subsurface temperature monitoring combined with skin surface infrared imaging. Presented at ASLMS, Boston, April 7, 2013.
17. Duncan D. Optimizing outcomes with Thermigen RF monopolar energy for nerve ablation, soft tissue tightening, and breast lifting. Presented at ASLMS, Boston, April 6, 2013.
18. Kinney B. Radiofrequency for facial rejuvenation. Presented at the premier Hot Topics Forum, American Society for Aesthetic Plastic Surgery Annual Meeting, New York, April 12, 2013.
19. Janis JE, Gharami A, Lemmon JA, et al. Anatomy of the corrugator supercilii muscle: part I: corrugator topography. Plast Reconstr Surg. 2007;120(6):1647-53.
20. Janis JE, Gharami A, Lemmon JA, et al. Anatomy of the corrugator supercilii muscle: part II: supraorbital branching patterns. Plast Reconstr Surg. 2008;121(1):233-40.
21. Cook BE, Lucarelli MJ, Lemke BN. Depressor supercilii muscle: anatomy, histology, and cosmetic implications. Ophthal Plast Reconstr Surg. 2001;17(6):404-11.
22. Bartolin C, Lalo J. The corrugator supercilii muscle: a review. Morphologie. 2008;92(299):145-53.
23. Chaiet SR, Williams EF 3rd. Understanding midfacial rejuvenation in the 21st century. Facial Plast Surg. 2013;29(1):40-45.
24. Centurion P, Romero C. Lateral brow lift: a surgical proposal. Aesthetic Plast Surg. 2010;34(6):745-57.
25. Saltz R, Ohana B. Thirteen years of experience with the endoscopic midface lift. Aesthet Surg J. 2012;32(8):927-36.
26. Iblher N, Manegold S, Porzelius C, et al. Morphometric long-term evaluation and comparison of brow position and shape after endoscopic forehead lift and transpalpebral browpexy. Plast Reconstr Surg. 2012;130(6):830e-40e.
27. Afifi AM, Alghoul M, Zor F, et al. Comparison of the transpalpebral and endoscopic approaches in resection of the corrugator supercilii muscle. Aesthet Surg J. 2012;32(2):151-6.
28. Knize DM. Limited-incision forehead lift for eyebrow elevation to enhance upper blepharoplasty. Plast Reconstr Surg. 1996;97(7):1334-42.
29. Honig JF, Frank MH, Knutti D, et al. Video endoscopic-assisted brow lift: comparison of the eyebrow position after Endotine fixation vs. suture fixation. J Craniofac Surg. 2008;19(4):1140-47.
30. Pascal M, Gualdi A, Bottini C, et al. An original application of the endotine ribbon device for brow lift. Plast Reconstr Surg. 2009;124(5):1652-61.

Section 4

Breast

Chapter Outline

- Stem Cell Fat Transfer for Mastoplasty using Vaser Ultrasound and Office Devised Stem Cell
- "Scarless" Mastopexy: Using Heat-Mediated Tissue Tightening to Lift the Breast
- Inverted "T" Superior Pedicle Technique with Inferior-Based Dermal Adipose Flap for Reduction Mammaplasty
- A Novel Approach in Male Breast Contouring after Massive Weight Loss: The Central Pedicled Breast Reduction Technique

9 Stem Cell Fat Transfer for Mastoplasty using Vaser Ultrasound and Office Devised Stem Cell

Alberto Di Giuseppe, Dennis Wolf

INTRODUCTION

The authors began using autologous fat transfer (AFT) or fat grafting procedures to provide lasting natural structure and contour changes 3 years ago. Vaser (Sound Surgical Technologies LLC, Denver, Colorado, USA) has been used since 2001, first in Europe, and then for all the lipoplasty procedures (Fig. 9.1). At the beginning Vaser was only used for body contouring purposes, then for breast reduction, neck-chin debulking and contouring, circumferential thighs and lastly axillary hyperhydrosis treatment. Just to mention few of the potential applications of this sophisticated device.

Recently, Vaser was used for fat harvesting, and AFT for breast enlargement and contouring, and adipose-derived stem cell (ADSC) treatments. After 3 years follow-up of this technique, it was concluded that the technique presents fewer side effects long term in comparison with traditional implants and is safe and effective if properly performed.

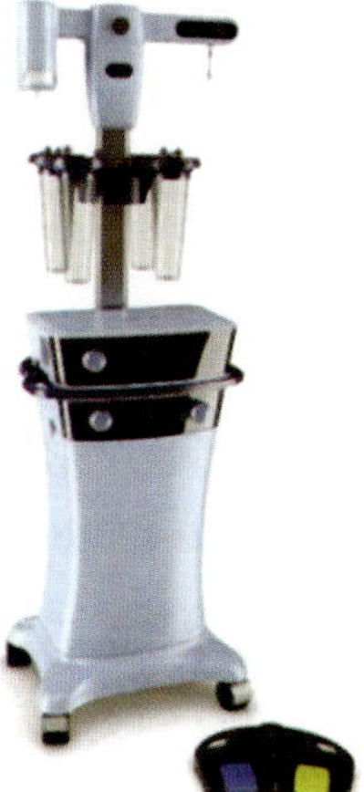

Fig. 9.1: Vaser system (Sound Surgical Technology, Denver, CO, USA).

Traditionally, physicians have used handheld syringes, following the Coleman technique. This method is both laborious and time consuming and depending upon the size of the needle and syringe used, may still disrupt fat cells.

To perform bilateral breast augmentation with AFT large amounts of harvest material is required (minimum 500 mL unfiltered material). In the last 3 years, the authors have used standard Vaser treatment, reducing the power to 60% of the total at continuous setting, followed by low-vacuum aspiration using the VentX system and achieved a raw fat viability of 83%. This high level of viability did not come at the expense of operative time or convenience. With experience, there was an average operating time of 3.5 hours, including Vaser to two to four areas for lipoplasty, fat harvesting, Pure-Graft washing and preparation, fat introduction into both breasts with small syringes. All treatments were performed under tumescent anesthesia and intravenous (IV) sedation. All patients were treated as day case with discharge few hours after surgery. A series of 120 cases, with regular follow-up to 3 years have been performed.

An important factor in the viability is the use of lower power Vaser to emulsify the adipose tissue before aspiration. Separating the adipose tissue into smaller clumps in situ permits the use of atraumatic cannulas and lower vacuum levels, which in turn, avoids traumatic injury to the fat during the aspiration. Also, by maintaining the overall cellular distribution and ratio of the lipoaspirate (mature adipocytes and the "loosely adherent" cell population (periadipocytes, stem cells, stromal cells, etc.) the retention rate of the implanted tissue matrix is enhanced. In addition to the use of harvested fat for immediate reinjection, adipose tissue is a significant source of stem cells for both enhancement of autologous fat grafts and for the use in often developing clinical treatments. As with direct

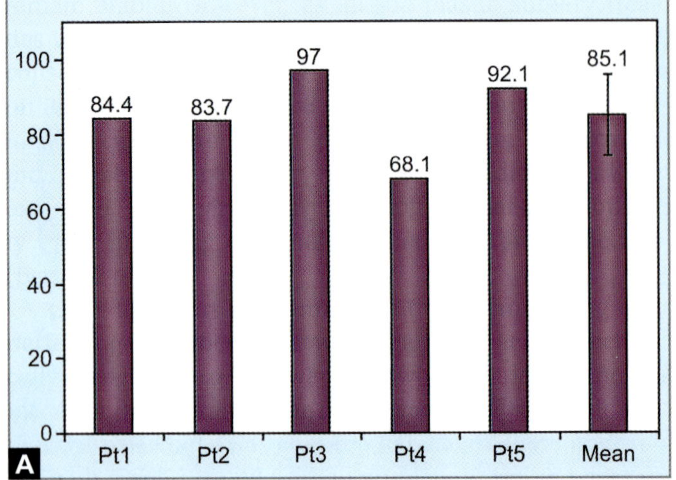

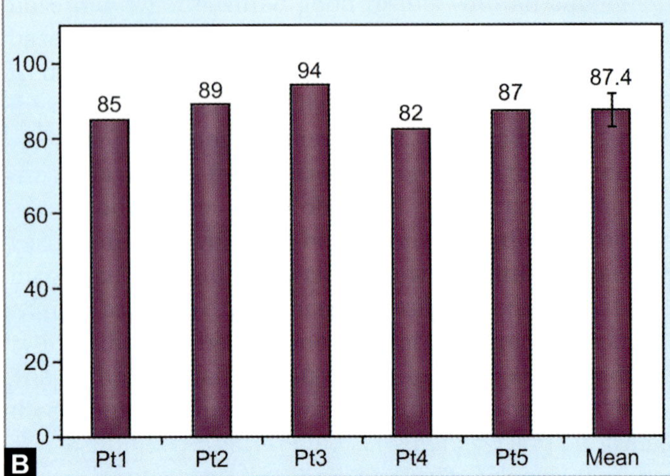

Figs. 9.2A and B: (A) Adipocyte viability: functional assessment by lipolysis assay. (B) ADRC viability.

autologous fat injection, the viability of the regenerative cells derived from the harvested adipose tissue is of primary importance, both as fresh tissue and after freezing.

The field of clinical treatments using adult stem cells continues to expand and patients undergoing liposuction are increasingly interested in storing tissue samples containing stem cells.

The tissue could then be thawed at some future date and utilized in the development of genetic and regenerative treatments. The viability of the ADSCs was higher than that for the overall tissue samples at over 87% (Figs. 9.2A and B). Even more importantly, the viability of the ADSCs was only slightly reduced to 75% after freezing using liquid nitrogen vapor.

In this application, the harvesting of the adipose tissue using Vaser system minimizes tissue damage and improves the viability of the harvested cells.

STEM CELL NICHE THERAPY USING ADIPOSE TISSUE

Adipose-derived stem cell niche refers to the complex relationships that ADSCs establish with all of the physiological or ectopic factors contributing to determine their identity and fate. The phenotypical identity of any cell and its reaction to a given stimulus are, therefore, not only determined by the genetic or epigenetic equipment of the cell, but also depend on the specific niche context in which it resides. A change in niche parameters or the transplantation of cells into other niches can have a considerable effect on cell physiology and alter its properties.

Research has shown that the signals controlling the embryonic origin of ADSCs and their differentiation in adult adipose tissue include the same pathways as those involved in the homeostasis of other adult and embryonic stem cell populations,[1] and their complex orchestration can have different effects depending on the concentration, stage of differentiation and extrinsic niche factors, such as cell-matrix and cell-cell interactions, the presence of vasculature, and the level and type of innervation. Despite extensive research into the intracellular signaling involved in ADSC homeostasis and differentiation, little is known about the role of cell-cell and cell-matrix interactions. Zannettino et al.[2] have suggested that ADSCs reside in perivascular niches, which prompts the speculation that perivascular structures (cells and extracellular matrix) may provide signals that balance the maintenance of ADSCs in an undifferentiated state and their commitment to differentiation.

It has recently been shown that in vitro culture and expansion significantly alter the transcriptional phenotype of ADSCs. Freshly isolated stromal vascular fractions (SVFs) express hematopoietic markers (CD34) that are lost within a few days of culturing.[3] In line with previously published findings,[4] the authors have found the increased expression of mesenchymal stem cell-associated markers in cultures of both in human and murine ADSCs, whereas the longer term loss of markers of undifferentiated status, such as undifferentiated transcription factor (UTF-1), indicated a shift toward differentiation. Prolonged culturing also significantly downregulated various isoforms of procollagen, matrix metallopeptidases and inflammatory cytokines, thus indicating adaptation to the artificial environment. Under extreme conditions, it has even been shown that prolonged in vitro culturing can induce the neoplastic transformation of ADSCs,[5] although it is still unclear whether these changes are reversible or how they may affect the therapeutic potential of the cell. However, ADSCs can be used in many clinical applications (particularly in the fields of plastic and reconstructive surgery) by means of transplantation without removing them from their fat niche.

In addition to molecular and cell biology, the dynamic and regenerative nature of fat grafts has been established in various areas of plastic surgery, and clinical practice that has shown that the long-term outcomes of fat grafting can include rejuvenation of skin texture,[6,7] adipocyte formation, and a large number of precursors at different stages of differentiation. Ultrastructural studies of centrifuged fat have revealed that mature adipocytes show interruptions in their cytoplasmic membrane and various degrees of degeneration including cell necrosis, but the SVF appears to be well preserved. Rigotti et al.[8] compared the ultrastructure of mammary radio-lesions before, and at different times after, fat grafting, and found clear signs of regeneration, with evidence of new the adipocyte phenotype. Before transplantation, almost all of the adipocytes were seriously damaged by centrifugation and in the radio-damaged recipient tissue. There were neither mature adipocytes nor differentiating preadipocytes. Reasonable interpretations of these findings are that the differentiating preadipocytes observed after treatment were either adipocyte-committed ADSCs originally embedded within the transplanted fat, or locally present endogenous adipocyte-committed ADSCs activated by the ectopically transplanted fat. The massive survival of ADSCs in fat transplants, despite liposuction and centrifugation procedures, strongly supports the first hypothesis, but the second may be equally valid as it assumes that transplanted fat enriched with ADSCs by centrifugation can behave as an atypical ectopic niche that orchestrates tissue regeneration by modulating endogenous tissue resources.

The term "atypical ectopic niche" could be used as a common paradigm of stem cell-based therapies. It is based on the idea of a "bystander" mechanism in which the stem cells ectopically transplanted into a generic lesion (radiolesion, myocardial infarction, cerebral stroke, etc.) do not replace tissue-specific cells by direct differentiation, but locally form an atypical stem cell niche that suppresses inflammation, promotes neoangiogenesis, and favors the activation of endogenous stem cell precursors by releasing trophic factors, such as cytokines, proangiogenic molecules, and growth factors. Therefore, adipose tissue can be considered as an ideal "biologic product."

The role of this essential component of the stromal fraction of the lipoaspirates argues for a regenerative theory based on angiogenesis imbued with various growth factors, not yet fully identified, released from stem cells. Thus, in addition to the traditional understanding that fat is an high-energy reservoir involved in homeostasis for its ability to bind large amounts of fluids and in the maintenance of thermoregulation it becomes apparent that it is also a regenerative organ providing the basis for soft tissue regeneration.

Adipose-derived stem cells have become one of the most popular adult stem cell populations for research in soft tissue engineering and regenerative medicine applications. Compared with other stem cell sources, ASCs offer several advantages including an abundant autologous source, minor invasive harvesting (liposuction), and significant proliferative capacity in culture and multilineage potential. To harvest the adipose tissue, a liposuction procedure is less invasive than bone marrow aspiration and the technique produces less patient discomfort and donor site morbidity. Small amounts of adipose tissue yields approximately 5×10^3 stem cells, which is 500-fold greater than the number of Mesodermal stem cells (MSCs) in 1 g of bone marrow.[9] Numerous preclinical studies have been pursued, with early clinical data appearing in the literature. Fat as a living, free graft does more than just fill the area into which it is placed. Grafted fat affects the tissue into which it is placed in many ways for the life of the patient. It can improve the quality of aged and scarred skin and heal radiation damage and chronic ulcers. Just how grafted fat causes these changes remains unanswered. We know that fat can perform amazing feats in a glass tube and in some animal models, but we have little insight into what happens to fat when it is grafted from one part of the human body to another part. The focus of the near future should be research to explain and expand on future clinical successes.

In addition to the outstanding results of lipotransfer for volume restoration, surgeons have become increasingly interested in the apparent rejuvenative effects on the skin itself. Coleman has noted improved skin quality, with softening of wrinkles, decreased pore size, and improved pigmentation during the first year post-treatment. In fact, analysis of clinical results following both reconstructive and aesthetic surgery reveals that after one or several repeated fat grafting procedures, the trophicity and quality of the recipient site is improved. These changes develop over several months following the fat grafting procedure, with an often variable expression, as improvements in skin texture, skin suppleness, skin color, and/or scar quality.

Topographical skin analysis systems such as the recently developed VISIA system (Canfield Imaging Systems) may determine whether the effect from fat grafting is an effective skin rejuvenation technique in comparison to chemical peels and laser resurfacing. Aside from effects on normal, aged skin, when fat has been grafted beneath depressed scars there was improvement not only in the depression but also in the character of the scar itself, with an apparent transformation to normal appearing skin. Other authors have reported adverse range of improvements in soft tissue conditions, including radiation damage, breast capsular contracture, damaged vocal cords, and chronic ulceration, as well as regrowth of calvarial bone. While many of the exact mechanisms for these effects remain to be described, what seems to be at the center of these changes is the presence of ADSCs in human adipose tissue. In fact, it has proven to be the most abundant source of stem cells in the body.

Benefits of stem cells in a fat transfer:

1. Grow new blood vessels to nourish the fat
2. Release anti-inflammatory agents to aid healing
3. Generate and release growth factors that support graft survival
4. Improve skin tightening and rejuvenation
5. No risk of allergic or adverse reaction
6. A cutting edge option used around the world today
7. The therapeutic target is the reconstruction of autologous niches, by simple moving stem cells niches from one connective tissue in which they are abundant into another in which they are scarce.[9]

PATIENT SELECTION

All the patients selected for bilateral breast augmentation to improve shape, contour, and volume using Vaser as primary source of fat harvest followed these criteria:

1. No significant Past medical history (PMH) or strong family history of breast cancer
2. Mammography
3. Preoperative as base line to exclude pathology. Patients with fibroadenoma, suspected cysts >1 cm, or significant calcifications are discouraged
4. Patients with moderate-to-severe glandular or skin ptosis are denied surgery (Figs. 9.3A to D)
5. Fat donor area (Figs. 9.4A and B)
6. Extremely slender patients are denied surgery (Fig. 9.5).

PATIENT ASSESSMENT

All candidates underwent:

1. Preoperative clinical evaluation
2. Photographs
3. Mammography (Fig. 9.6) or ultrasonography (Fig. 9.7) in younger patients.
4. Some patients had three-dimensional imaging pre- and postoperatively to assess fat survival and fat distribution in long-term follow-up.
5. In preparation for surgery, standard electrocardiography, and blood test.
6. All patients operated were American Society of Anesthesiologists (ASA) 1–2 category.
7. Patients were warned to maintain their weight in the postoperative period.
8. Weight loss could severely influence fat retention.
9. Hormonal changes, as in pregnancy and menopause, may affect fat retention, decreasing the breast volume.
10. Patients with unrealistic expectations of large volume were denied surgery.

Selection of site of fat harvesting (Fig. 9.8):

1. Abdomen
2. Flanks
3. Anterior thighs
4. Outer thighs
5. Arms
6. Buttocks

SELECTION OF ANESTHESIA

All the patients in this series were operated office-based surgery, with local tumescent anesthesia and intravenous (IV) sedation. Tumescent anesthesia consisted of 1,000 mL normal saline (0.9%), 1 mL adrenaline (1:1,000), and 500 mg lidocaine. Author DW uses routinely 600–800 mg of lidocaine in his tumescent anesthesia. Breast tumescence infiltration ranges 100–300 mL (Fig. 9.9).

Intravenous sedation is given by an anesthetist with a fully monitored patient, consisting mainly of propofol, fentanyl, midazolam, and IV paracetamol. Sedation was mainly light in the majority of patients remaining conscious and conversant. Fentanyl and/or Fentamest were

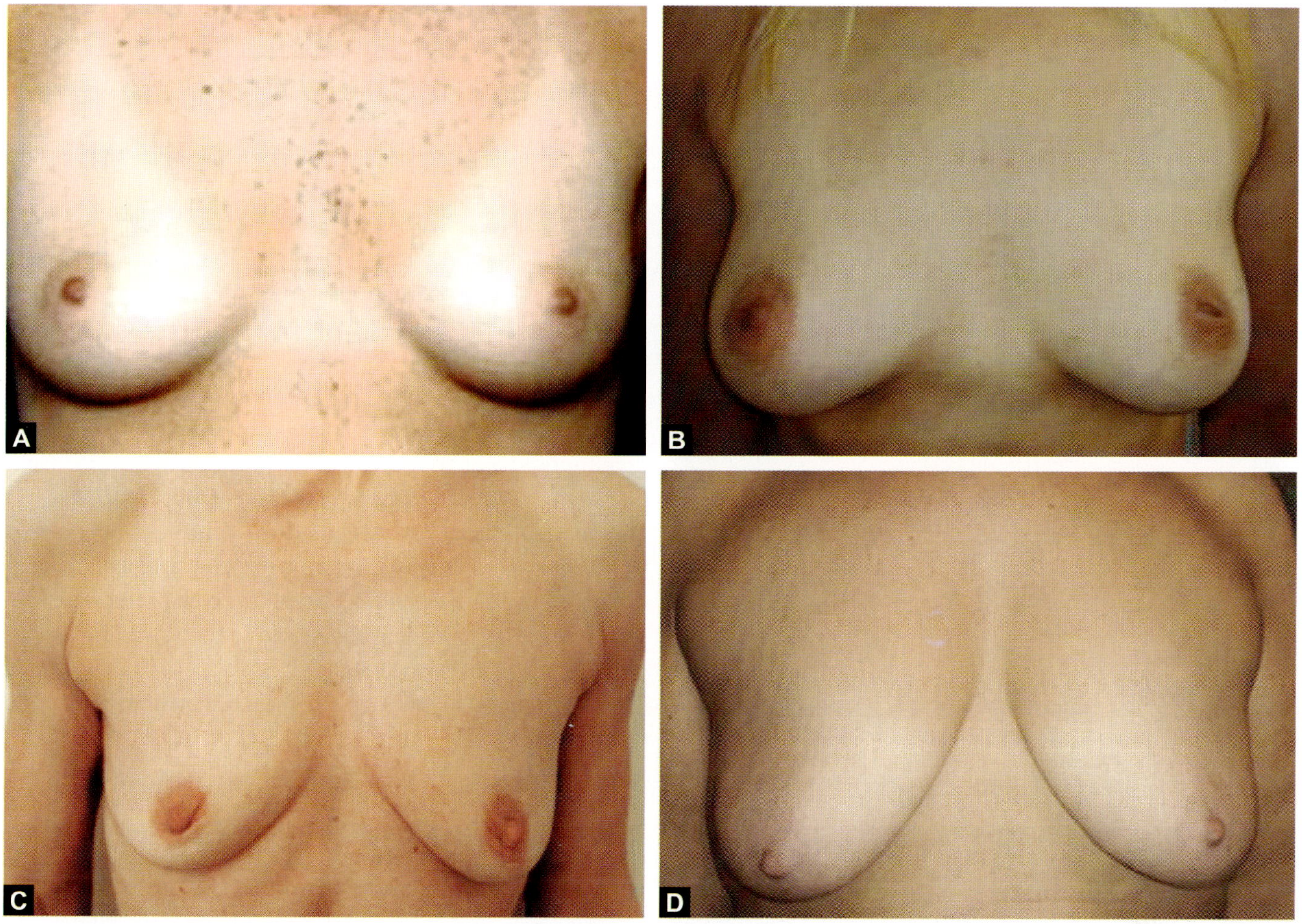

Figs. 9.3A to D: (A) Good candidate for fat transfer (good skin tone, elasticity, nipple position). (B) Good candidate for fat transfer (mild ptosis). (C) Poor candidate (breast ptosis, poor skin tone, no projection). (D) Contraindication to fat transfer for breast enlargement (severe breast ptosis).

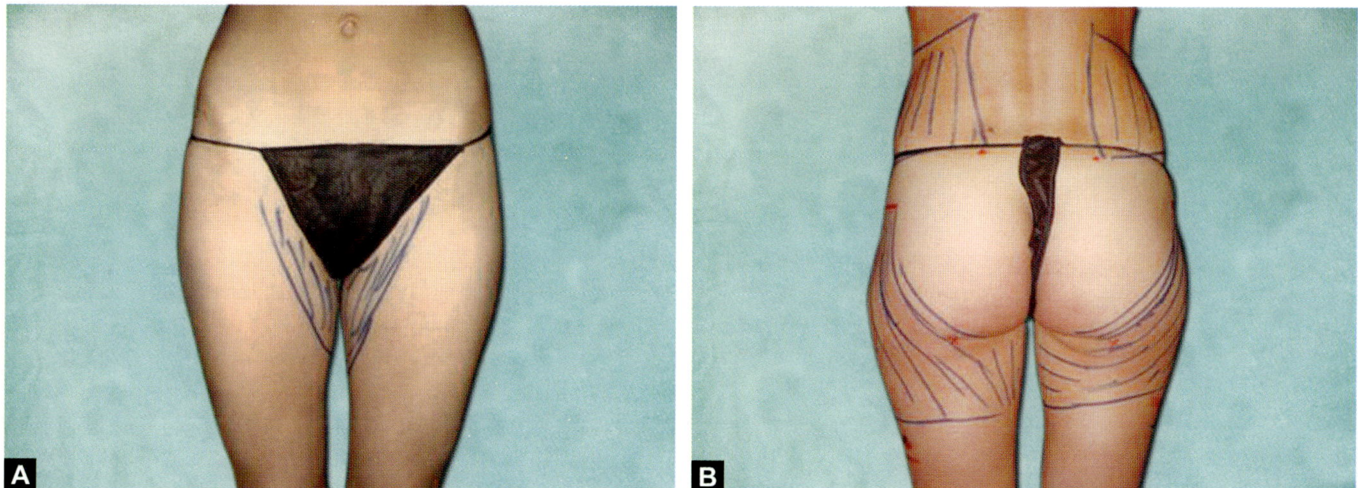

Figs. 9.4A and B: Preoperative donor area for fat transfer: trochanters, inner thighs, and flanks. From this patient, a total of 1,800 mL emulsion was removed and 600 mL of pure graft was transferred.

added following patient's analgesia requirement and according to anesthetist protocol and indications.

Harvest sites infiltration ranges from 2,000 to 4,000 mL, aspirate ranges from 800 to 3,000 mL.

Pure graft ranges from 280 to 400 mL.

All patients had intraoperative antibiotics. Author ADG uses metronidazole IV (400 mg) and cefotaxime (1 g) followed by 5 days of oral course of the same antibiotics, while author DW uses coamoxiclav 1.2 g IV and 5 days oral postoperatively. Antiemetic drugs and gastroprotectors were given by author ADG routinely.

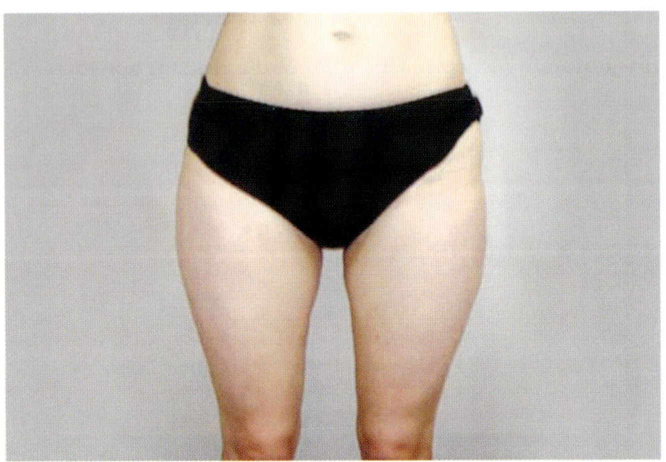

Fig. 9.5: Extremely slender patient. Nonindication for fat transfer.

Typical dressing includes compression garment [apart from breast, where a light support bra (impact level III) or brasserie is advised]. Absorbable pads were used for postoperative leakage. Soft silicone drains (corrugated) were positioned at the lower abdomen. Analgesics were used (if needed). All patients were discharged 1–2 hours average after surgery.

Follow-up was on the first and second days postoperatively. Manual lymphatic drainage starting third day postoperatively, followed by LPG (Endermologie or similar) or VelaSmooth program postliposuction, for 6–8 weeks on areas treated. Breasts need no compression for first 3–4 weeks (i.e. sleeping in supine position). Swelling normally lasts about 3 weeks. Two pillow elevation of the thorax for first 2–3 weeks is advised to reduce swelling as well as a light bra for few weeks.

Postoperative photographs were taken at 3, 6, and 12 months postoperatively (Figs. 9.10A to C).

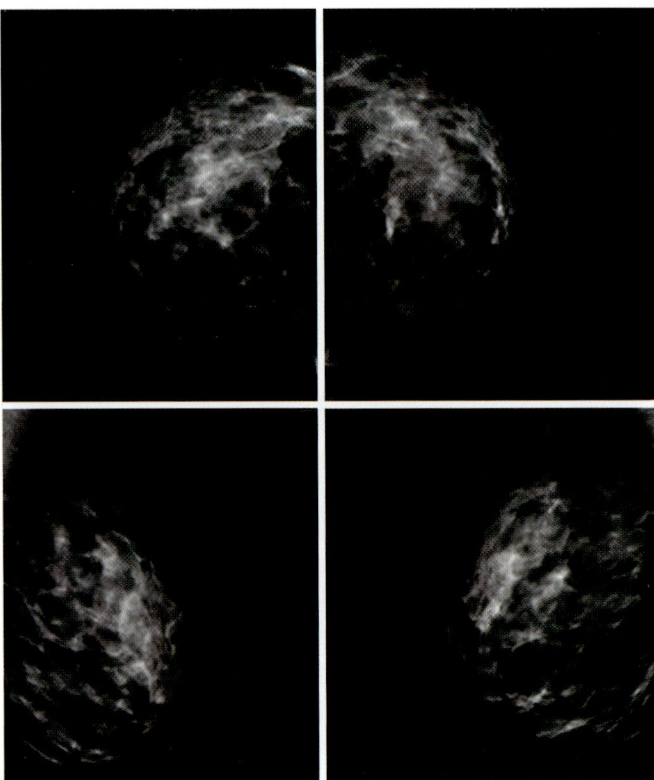

Fig. 9.6: Mammography.

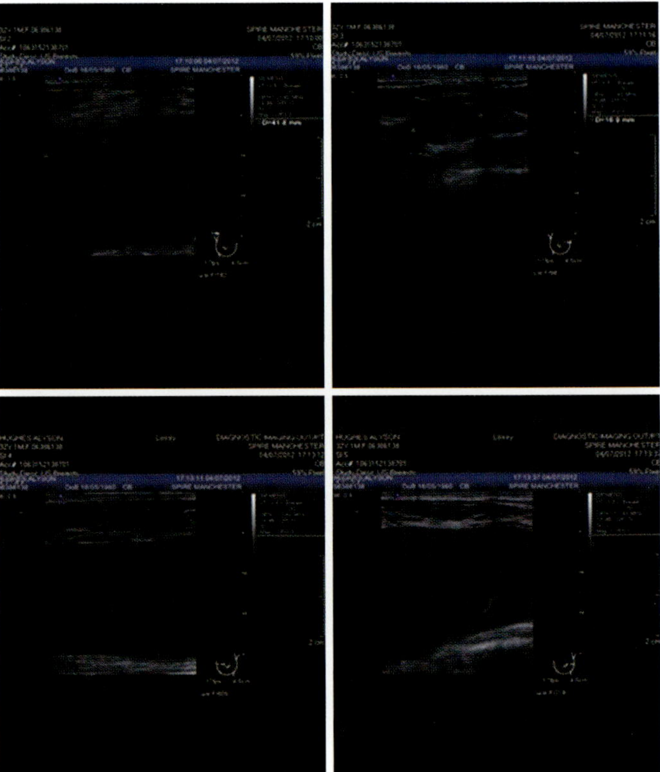

Fig. 9.7: Ultrasound of breast.

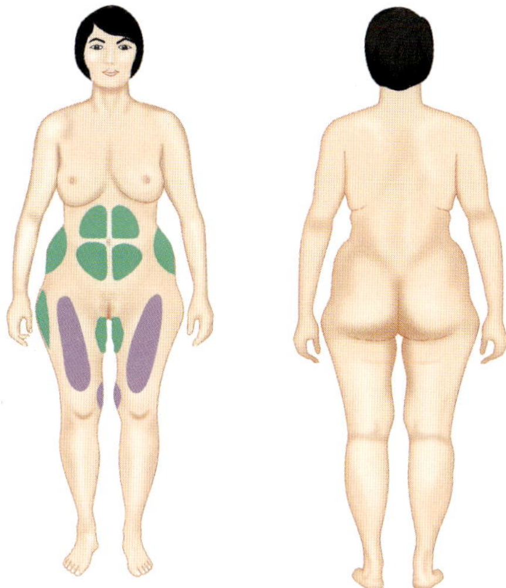

Fig. 9.8: Sites for fat harvesting.

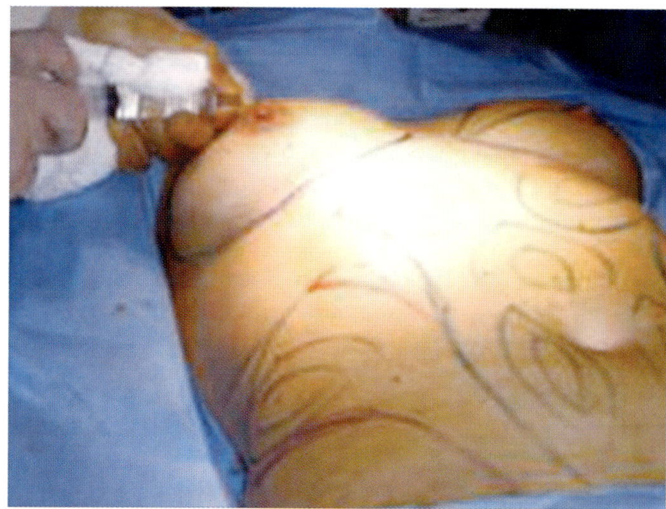

Fig. 9.9: Local anesthesia in periareolar incision.

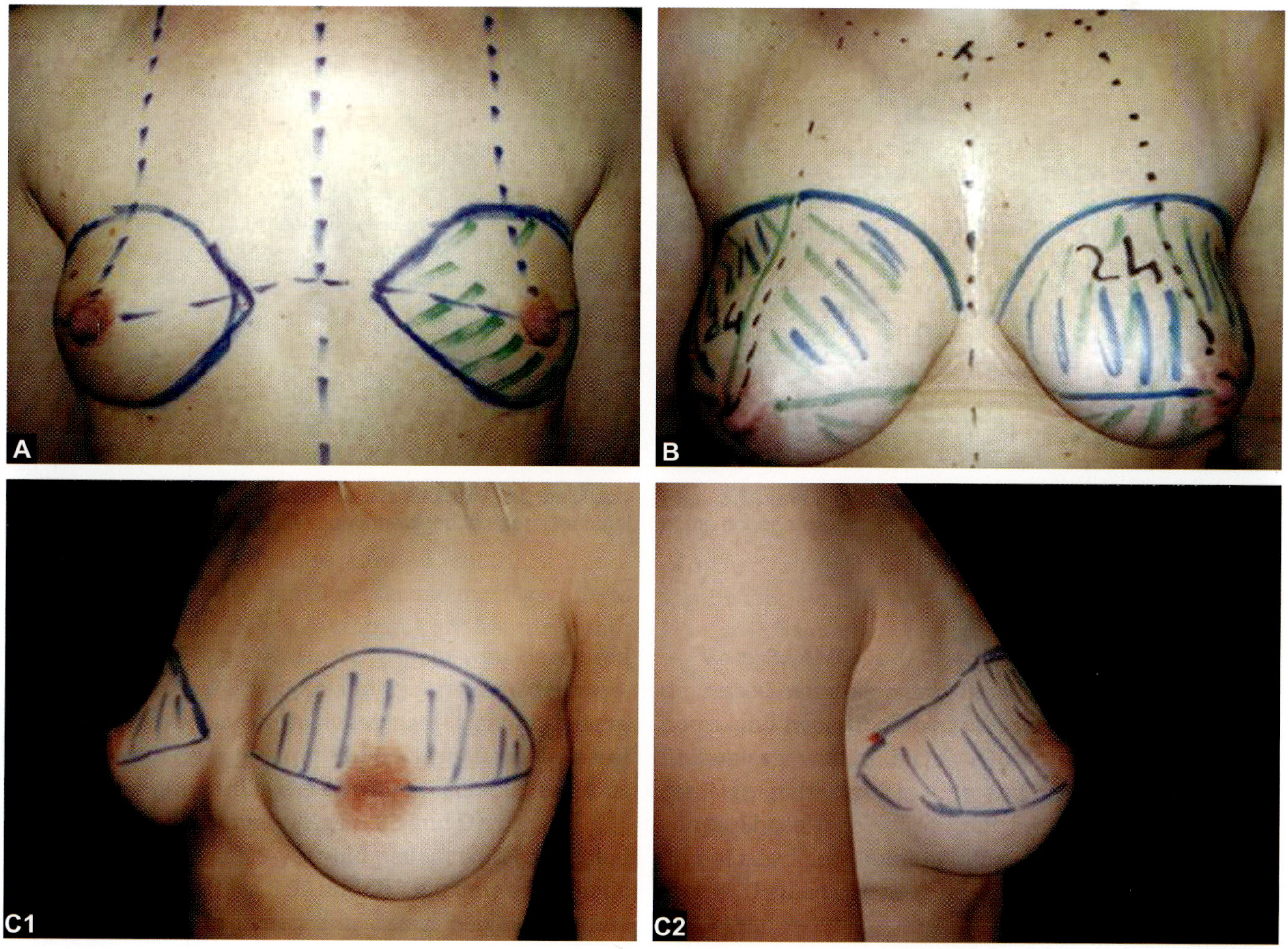

Figs. 9.10A to C: Markings are different depending on breast size and area to be filled. Breast is normally divided in four quadrants. (A) Augmentation in small breast. (B) Augmentation and breast ptosis correction. (C) Postremoval of breast implants: upper quadrants deficiency.

Markings were done in the standing position with the arms down. Preoperative markings and drawings are similar to the standard breast augmentation care:

1. Tridimensional point is marked bilaterally
2. Nipple alveolar complex distance is marked bilaterally with distance from clavicle and clavicular notch:
   a. Inframammary crease is marked bilaterally
   b. Straight line is drawn from clavicular notch to umbilicus
   c. The four breast quadrants are marked
   d. Nipple dimension and areola dimensions are marked
   e. Asymmetries of position of nipple, of the areola, and breast volume are determined
   f. Consistency of breast tissue is noted
   g. Areas of volume deficiencies are marked
   h. The outer margins of the volume deficient areas are marked, similar to the standard breast augmentation, where the limits of pockets undermining before implants placement are marked.

Markings are different depending on breast size and area to be filled. Breast is normally divided in four quadrants:

1. Augmentation in small breast
2. Augmentation and breast ptosis correction
3. Postremoval of breast implants: upper quadrants deficiency
4. Postremoval of breast implants: upper quadrants deficiency; upper lateral lack of fullness.

INCISIONS FOR INFILTRATION

The incisions for infiltration are marked in each breast (Fig. 9.11):

1. Periareolar
2. Axillary
3. Inframammary areas: Two of these incisions (3 mm large for allowing blunt cannula for infiltration, and 17-gauge needle for fat placement) are always utilized:
4. Midclavicular
5. Axillary
6. The medial incision is utilized when central sternal deficiencies need to be filled with fat, or to decrease the distance between the breasts.
7. The lateral incision is utilized when a major filling is necessary in the lateral quadrants.
8. The periareolar incision (to leave an inconspicuous scar) is utilized when the upper quadrant needs to be filled.
9. All incisions will leave inconspicuous scars.

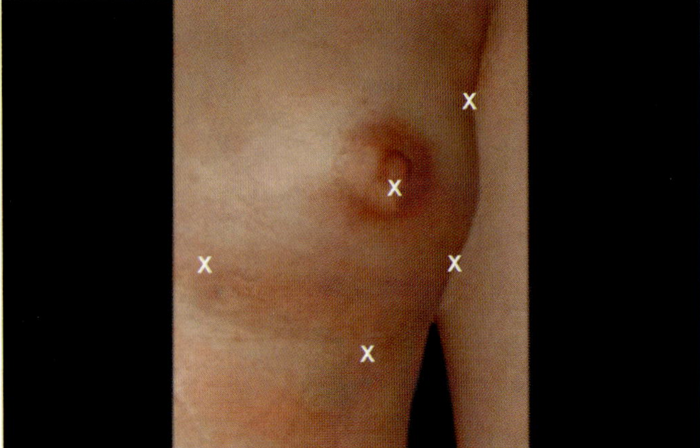

Fig. 9.11: Incisions sites.

LEVELS OF INFILTRATION

The breasts are shaped by layering the fat into different levels until the desired contour is achieved (Figs. 9.12A and B). Although a breast implant augments by expanding the retromammary or retropectoral space, the structural fat grafting technique allows selective augmentation and contouring from the chest wall to the skin. Shaping off the breast is achieved by placing aliquots (microdroplets) subcutaneously into the superficial breast tissue. Placement of fat into the parenchyma of the breast should be limited, but is necessary at times to increase projection.

There is no infiltration of fat into the pectoralis major space for the following reasons:

1. Increase the possibilities of complications, such as bleeding, hematoma, and hemo/pneumothorax.
2. Volumes located close to the chest wall provide a diffuse increase in the chest size without a specific shaping of the breasts.

METHOD OF INFILTRATION (FIGS. 9.13 AND 9.14)

The key to success in fat grafting is to preserve as much fat tissue as possible. So, minimizing trauma during fat harvesting, filtering and placing the living tissue in a way that optimizes the potential for neovascularization. When fat is placed into the recipient site in large volumes, some clusters of adipose cells may be too far from a blood supply. This can lead to fat necrosis, causing not only lumps and calcifications, but also the formation of liponecrotic cysts.

Ten-milliliter syringes and 17/18 gauge cannulas are used to place fat in small aliquots, in different layers, and

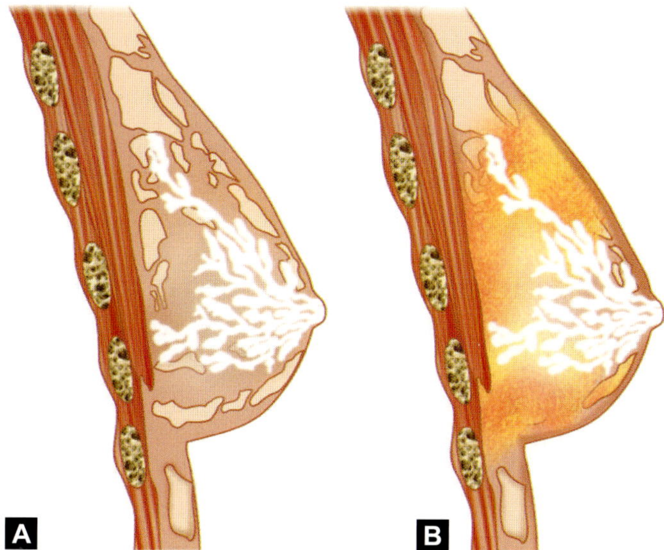

Figs. 9.12A and B: Fat graft placements. (A) Prefat grafting. (B) Postfat grafting.

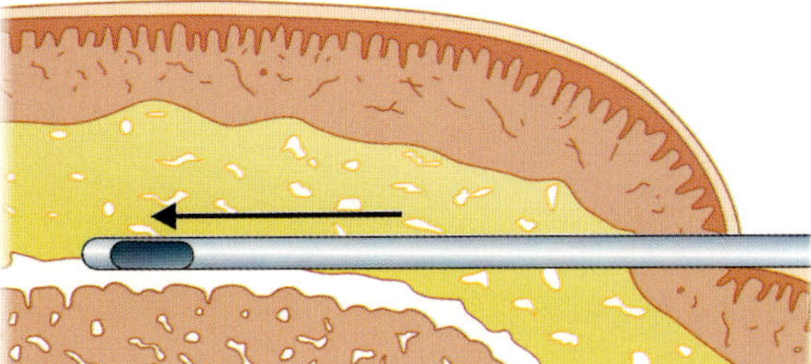

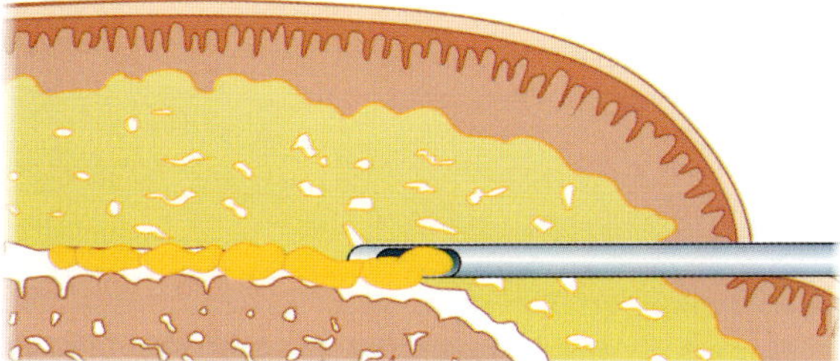

Fig. 9.13: Fat is deposited with a back forward movement in small little pearls.

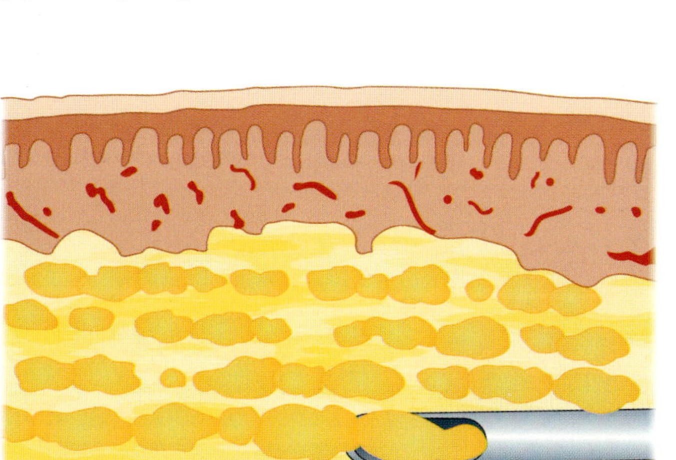

Fig. 9.14: Fat infiltration. Multiple layers fat deposit.

in a fan pattern. Pressure at infiltration is diminished by using special SoftJet syringes by Citori, and a CellBrush infiltration system, which decreases the pressure by 80% at site of infiltration.

Blunt 17/18 gauge infiltration cannulas vary from 9 to 15 cm in length. The fat is infiltrated only while the cannula is being withdrawn, not during the advancement of the cannula. Approximately 0.1–0.2 mL is placed with each withdrawal of the cannula. This approach maximizes the surface areas of contact between the surrounding tissue to blood supply, plus maximizing the potential for survival and minimizing the possibility of fat necrosis.

VOLUME RANGES

The authors utilized a range of as little as 90 mL (Figs. 9.15A to F) per breast to 500 mL per breast (total of 180–1,000 mL). The amount placed depends on the amount taken and successfully harvested:

1. You can never have enough fat.
2. Take as much as you can, and never throw it out.
3. You will regret not having taken enough fat or that there was not more available to be taken.
4. Never regret to have placed too much.
5. You will recognize good-quality fat—no connective tissue strands. This should be removed by the PureGraft filtration.

DONOR AREAS FOR FAT HARVESTING

Patients who are candidates for breast enlargement with AFT undergo a double procedure:

1. Fat extraction from multiple areas with body sculpting (Fig. 9.16).
2. Breast augmentation with harvested fat.

Fat extraction/fat harvesting/body sculpturing.

Full-body naked photographs (when possible) are taken in frontal, back, oblique, and lateral views, bilaterally.

Body is studied in order to plan the area to treat in order to remove fat, but contouring at the same time.

Lines of concavity and convexity are drawn (see preoperative plan) as in classic liposculpting in order to figure

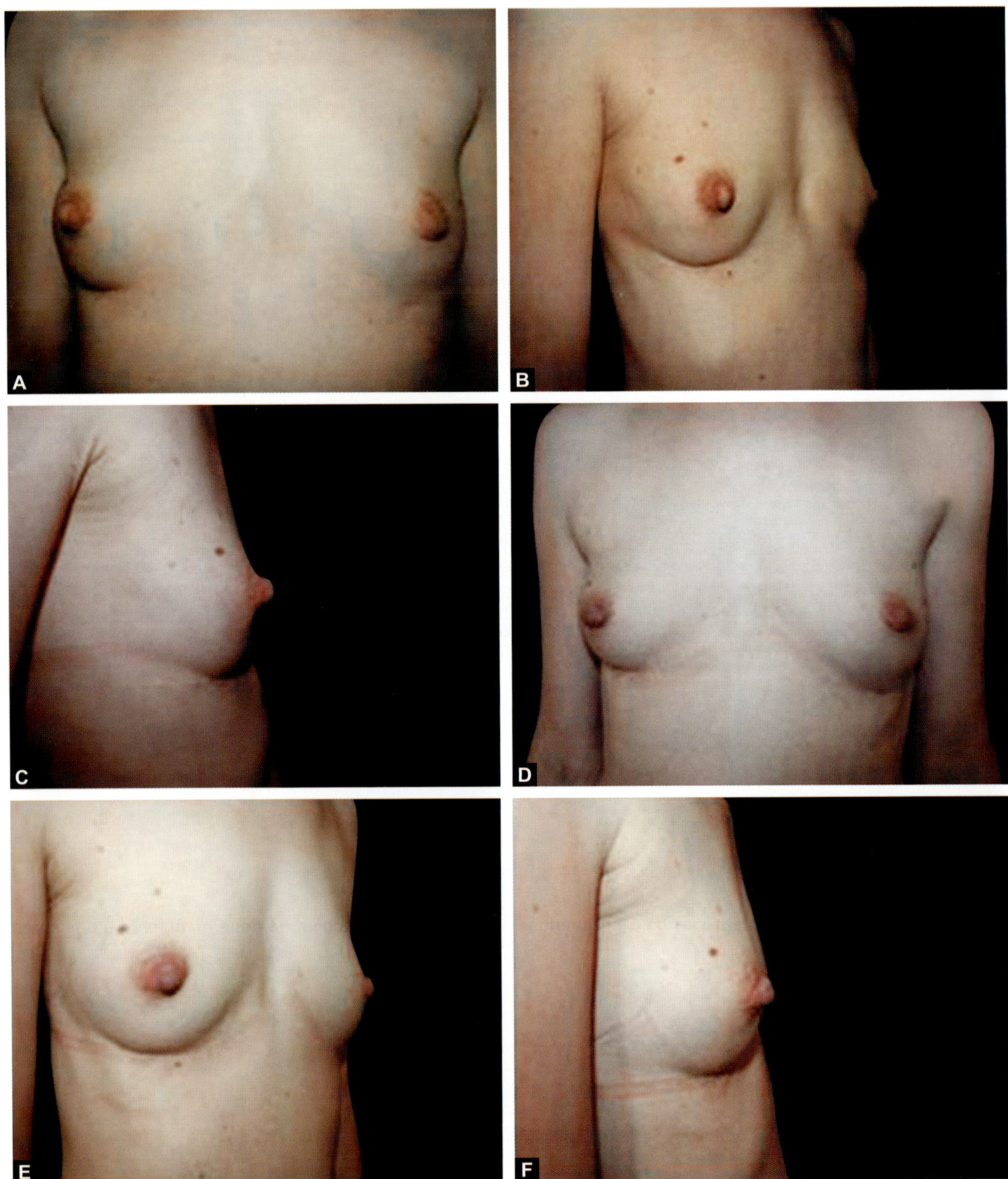

Figs. 9.15A to F: (A to C): Preoperative 41-year-old female. Extremely slimy woman with associated mild form of pectus excavatum. (D to F) Postoperative following PIP implant removal and 90 mL fat transfer to each side.

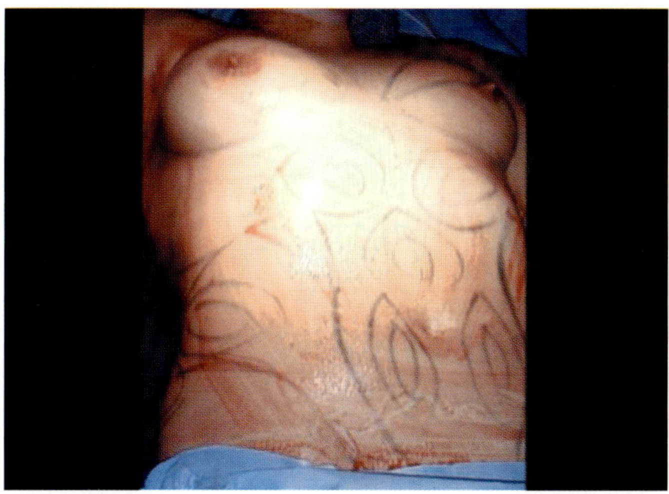

Fig. 9.16: Marking donor areas for fat harvesting: upper/lower abdomen and upper/lower flanks.

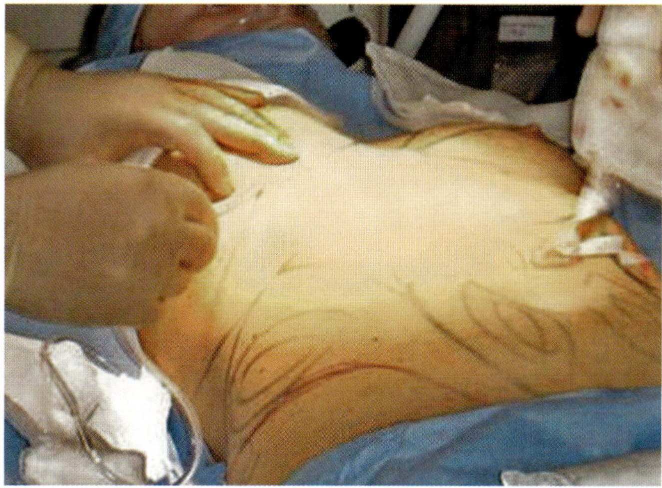

Fig. 9.17: All surgery is performed under tumescent anesthesia and conscious EV sedation.

the new ideal body shape. Areas of volume reduction are marked, lines of muscle sculpting and definition is drawn, using permanent marker pens of different colors.

All the patients in the authors' series were performed under local tumescent anesthesia and IV sedation (Fig. 9.17). Surgeons must calculate the maximum amount of lidocaine concentration per body weight permissible. Both authors remain within the safety level of 35–40 mg/kg bodyweight. In most cases, harvesting is performed on the flanks, abdomen, and outer thighs, as the adipose deposits are most consistent. It obviously depends on the amount available and also the amount required to augment the breasts. The aim of this procedure is to sculpt the torso as well as remove as much material as possible for harvesting.

TECHNIQUE

Small puncture holes are created with an 18-gauge needle or a 1-mm punch after injecting a tiny bleb of local anesthesia. A small amount of local anesthesia is infiltrated into subcutaneous and subglandular space.

Local anesthesia of 40–100 mL is sufficient to anesthetize this area. Once the breasts are infiltrated the harvesting sites can be prepared. This gives the local anesthesia time to take effect in the breasts. The surgeon will return to this area (usually in 2.5 hours) once harvesting is complete. Tumescence is then infiltrated in all the harvest sites following typical Vaser protocol (ultrawet solution).

After waiting 15–20 minutes for anesthesia to set in, the Vaser setting is placed at 50% of Vaser power, to decrease the emulsifying intensity of the probe thus allowing for greater survival of adipocytes (Fig. 9.18). When using the Vaser probe at 50% of full power, emulsification takes longer especially in more fibrotic areas (Fig. 9.19). Once the end point has been reached with the Vaser in the harvest sites, aspiration is commenced. The VentX aspiration system is used. Suction intensity is decreased to 30% in order to minimize damage to the emulsified fat and the live fat cells.

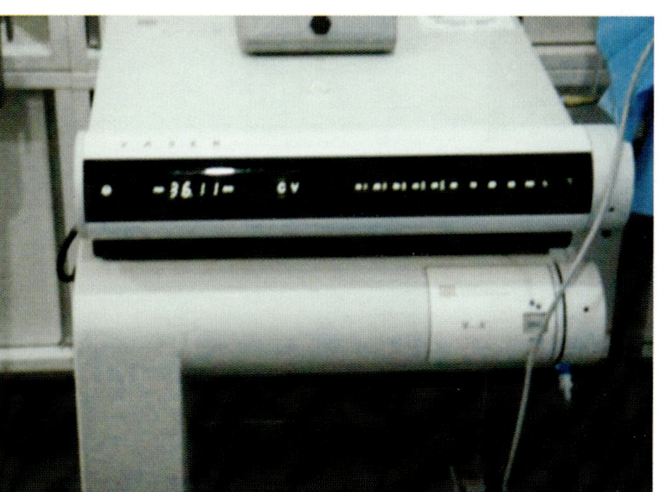

Fig. 9.18: Vaser system setup at 50% of power to decrease fat lobule destruction.

The 3-mm diameter VentX cannula (Mercedes type) is used to minimize trauma to the adipocytes (Fig. 9.20). The extracted emulsion is collected in a sterile closed system (Aquavage or Origins), with a part for fluid extraction. Aquavage is a disposable plastic canister, with a steel

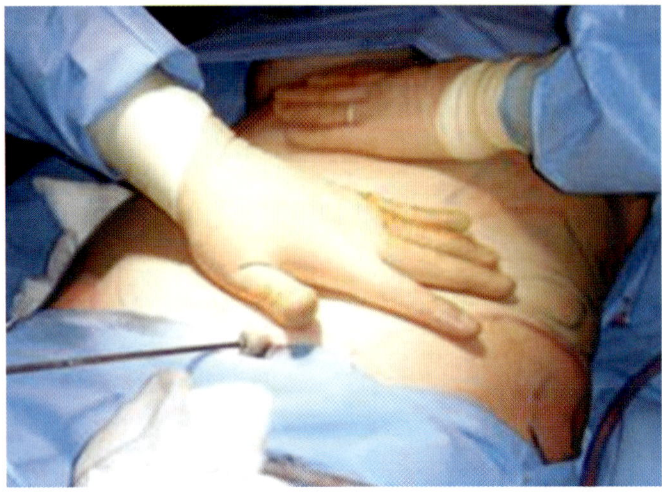
Fig. 9.19: Vaser in action for fat emulsification in lower abdomen. Two rings probe.

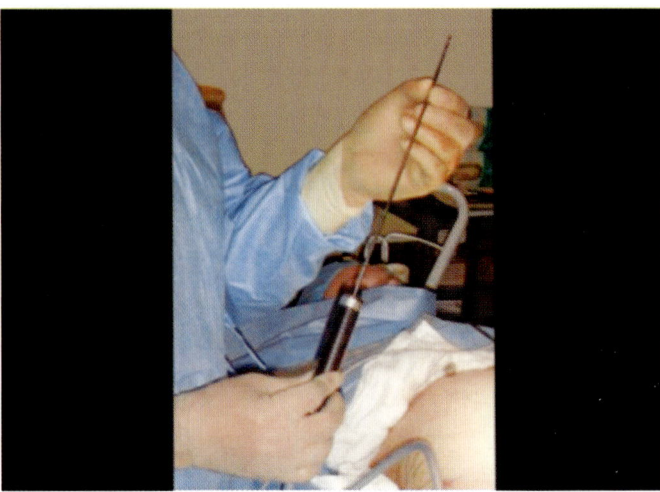
Fig. 9.20: 3-mm diameter VentX cannula.

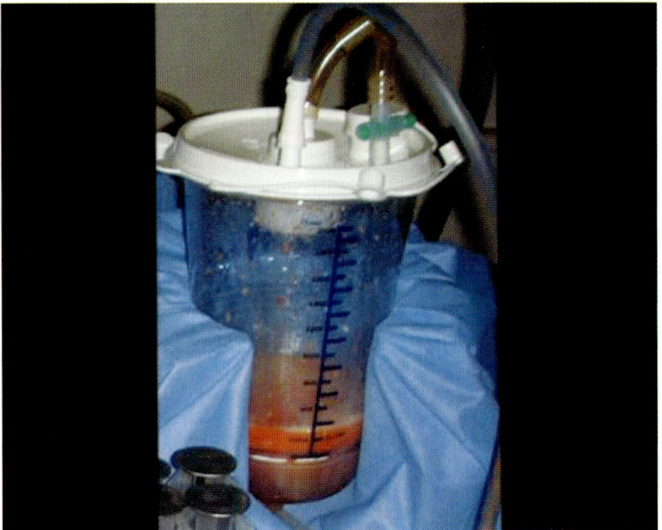
Fig. 9.21: Aquavage canister disposable (plastic).

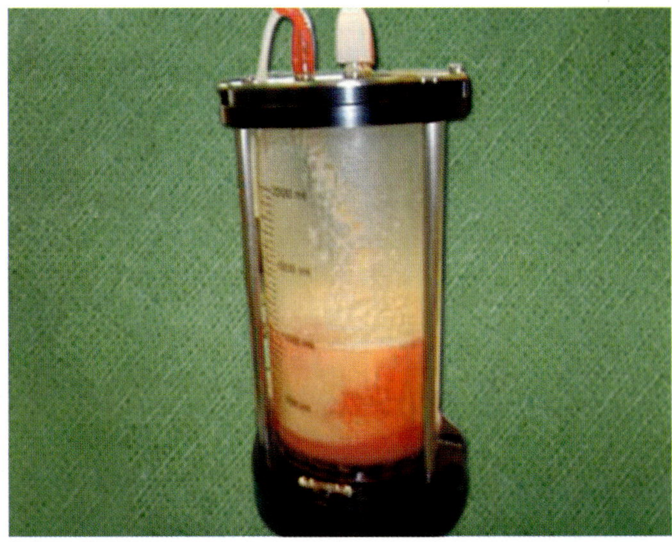
Fig. 9.22: Origins canister autoclavable (glass).

support (Fig. 9.21). It contains up to 1,200 mL. Origins is a glass canister that can be sterilized and contains up to 2,000 mL (Figs. 9.22 and 9.23).

Whichever closed system is used is not relevant, as the technique does not change. Once the canister contains at least 500-mL, Toomey syringes are used to aspirate the infranatant fluid that is discarded (Figs. 9.24 to 9.26). Once fatty material is aspirated in the Toomey syringes, this material is then retained and injected into the PureGraft bag.

The fat is immediately transferred via a connector into the PureGraft 250 bag (Fig. 9.27).

PureGraft 850 is also available for larger volume procedures. The material is then washed twice with 150 mL of Hartmann solution (Fig. 9.28). The aspirate is allowed to drain via gravity until no further drainage occurs. The PureGraft bag is gently "massaged" with a spatula several times. The material is then ready to be removed (Fig. 9.29), by using the 60-mL Toomey syringes (Fig. 9.30). The syringes have a connector the same size as the PureGraft bag, to minimize trauma to live adipocytes. The filled syringes are then transferred to a sterile syringe rack (Fig. 9.31). It is important to note the total amount of material harvested as it allows the surgeon to estimate the volume that can be infiltrated per breast.

BREAST FAT AUGMENTATION

To prepare for the infiltration the Toomey syringes are attached to a metal connector that has a male Luer lock

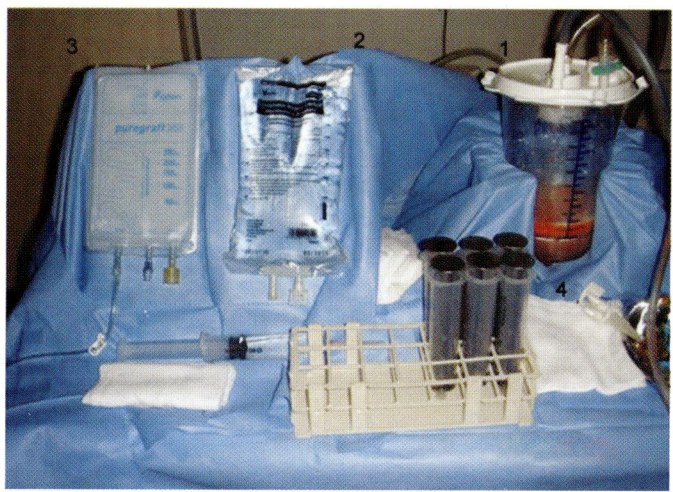

Fig. 9.23: Console: (1) Aquavage canister; (2) physiologic solution; (3) pure graft bag; and (4) Toomey syringes.

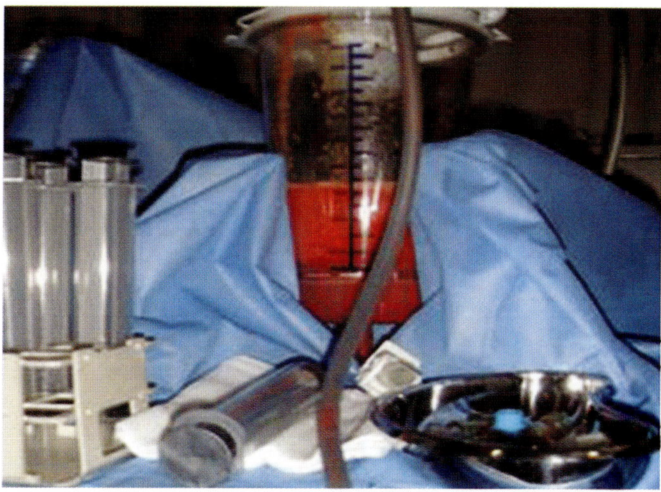

Fig. 9.24: The infranatant aspirated in the Aquavage canister.

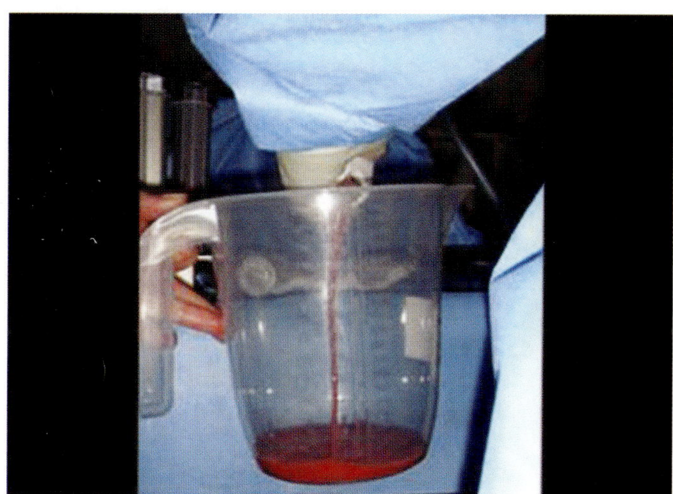

Fig. 9.25: Eliminating bloodstream from canister.

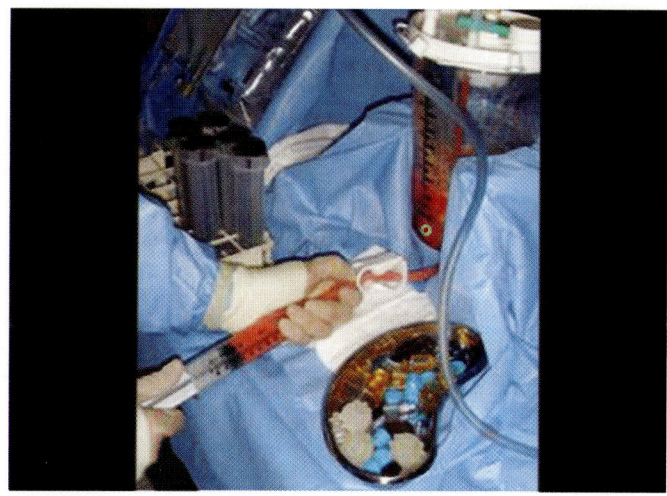

Fig. 9.26: Fat aspirated with Toomey syringe.

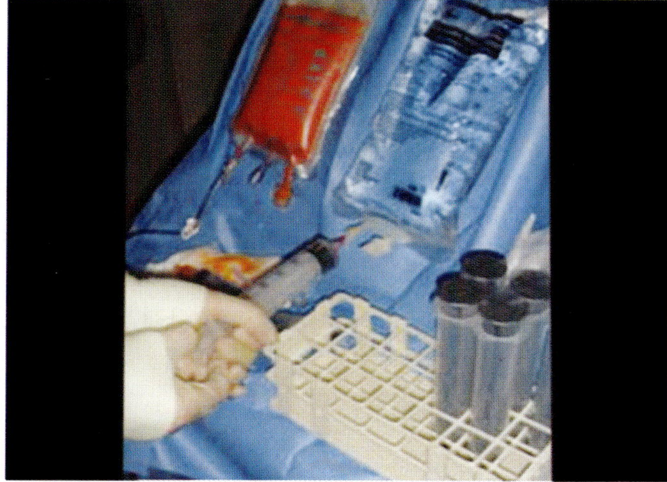

Fig. 9.27: Saline solution aspirated for fat washing.

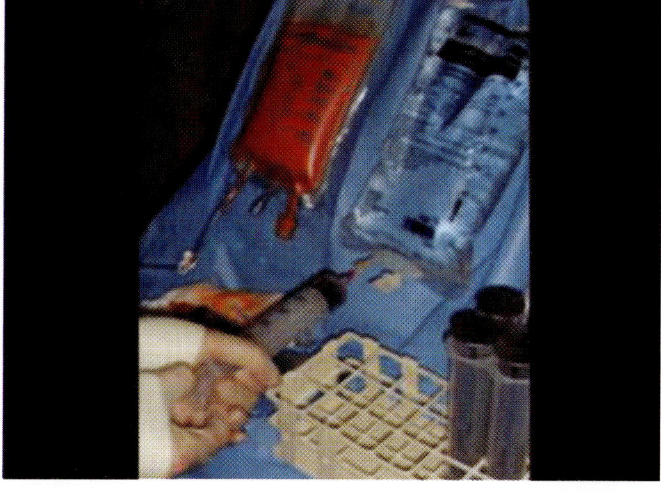

Fig. 9.28: 200 mL of saline solution for each bag of pure graft.

at one end. A Cytori SoftJet 10-mL syringe is loaded into the Cytori CellBrush injector (Fig. 9.32). This allows for accurate microdroplet deposits. The Toomey syringe is connected via the Luer lock adaptor and material is transferred to the 10-mL syringe. A 17-gauge Byron cannula is used for infiltration (Fig. 9.33). The SoftJet syringes minimize the pressure on the plunger and thus minimize damage to the adipocyte.

The patient is positioned with thorax elevated by 45° in order to create the natural gravitational forces on the breasts. At this stage, if there are two surgeons working, the fat transfer is started bilaterally. The 17-gauge cannula can be used to undermine the overlying tissue.

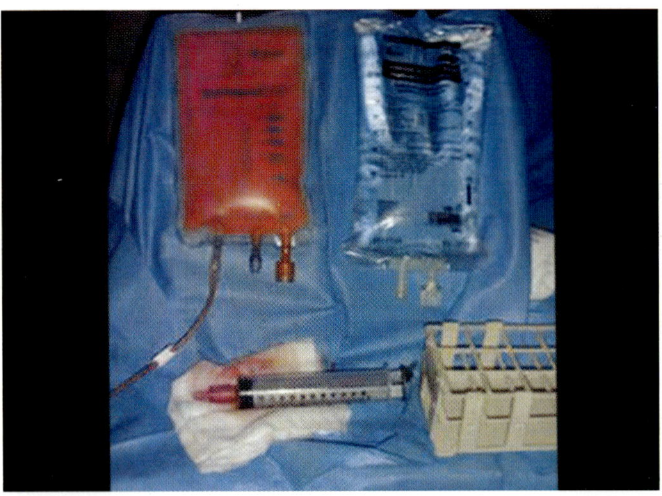

Fig. 9.29: 300 mL pure graft ready for transferring in Toomey syringe.

Small aliquots of fat are deposited in stages in a radial- and fan-shaped pattern. Accurate counts are vital to ensure symmetrical infiltration of volume. Preoperative photographs and three-dimensional imaging of the breasts are always kept in the operating room to allow for comparison. Preoperative asymmetry of volume, position, inframammary crease can be corrected. Fat is placed subcutaneously and subglandularly. Subcutaneous placement gives consistency of the tissue and also helps with skin rejuvenation. Subglandular placement gives projection. The initial preoperative markings are adhered to. The reuse of artistry and proportion of the surgeon is essential to increase volume of breast respecting shape and natural looking and appearance of the breasts (Fig. 9.34). In the authors' series, all the fat harvested has been infiltrated to enhance breast volume.

The incisions are sutured with 6-0 nylon. Dr Wolf uses only puncture holes that do not require suturing and are only covered with Steri-Strips. A light support bra is applied at the end of the surgery, while for the rest of the body a compression garment is utilized. At the end of the surgery, the breasts will appear swollen and edematous. The patient is to be reminded that the size will diminish (Fig. 9.35).

All surgical data are recorded:

1. Infiltration of tumescence
2. Total minutes of Vaser
3. Total lidocaine given per area
4. Vaser setting
5. Total aspirate
6. Total fat harvested
7. Total infiltrated for side

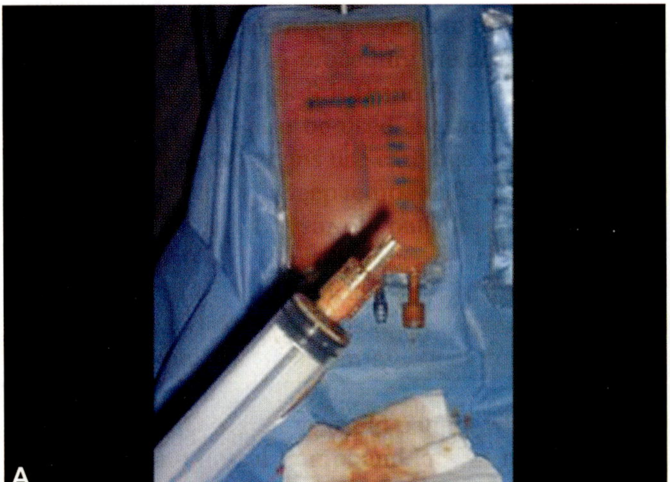

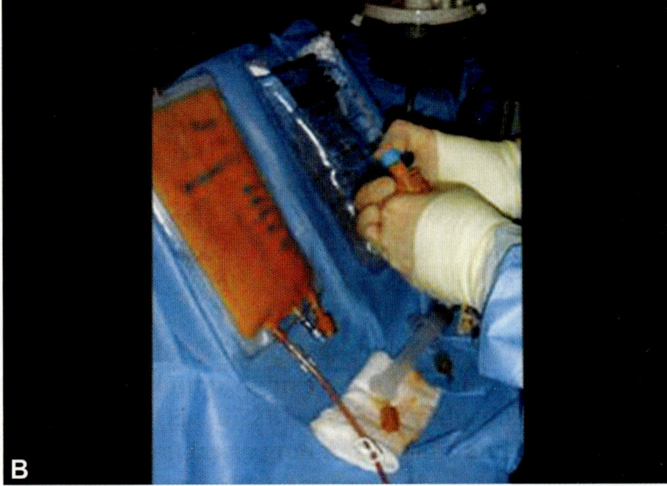

Figs. 9.30A and B: (A) Toomey syringe. (B) Fat transferred from pure graft bag to Toomey syringe.

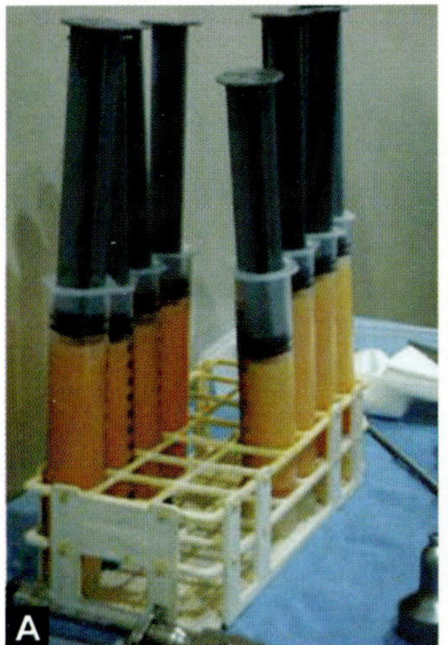

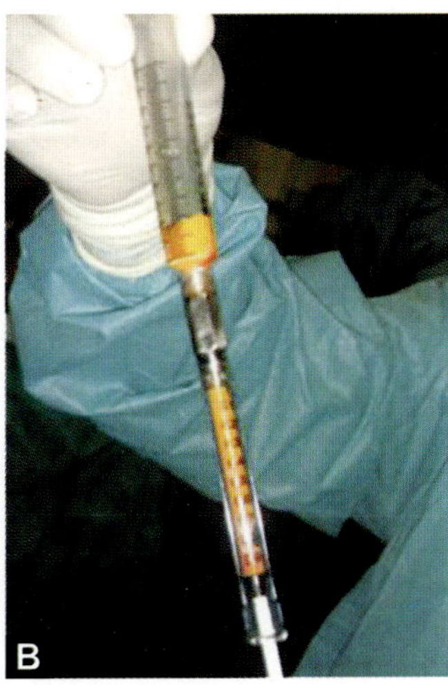

Figs. 9.31A and B: (A) 60-mL syringes ready for transferring. (B) Fat transferred into smaller syringes through connector (from 60 to 10 mL or from 10 to 2 mL).

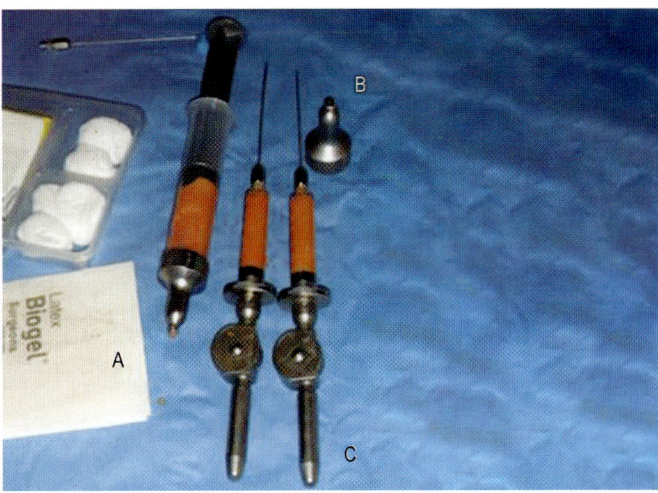

Fig. 9.32: (A) Toomey syringe; (B) connector; (C) Cytori 10-mL syringes with 17-gauge needle for implant.

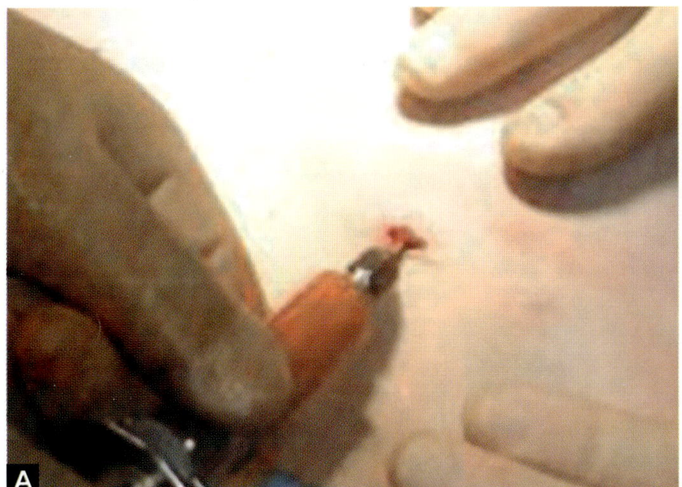

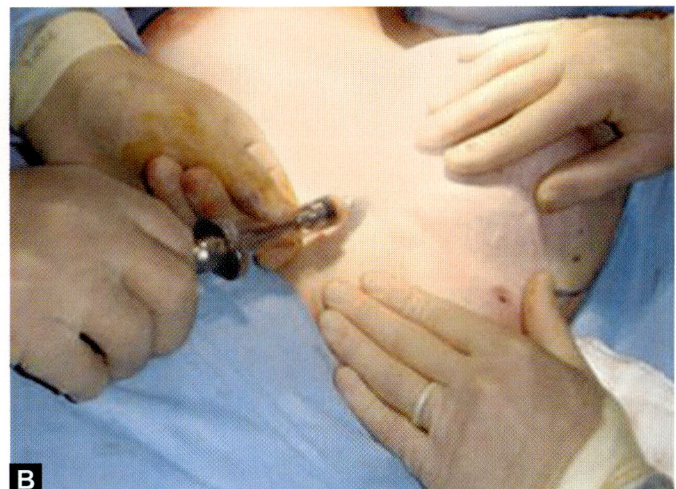

Figs. 9.33A and B: (A) Infiltration trough upper lateral chest incision. (B) Infiltration trough upper medial chest incision.

Placement of fat begins into the lower pole through the middle inframammary incision.

With the lateral inframammary incision, further fat is added in the lower lateral pole of breasts.

Ideally, some amounts of fat (as 10–20 mL) are placed in the four quadrants. Through the three incisions, fat is placed on the entire lower and upper quadrants. Once the central and lateral quadrants are full, we improved the medial ones. We leave the stern on medial quadrants (the so-called décolleté) to the last amount of fat infiltration. It is possible to reshape the thorax, and even in presence of large deficiency of fat.

LIMITS OF TECHNIQUE

1. *Weight*: The patients are instructed to maintain their body weight. Fat added to breast behaves as fat from where it was harvested. If there is any weight loss, then there will be a loss of volume in the breasts.
2. *Pregnancy/menopause*: Hormonal changes connected to menopause and pregnancy will influence the breast fat appearance and volume. During pregnancy, there is initial growth and increase of the glandular tissue, then followed by atrophy. In menopause, the glandular tissue becomes fibrotic, and diminishes in quantity.

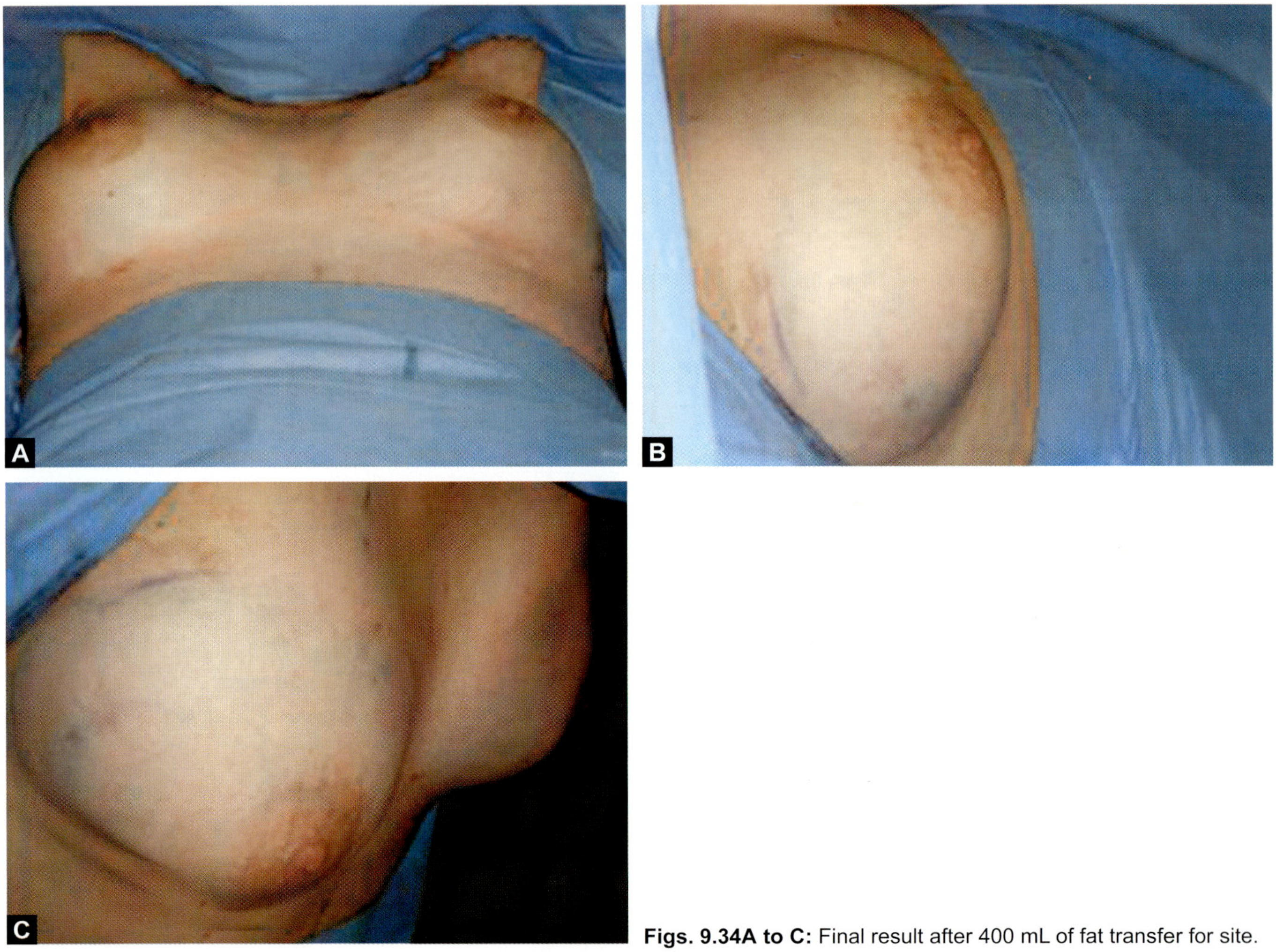

Figs. 9.34A to C: Final result after 400 mL of fat transfer for site.

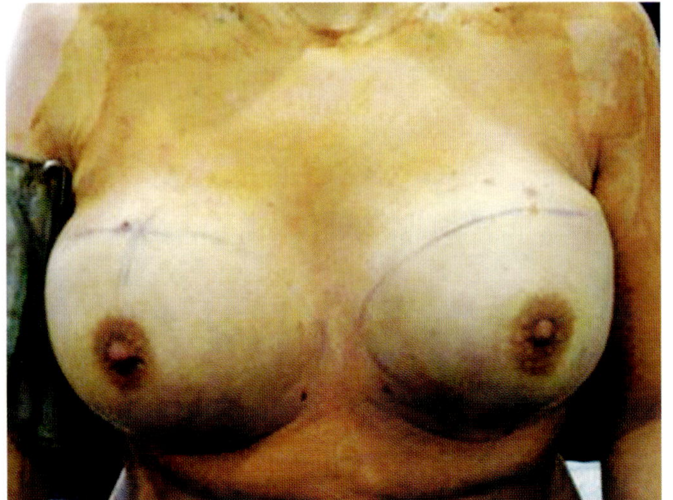

Fig. 9.35: Patient standing at the end of the procedure.

3. *Large volume changes*: The large volume changes obtained with implants are not possible using structural fat grafting. Even with multiple donor sites, the maximum volume the authors obtained was a two cup volume increase (typically cup A to B; or cup B to C).
4. *Type of volume changes*: The effect of volume change with fat is different from the change achieved by placing an alloplastic implant. With implants, a discrete volume is placed into an anatomically limited space. In the technique for fat augmentation, the surgeon infiltrates fatty tissue diffusely along the chest wall, under the skin envelope, and into surrounding areas of the sternum and/or the axilla. Such an integrated and dispersed fullness does not translate into the same visual change in volume as the localized change afforded by

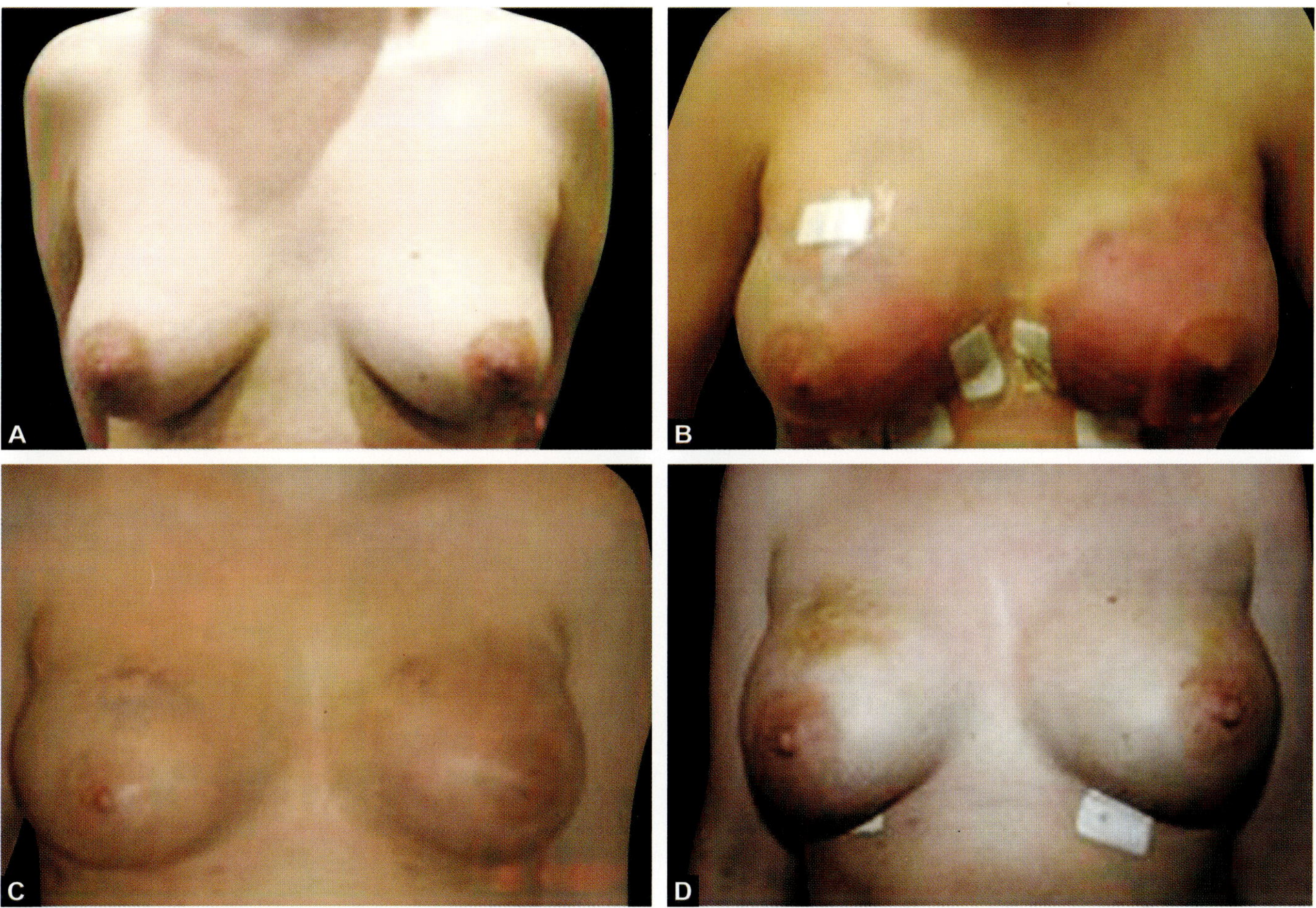

Figs. 9.36A to D: (A) Preoperative, (B) 24 hours postoperative with breast inflammation, more pronounced on the left breast, (C) Postoperative 48 hours, (D) Postoperative 3 weeks.

alloplastic implants. The effect is a moderate, natural looking increase of volume, without the classic feature and "stigmata" of the implants.

5. *Length of procedure*: Two aesthetic surgery operations are performed with this technique. Body lipsosculpting with Vaser and breast augmentation. So, 3.5 hours for completing two combined surgeries is not a larger operation, if compared with a Breast Augmentation + Lipoplasty of multiple areas. It is a larger operation if compared with breast implant augmentation.
6. Costs: Two operations cost more than one. Monsieur de Lapalisse clarified this obvious point centuries ago: Costs are connected with two surgeries, not one. But if costs are abused, also benefits are. But in only one stage.
7. *Retouch*: All patients are warned of the possibility of a secondary minor fat transfer in the future (minimum after 1 year) if not pleased about results, or just requiring more volume added.
8. Only 2 in 120 cases treated required a touch-up procedure in a second stage.

COMPLICATIONS

1. *Edema and bruising*: Normally least 3 weeks.
2. *Inflammation*: One case of redness occurred on the first postoperative day. The patient had followed the standard antibiotic intra- and postoperative protocol (cephalexin † metronidazole). Blood tests (full blood count, white cells, γGT, CRP, blood cultures) revealed no significant change in comparison to preoperative assessment. The clinical picture increased in second day after surgery, and disappeared progressively in days 3–5 postsurgery (Figs. 9.36A to D).
3. *Infection*: The authors had no infections.

4. *Calcifications*: Bircoll reported a 1.4% of incidence of calcifications over >600 breast implantations with injected fat. There is no evidence that fat grafting should cause greater concern than any other breast augmentation procedure (Fig. 9.37). Fat necrosis and calcifications occur in patients with every type of breast surgery. The incidence of calcifications varies (including all types of breast surgeries) and has been reported to be as high as 50% of patients after 2 years (Fig. 9.38).[10] Newer imaging techniques allow for radiologists to distinguish calcifications associated with malignant lesions from benign calcifications.

By using blunt, tiny cannulas, the possibility of damaging nerves, vessels and ducts are minimal. The possible complications associated with fat grafting to breast are similar to all other breast augmentation procedures. The most important benefits, however, are as follows:

1. Local anesthesia + sedation day case procedure
2. Liposculpting + breast augmentation in one procedure
3. Natural look and texture of the breast
4. No risk of capsule formation and contracture
5. Autologous

See clinical cases (Figs. 9.39 to 9.42).

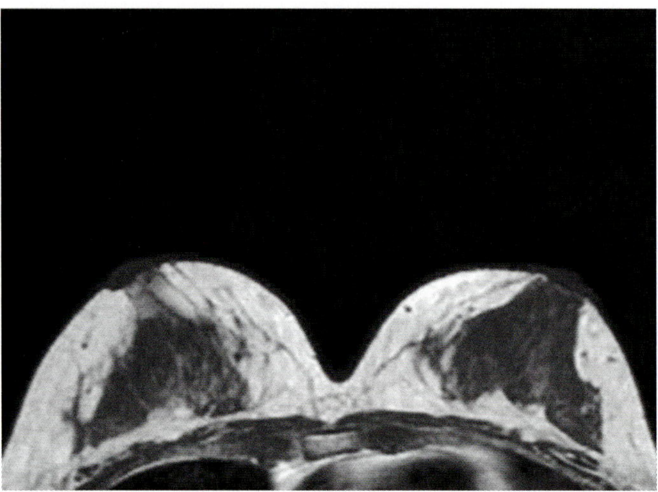

Fig. 9.37: MRI at 12 months revealed that transplanted adipose tissue had largely survived and formed thick layers around and under the mammary gland.

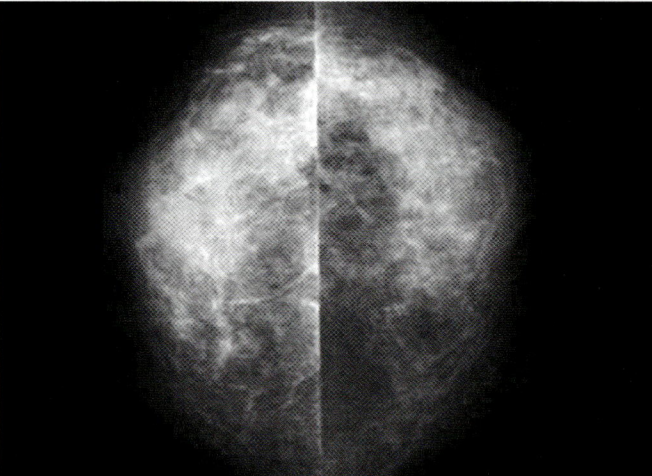

Fig. 9.38: Mammograms showed no calcification or other abnormal signs in either breast at 12 months.

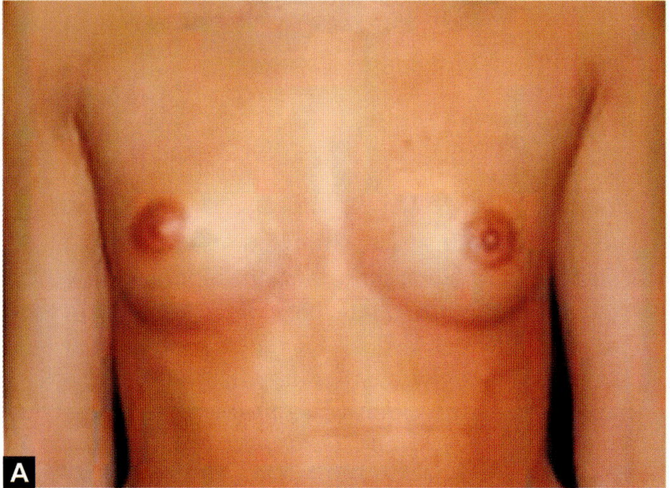

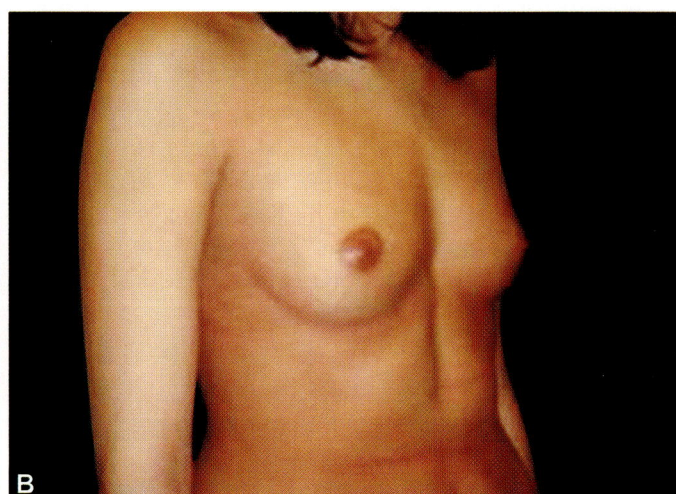

Figs. 9.39A and B

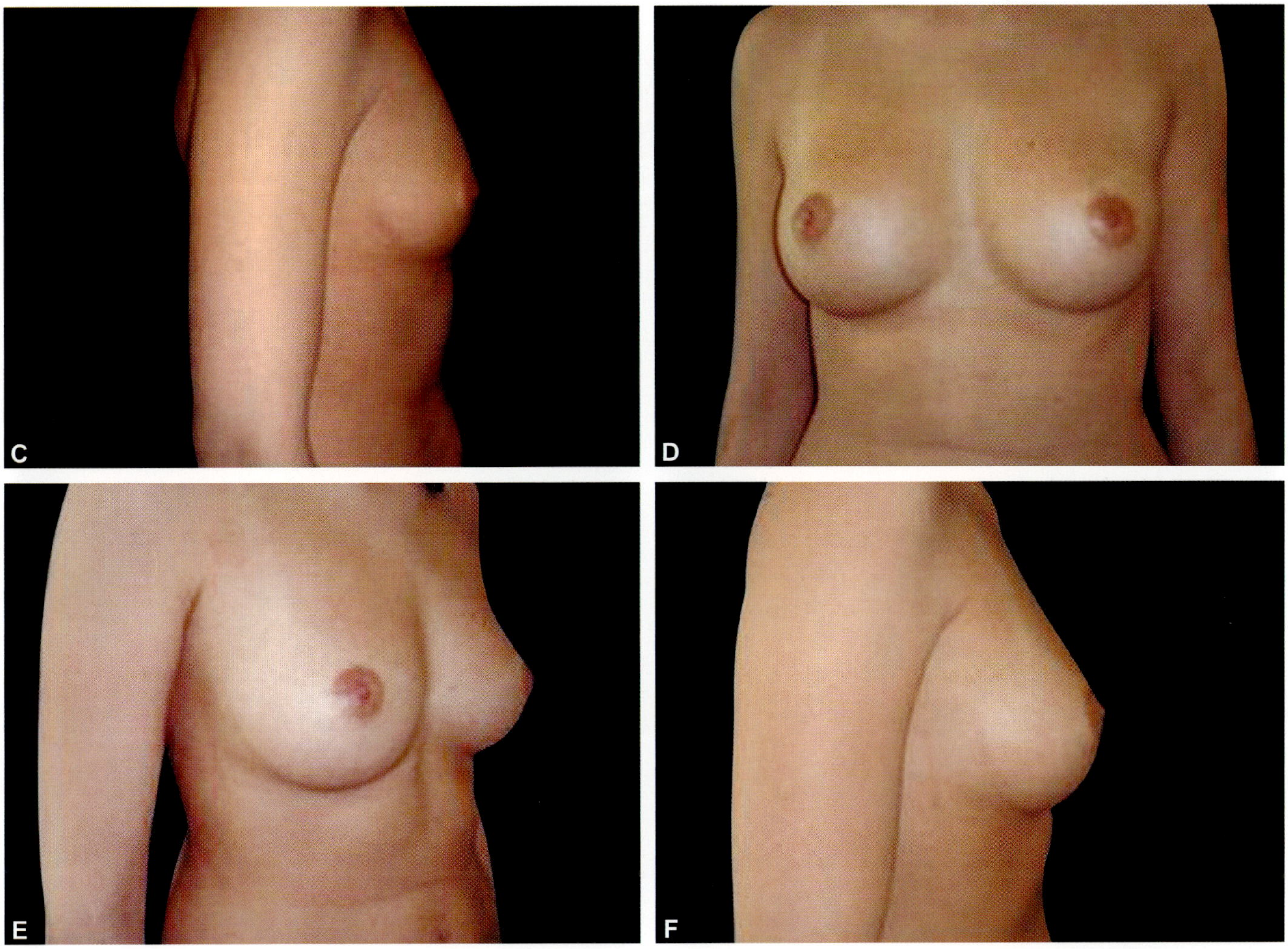

Figs. 9.39A to F: (A to C) Preoperative 28-year-old female. (D to F) Postoperative after 360 mL fat transfer to each side.

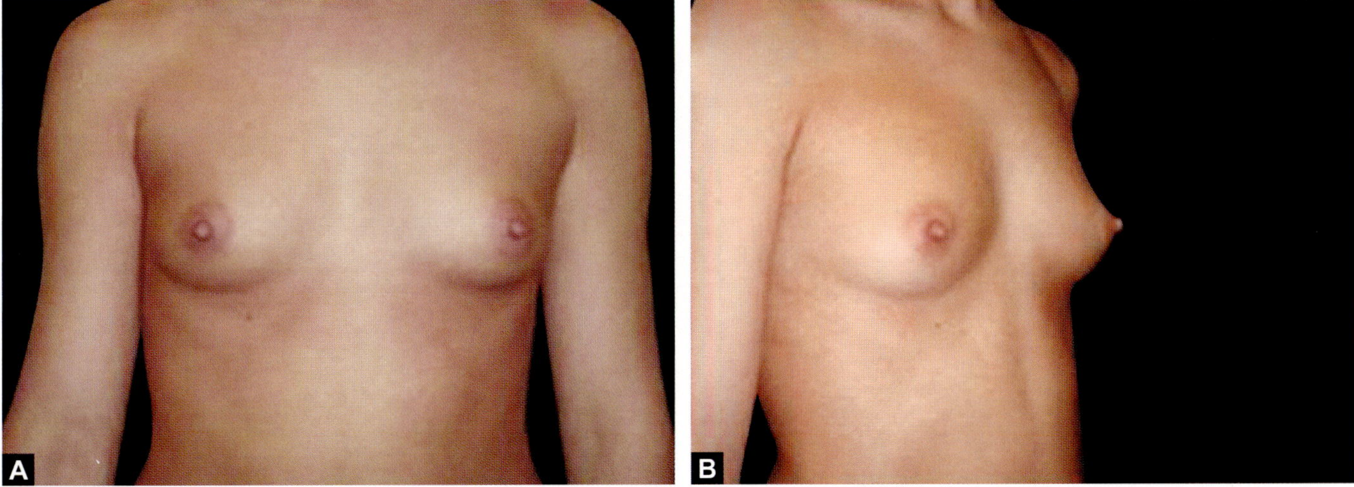

Figs. 9.40A and B

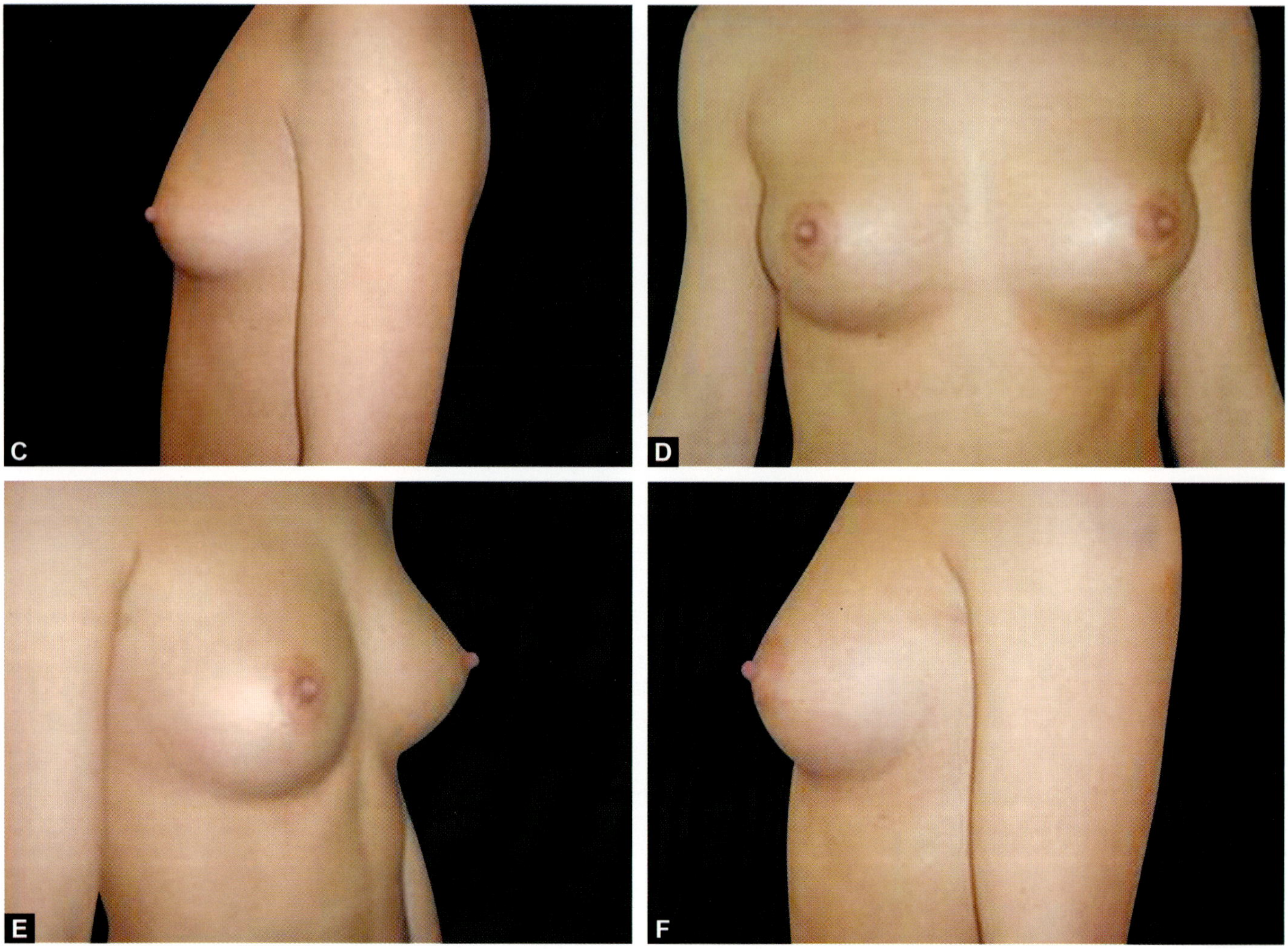

Figs. 9.40A to F: (A to C) Preoperative 24-year-old female. (D to F): Postoperative following 355 mL fat transfer to each side.

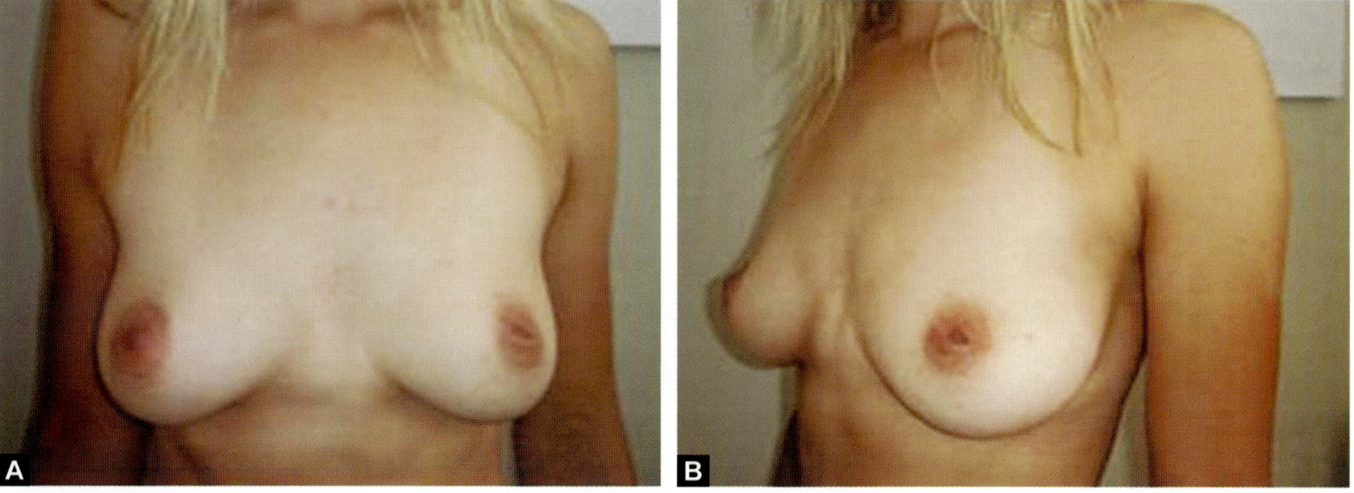

Figs. 9.41A and B

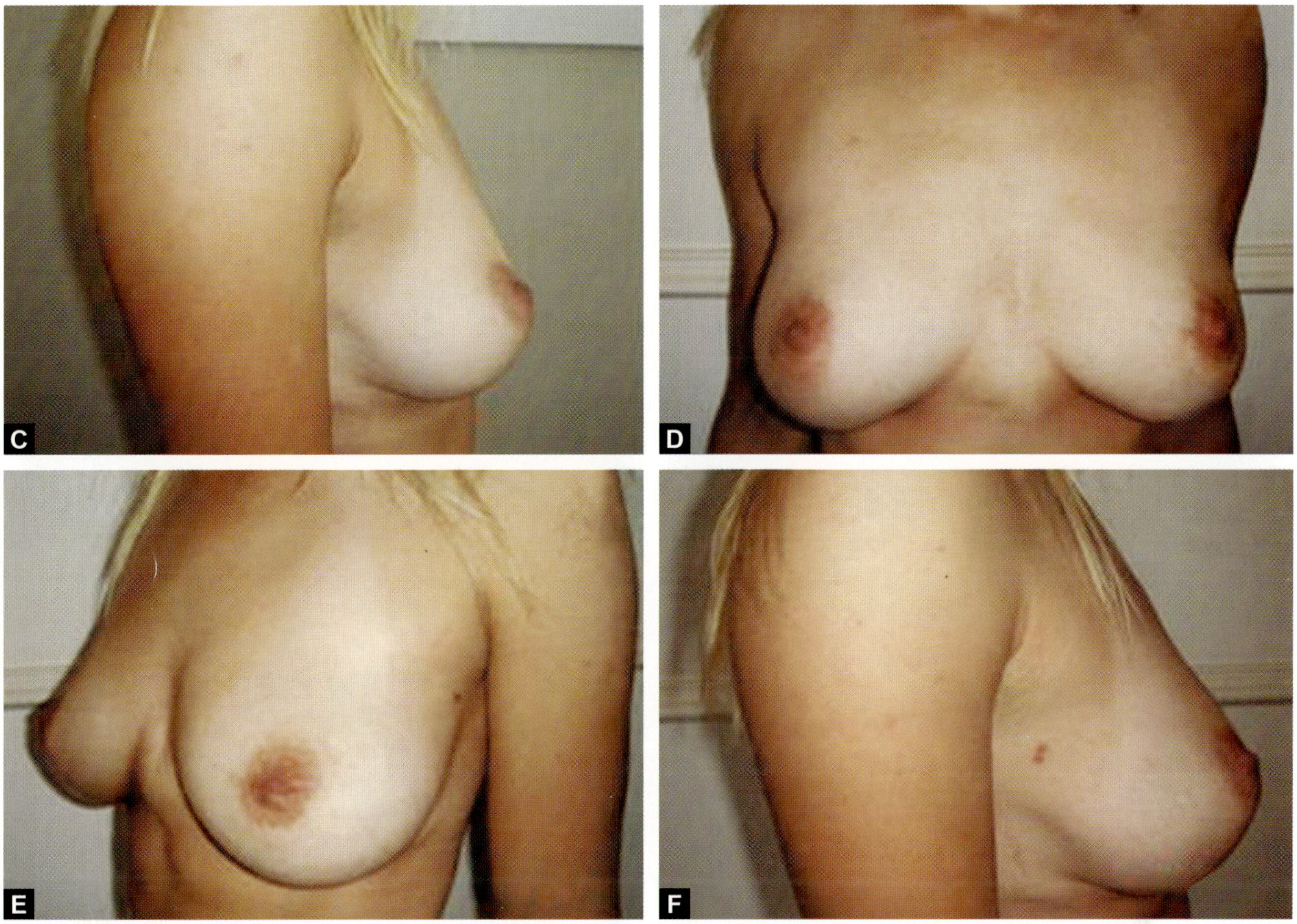

Figs. 9.41A to F: (A to C) Preoperative 27-year-old female who had two breast augmentation with implants and wanted them removed. There was mild breast ptosis. (D to F) Ptosis corrected with 300 mL fat transfer to each side.

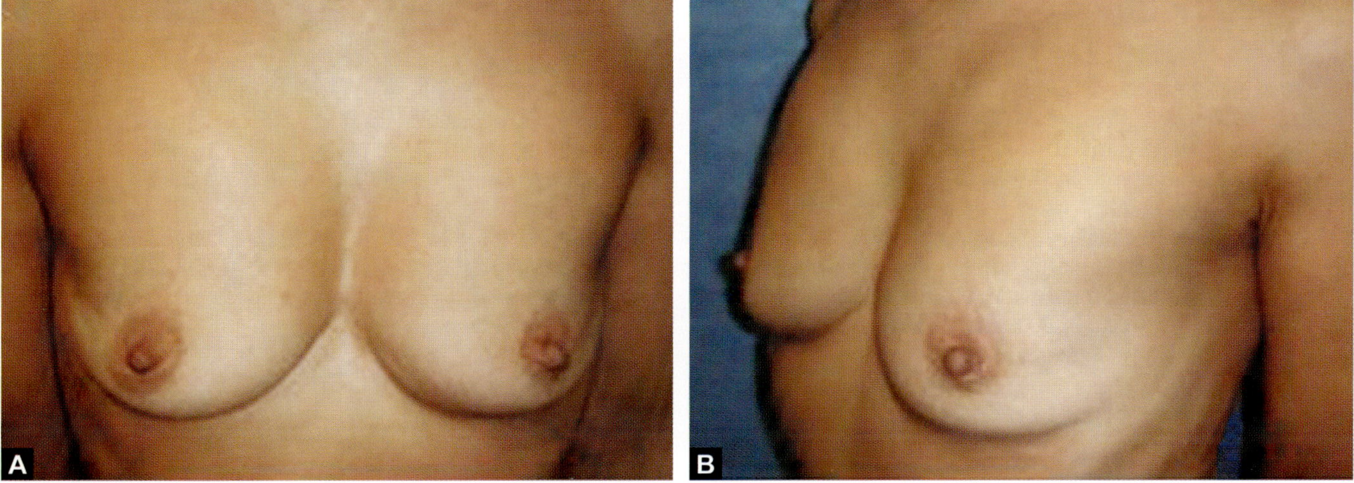

Figs. 9.42A and B

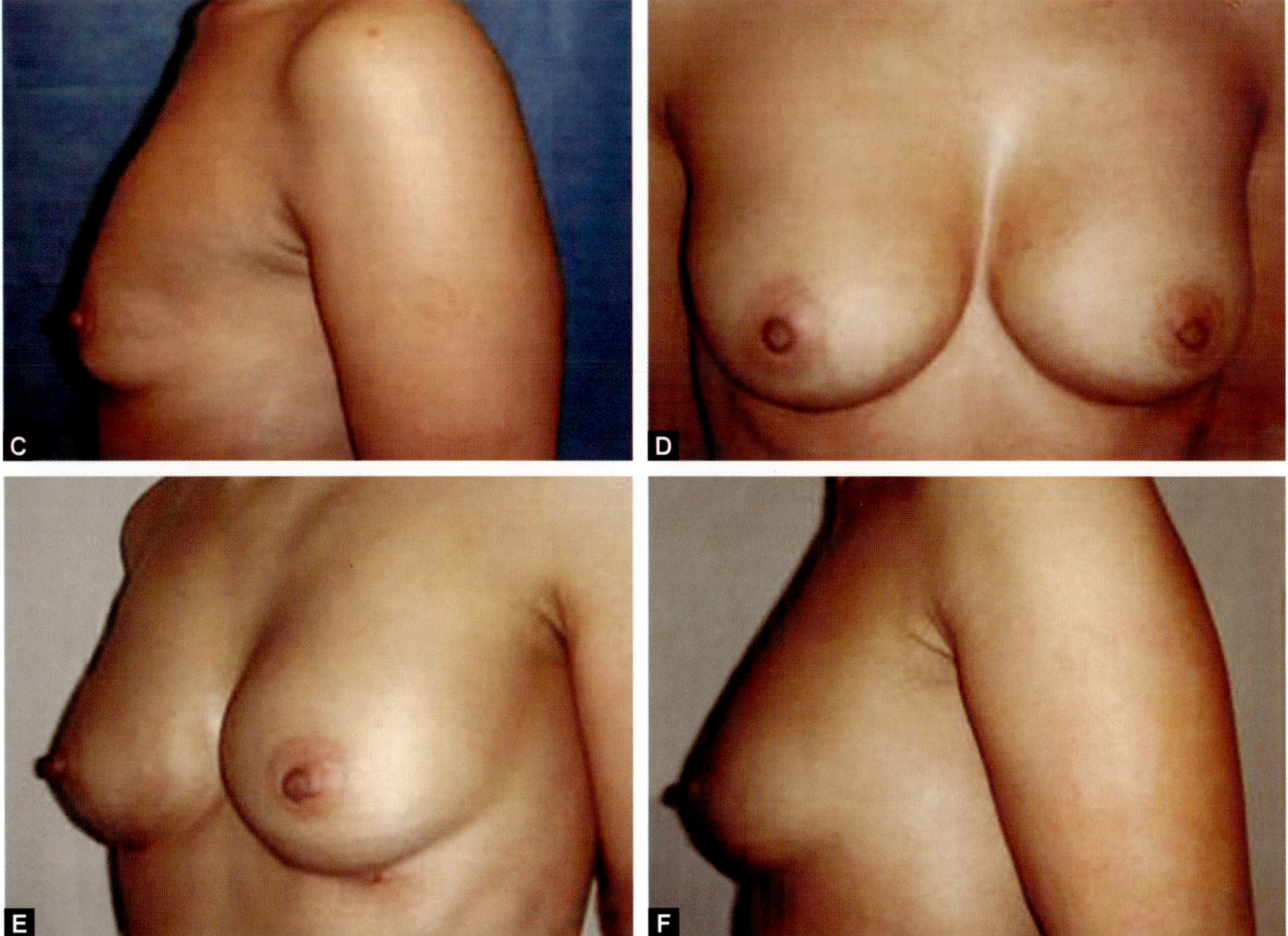

Figs. 9.42A to F: (A to C) Preoperative 52-year-old female. (D to F) Postoperative following 250 mL fat transfer to each side.

REFERENCES

1. Gesta S, Tseng YH, Kahn CR. Developmental origin of fat: tracking obesity to its source. Cell. 2007;131(2):242-56.
2. Zannettino AC, Paton S, Arthur A, et al. Multipotential human adipose-derived stromal stem cells exhibit a perivascular phenotype in vitro and in vivo. J Cell Physiol. 2008;214(2):413-21.
3. Miranville A, Heeschen C, Sengenes C, et al. Improvement of postnatal neovascularization by human adipose tissue-derived stem cells. Circulation. 2004;110(3):349-55.
4. Yoshimura K, Shigeura T, Matsumoto D, et al. Characterization of freshly isolated and cultured cells derived from the fatty and fluid portions of liposuction aspirates. J Cell Physiol. 2006;208(1):64-76.
5. Rubio D, Garcia-Castro J, Martin MC, et al. Spontaneous human adult stem cell transformation. Cancer Res. 2005;65(8):3035-9.
6. Tzikas TL. Lipografting: autologous fat grafting for total facial rejuvenation. Facial Plast Surg. 2004;20(2):135-43.
7. Boschert MT, Beckert BW, Puckett CL, et al. Analysis of lipocyte viability after liposuction. Plast Reconstr Surg. 2002;109(2):761-5.
8. Rigotti G, Marchi A, Galie M, et al. Clinical treatment of radiotherapy tissue damage by lipoaspirate transplant: a healing process mediated by adipose-derived adult stem cells. Plast Reconstr Surg. 2007;119(5):1409-22.
9. Strem BM, Hicok KC, Zhu M, et al. Multipotential differentiation of adipose tissue-derived stem cells. Keio J Med. 2005;54(3):132-41.

10. Brown FE, Sargent SK, Cohen SR, et al. Mammographic changes following reduction mammaplasty. Plast Reconstr Surg. 1987;80(5):691-8.

FURTHER READING

1. Shiffman MA, Di Giuseppe. A Liposuction: Principles and Practice. Berlin: Springer; 2006.
2. Shiffman MA, Di Giuseppe. A Body Contouring, Art, Science, and Clinical Practice. Berlin: Springer; 2010.
3. Shiffman MA, Di Giuseppe. A Cosmetic Surgery: Art and Techniques. Berlin: Springer; 2013.
4. Coleman S. Structural Fat Grafting. St. Louis, MO: Quality Medical Publishing, Inc; 2004.
5. Coleman S, Mazzola R. Fat Injection: From Filling to Regeneration. St. Louis, MO: Quality Medical Publishing, Inc; 2010.
6. Rubin P, Jewell M. Body Contouring and Liposuction. Philadelphia, PA: Elsevier Saunders; 2012.
7. Spears S. Surgery of the Breast: Principles and Art. Philadelphia, PA: Lippincott Raven; 1998.

10 "Scarless" Mastopexy: Using Heat-Mediated Tissue Tightening to Lift the Breast

Diane I Duncan

INTRODUCTION

Mastopexy has been frequently turned down by patients with breast ptosis because of the unattractive scarring associated with procedures that excise skin. Many surgeons are reluctant to perform mastopexy, as it is difficult to meet patient expectations. Limitations of current mastopexy techniques include unattractive scarring, numbness, or hypersensitivity, residual or recurrent ptosis, and an unattractive shape post-treatment. Patients comment that they have "just traded one problem for another," and a small but significant number state that they wished they had never had the mastopexy done. Goals listed by patients seeking treatment include a permanent improvement in the flabby, saggy character of the breast, filling in of upper pole hollowing without the need for an implant, correction of bottoming out, and correction of breast dislocation into the armpit while sleeping. These goals are rarely achieved with traditional excisional treatment.

EVOLUTION OF TECHNIQUE

In 2008, the author was involved in an IRB study of the Invasix BodyTite device. A study completed in 2010 showed that with abdominal tattoo-defined surface area measurements taken with the Canfield Vectra system,[1] there was a measured 26% skin surface area reduction at 6 weeks post-treatment when radiofrequency (RF)-assisted heating was performed in conjunction with suction assisted lipectomy (SAL). This prospective randomized study showed that the side treated with SAL only had a measured 10% skin surface area contraction at the same post-treatment interval. At one year following treatment, the RF plus SAL side showed a mean surface area contraction of 34.5%, while the SAL only side had a mean surface area contraction of 8.5%. Multiple studies confirm an increase in tissue tightening with overlying skin contraction with RF- and laser-assisted tissue heating.[2-4]

Many regions of the body, neck, and lower face were treated with this device over a 4-year period. While Blugerman[5] reported the use of the device for Gynecomastia, no treatments for the purpose of breast lifting have been reported.

Several of the author's patients who had undergone radiofrequency-assisted liposuction (RFAL) of other body regions began requesting similar treatments for breast ptosis. Most had grade I–II glandular ptosis, and none would accept a scar. The development of a study protocol was initiated. Indications included patients between the ages of 17 (with parental permission) and 65 with grade I–II plus ptosis. Preoperative mammograms were required, and a pretreatment high-resolution ultrasound of each breast was performed. Standardized two-dimensional and three-dimensional photography was performed prior to treatment and at each visit. Patients were required to sign both treatment consent and study consent, including permission to publish before and after treatment photographs. Follow-up was performed at 1 week, 6 weeks, 3 months, 6 months, and 1 year. The RF energy was only applied to the subcutaneous tissue, and was not used within the breast gland itself.

In September 2011, the author began an Institutional Review Board (IRB)-sponsored study of the use of RF-assisted tissue tightening for the purpose of breast lifting. This study, presented at ASLMS in Boston during the 2013 annual meeting,[5] showed the results of the 50-patient study.

TECHNIQUE

The procedure was performed under local anesthesia in 22% of patients. The remainder of procedures was performed under general anesthesia, frequently in conjunction with other procedures. Local anesthesia was injected intradermally within each of three access ports. Technically these do leave a scar. However, with the use of a 16-gauge needle, a small tumescent infusion cannula, and the FaceTite device from Invasix, the access openings remain very small. Access ports typically were located within the areola above and below the nipple, and at one lower pole position.

Tumescent fluid was injected into the subcutaneous tissue only, except in one patient who underwent simultaneous liposuction for breast reduction. Tumescent infusion was followed by radial heating of the subcutaneous tissue with the RF cannula. More time was spent in regions of need. While the procedure first began with a focus on the upper pole of the breast, attention quickly shifted to the entire breast when improvement of bottoming-out, lateral splay, and nipple-areolar asymmetry was noted. The technique was subjective, as the treatment endpoints are subtle. Endpoints include a subjective improvement in the skin laxity, warmth, and slight erythema at the treatment region, and a visible tissue contraction as each treatment region was heated. Checking of contour in the upright position was performed before moving on to the opposite side.

Device settings included a maximum skin temperature of 37° in order to have no patients with burns. The energy setting of 35–45 W was able to be consistently used. Between 9 and 22 kJ of energy were used on each breast.

Following completion of radial heating, the access points were sutured and microfoam tape was used to help support the nipple-areolar elevation. Other than recommending reduced activity for 24 hours while the tumescent fluid was absorbed, no activity restrictions were given.

RESULTS

While all patients noted some improvement, the results varied from one individual to another, as expected. Patients were warned that a second treatment session or surgical revision might be needed, as results are dependent on tissue quality and compliance with the tape and underwire support bra. Younger patients responded better, in general, than older patients did.

Case 1 (Figs. 10.1A and B)

The first study patient was a woman with grade II glandular ptosis after breast feeding. She was offered a traditional mastopexy, but declined. Pretreatment measurements showed that with a proper implant size, her nipple-areola and inferior breast tissue would hang below the inferior implant border following augmentation. Once the study protocol was established, this patient volunteered to undergo the described procedure. A two-stage process was offered. The patient requested simultaneous procedure performance, with a written understanding that if the RF-assisted lift was unsatisfactory, she would be allowed to have a later surgical lift. Postoperative measurements with the Canfield 3D Vectra showed a mean 5.1-cm nipple elevation with the combined procedure.

Case 2 (Figs. 10.2A to C)

This patient was even more challenging. She had grade II plus ptosis, and desired a similar procedure to patient 1.

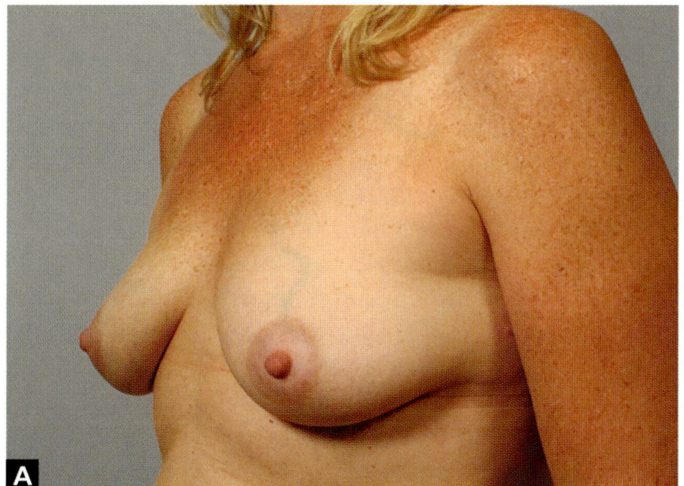

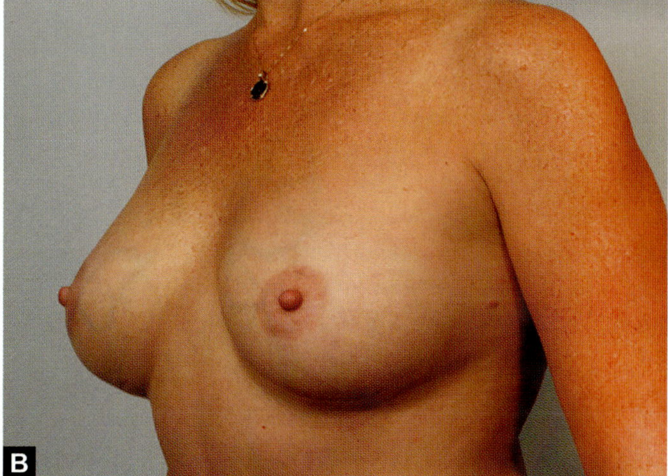

Figs. 10.1A and B: (A) Preoperative 35-year-old female after breastfeeding two children. (B) Two months following subpectoral augmentation plus RF-assisted breast lift.

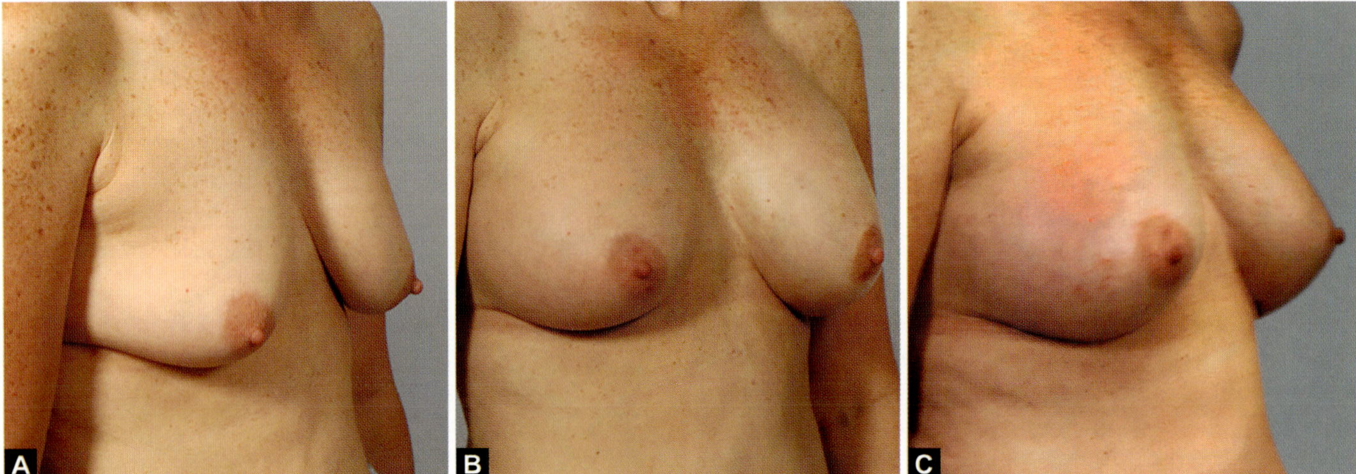

Figs. 10.2A to C: (A) Preoperative 47-year-old female. (B) Six weeks following augmentation and RF-assisted lift. (C) Three months postoperative.

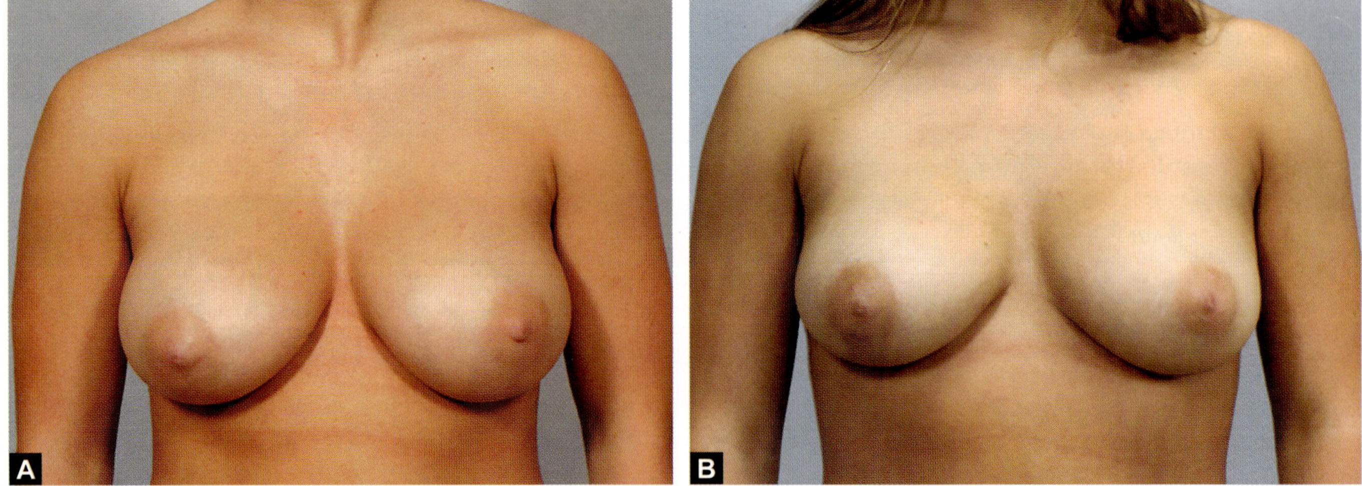

Figs. 10.3A and B: (A) Preoperative 17-year-old female athlete with 34 DDD. (B) Two months following SAL breast reduction and RF-assisted lift. Note asymmetry improvement.

She was told that she did not have a good chance of a single-session success. She opted for a simultaneous augmentation plus RF lift. At 6 weeks, bilateral nipple-areolae were still low. The punctate access marks can be clearly seen. The patient was requested to return at 3 months post-treatment, in order to discuss further improvement. At 3 months, further nipple-areola lifting was noted. No further surgery was indicated.

Case 3 (Figs. 10.3A and B)

This patient was a 17-year-old athlete. She requested a breast reduction, as she was very self-conscious about her breast size while on the playing field. She was asymmetric, with the right breast being larger and more ptotic. She requested a significant reduction in order to be able to play sports unimpeded. Close examination of the areola post-treatment shows a faint mark where the liposuction cannula and RF cannulas were inserted. The patient noted significant improvement and no more self-consciousness while playing sports. Liposuction-only breast reductions have lost popularity because of poor shape and residual ptosis after treatment. By adding RF-assisted tissue tightening, this approach can be revived in younger patients with grade I and II ptosis and a need for mild to moderate reduction.

ASYMMETRY TREATMENT

Many patients complain of asymmetry but will not pursue a surgical correction unless the deformity is extreme. The RF-assisted lift is ideal for treatment in those patients. Although perfect symmetry can never be achieved, significant improvement is a reasonable expectation when proper treatment parameters are used.

Case 4 (Figs. 10.4A to D)

This 38-year-old patient presented with a very common condition: postchildbearing ptosis with asymmetry. She breast-fed more frequently on the left side. While she had a mild pre-existing asymmetry, now the problem was magnified and noticeable, especially in a tank top or swimsuit. While the left breast was attached to the chest wall in a lower position than that of the right, significant improvement in asymmetry was able to be achieved with an RF breast lift alone. The patient also noted correction of the upper pole hollow on the left side.

Case 5 (Figs. 10.5A and B)

Occasionally, patients with difficult problems present for treatment. This 48-year-old had undergone breast augmentation surgery in a different city 2 years prior to her visit. Her left breast appeared quite a bit longer than the right. Both had severe ptosis. She was treated with implant exchange and extensive RF-assisted breast lift bilaterally with good results.

THE MODEST RESULT

With most procedures, there is some variability in the level of improvement following treatment. Not all patients will experience the same outcome as those posted on the website.

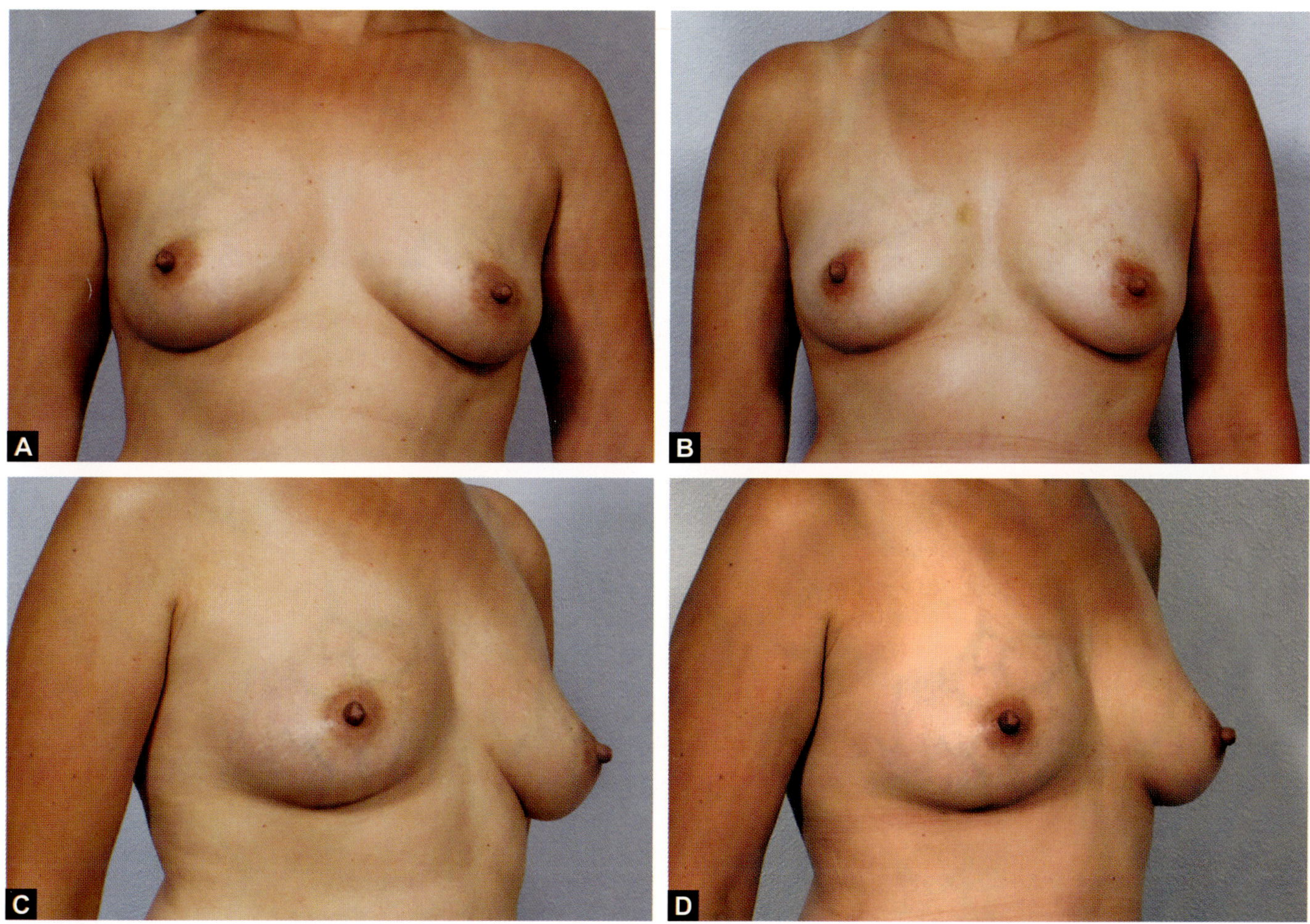

Figs. 10.4A to D: (A and B) Preoperative 38-year-old mother after breastfeeding. (C and D) Six weeks following RF-assisted lift only.

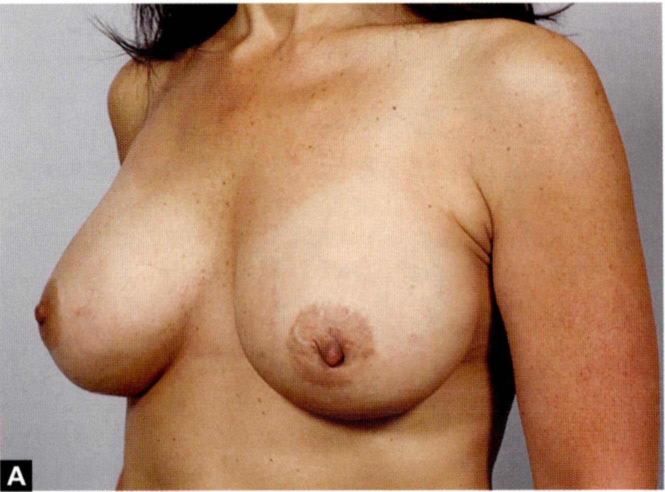

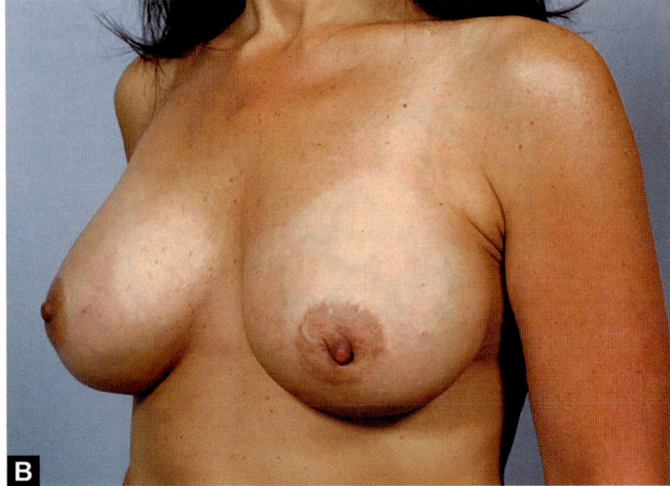

Figs. 10.5A and B: (A) Preoperative 48-year-old female 2 years after asymmetric augmentation. (B) Two months following implant exchange and extensive RF-assisted breast lift bilaterally.

Ethical surgeons will show a variety of outcome photographs to prospective patients in order to demonstrate the variable nature of results in a variety of patients.

Case 6 (Figs. 10.6A to C)

This middle-aged patient presented with severe ptosis, upper pole hollowing, and lateral splay of her breasts while in the recumbent position. She stated that she was very interested in improving this condition, but declined a traditional mastopexy. In addition to disliking the scars, she stated that she had no down time and wanted to be able to return to work within 48 hours. She had an RF-assisted breast lift with very good results including filling of the hollow upper pole.

DISCUSSION

While the indexed plastic surgical literature is filled with descriptions of various types of breast lifts, there are no references to scarless mastopexies. Interestingly, an online search shows numerous references for scarless breast lifts. Most of these are not actually scarless. Dissatisfaction with the sagging and volume loss that occurs with aging and post-childbearing has caused women to seek improvement in breast contour on a regular basis. Breast augmentation with implants of with fat grafting can improve the volume problem, and, in many cases, can create enough of a lift for many patients to be satisfied with these restorative procedures.

However, with moderate-to-severe ptosis, excisional breast lifting is generally indicated. In years past, patients were told that if they wanted to avoid the scars of a traditional mastopexy, much larger implants would be needed in order to fill out the skin envelope. If patients declined large implants, the only option has been excisional mastopexy. Various scar patterns and reshaping options exist.

Mastopexy preferences were studied by Rohrich.[6] A total of 487 surgeons responded to his survey. He noted that the inverted T skin pattern was most popular. However, patient satisfaction was higher with a short-scar periareolar technique with inferior pedicle reduction.[7,8] Spitting sutures, bottoming out, and unsatisfactory scarring were the most common complications. Interestingly, the most minimal scar procedure—the periareolar approach—had the highest incidence of revision.

The "upside down" mastopexy was developed by Migliori[9] to correct breast ptosis in the massive weight loss patient. This procedure uses an implant placed subpectorally in the upper pole to fill out the hollow, or in the usual position to fill out the entire glandular contour. An unusual approach to breast lifting is described by de la Plaza.[10] In this procedure, a superior pedicle is used. The medial and lateral inferior breast tissue is elevated and is fixed to the upper pole in the shape of a hammock. Rubin[11] noted that the shape of the breast is dictated by the shape of the gland. His results with dermal suspension and reshaping of the breast glandular tissue are quite good; aesthetic outcome with parenchymal reshaping offers a more attractive shape than can be achieved with skin resection alone.

In recent years, great attention has been given to the limited scar mastopexy. Pioneered by Benelli,[12] Lassus,[13] and Lejour,[14] the periareolar and "lollipop" type approaches have become more popular in recent years.[15] A variation

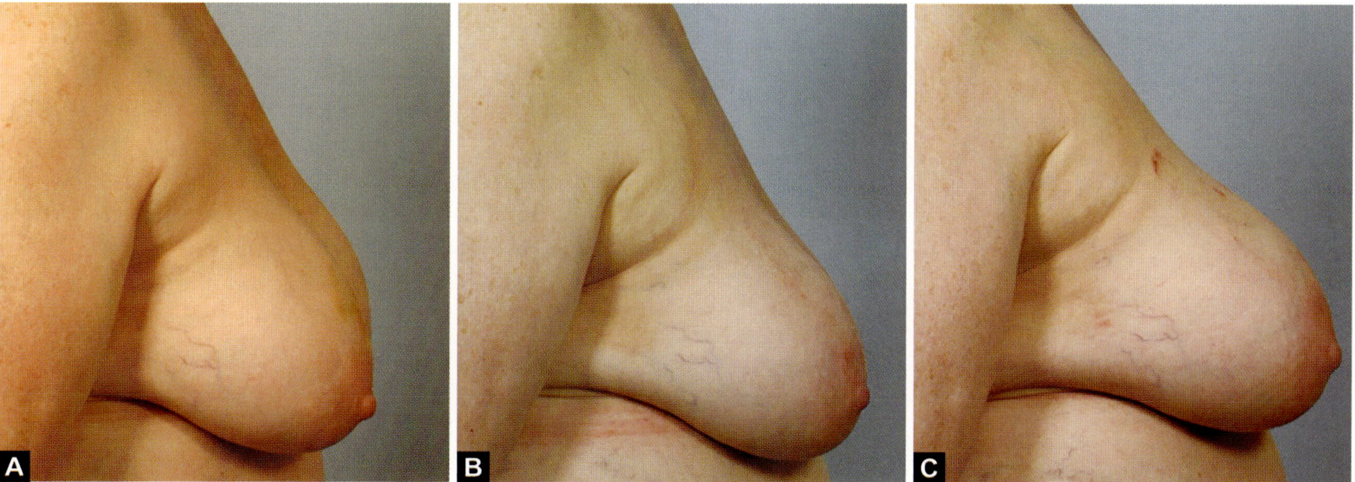

Figs. 10.6A to C: (A) Preoperative 53-year-old female with grade II + ptosis. (B) Six weeks following RF-assisted breast lift. (C) Three months post-treatment. Note fill of upper pole hollow.

on the minimal scar technique is offered by Keskin,[16] who avoids the vertical scar but utilizes both a periareolar and an inframammary scar.

Other methods of minimizing scarring are offered by Marcon,[17] who advocates a dermal inframammary purse string scar. Gryskiewicz[18] feels that the traditional periareolar scar looks artificial. If a "zigzag" or wavy line is created in the periareolar space, he argues that this appears more natural and less like an actual scar. The "Owl" technique[19] is another modification of a shorter scar mastopexy, which combines a periareolar component with a vertical scar. More focus on glandular reshaping plus skin excision is demonstrated in Honig's treatise on an autoaugmentation mastopexy.[20] Botti[21] also utilizes autoaugmentation using a superior pedicle. Both techniques improve central projection and glandular shape. Gonzalez[22] recommends a combination procedure in which a circumareolar incision is used to place an implant with detachment of the lower dermal areolar attachment.

A frequent deficit of traditional mastopexies is the residual upper pole hollow. The teardrop augmentation plus mastopexy[23] creates an upper pole elevation through a periareolar approach. Kelemen[24] also addresses the restoration of upper pole fullness by repositioning the parenchyma.

While the articles published in the peer-reviewed medical literature tend to be more scientific, online resources for breast lifting information are more commercial. A close look at over thirty claims for scarless breast lifting found online shows that almost all of these do leave scars. The two claims for a true scarless lift with noninvasive devices originate from Sanctuary Medical Center in Boca Raton.[25] In 2008, Pozner posted a You Tube video demonstrating the Accent laser breast lift, purportedly targeting collagen remodeling. In 2012, Pozner (personal communication July 4, 2012) stated that he was no longer using the procedure due to inconsistent results. In 2012, the same clinic posted a You Tube video lauding the effects of the Tripollar Apollo device, another RF device that they claim reduces the flabby appearance of aging breasts.

While results may be modest, the claims of a scarless lift are true with the totally noninvasive devices. In 2011, Duncan[26] showed a mean 1.5 cm nipple to sternal notch lift with the use of Ulthera for treatment of the décolleté. "Almost scarless" lifts utilize minimally invasive techniques, sometimes combining liposuction with some type of energy assistance. The "scarless breast reduction"[27,28] was popular a decade ago when a liposuction-only approach was used. Unfortunately, some patients noted devolumization without an apparent lift when pre-existing ptosis was moderate to severe.[29] Gynecomastia[30,31] is another area in which SAL or SAL plus energy assisted tissue heating has been utilized for male breast reductions with minimal scarring. "Twists" on scarless breast lifting are claimed by surgeons who perform an "internal lift" during augmentation,[32] or a simple augmentation that produces an expected lift.[33] Another surgeon, Becker,[34] claims to offer a scarless lift, when the "after" photographs clearly show bilateral periareolar scars.

The development of heat mediated tissue tightening has added a new tool to the armamentarium of the body contouring surgeon. A variety of devices have been scientifically shown to reduce skin surface area more than the baseline 8–10% that occurs with SAL alone.[1] These include Smart Lipo,[35] the BodyTite,[36,37] and the Thermigen device.[38] Sadick[39] notes that RF is the optimal energy type for producing skin and soft tissue tightening. The coagulative effect draws the subcutaneous fibroseptal collagen matrix together. The overlying skin accommodates, but there is a limit to the amount of skin surface area reduction that can be achieved using this method.

Blugerman's study[5] presented a review of 59-patient treatments under tumescent anesthesia. Twelve of these patients underwent RFAL plus resection of glandular tissue, while 47 were treated with SAL plus RF heating (RFAL) alone. The mean aspirated volume was 625 mL. Patient satisfaction was rated as a mean of 8.13 out of 10. A mean of 28 kJ of energy per breast was used.

Duncan first presented this technique in 2012 as a new use for RF-assisted tissue tightening.[40] A 50 patient prospective study was presented in Boston at the annual ASLMS meeting of the American Society for Laser Medicine and Surgery[41] where one year results were reviewed. Lift, as measured with the Canfield Vectra system, ranged from 2.3 to 6.7 cm. Improvement parameters that cannot be measured included filling of the upper pole hollow, improvement of bottoming out, and improvement of lateral splay with the patient in the supine position.

COMPLICATIONS

In the author's series, one patient sustained a traumatic postoperative hematoma with no long-term residual effect. There were no burns. Two patients had persistent nodularity of the subcutaneous tissue of the breast. These were successfully treated with collagenase injections. Two patients stated they had a less than expected improvement, but none opted for the offered complimentary revision.

Limitations of this technique include the variability of outcomes, and difficulties in meeting patient expectations. This technique is not indicated for patients with multiple striae or severely damaged skin, or for patients with grade III ptosis. Radiofrequency-assisted breast lifting will not be a substitute for skin excision when used in conjunction with liposuction for breast reduction in patients who need a large volume removed, or in those with severe pre-existing ptosis. When considering this option as a treatment modality for patients with breast ptosis, it is important to advise each patient of the variable nature of the outcome, with a possible need for a second stage touch-up.

CONCLUSION

Improvement of breast ptosis with RF-assisted tissue tightening is an exciting new option for treatment of sagging, asymmetry, upper pole hollowing, lateral splay, and inferior bottoming out.

While not technically scarless, the three 16-gauge needle punctures do leave extremely minimal scars.

This procedure can be performed under local tumescent anesthesia, with minimal down time. Best results are obtained in younger patients with grade I–II ptosis. Limitations include meeting patient expectations (this is not a "magic wand"), variability in patient outcome, and a modest result in those with more severe ptosis and damaged skin. Risks other than a less than hoped for improvement were minimal.

The large number of available mastopexy options available infers that none is superior in all situations. Radiofrequency-assisted breast lifts can offer truly minimal scars with very little down time, but it is only effective in a limited number of patient situations.

REFERENCES

1. Irvine Duncan D. Nonexcisional tissue tightening: creating skin surface area reduction during abdominal liposuction by adding radiofrequency heating. Aesthetic Surg J. 2013;33 (8):1154-66.
2. Sasaki GH. Quantification of human abdominal tissue tightening and contraction after component treatments with 1064-nm/1320-nm laser-assisted lipolysis: clinical implications. Aesthet Surg J. 2010;30(2):239-45.
3. DiBernardo BE, Reyes J, Chen B. Evaluation of tissue thermal effects from 1064/1320-nm laser-assisted lipolysis and its clinical implications. J Cosmet Laser Ther. 2009;11(2): 62-9.
4. Waldman A. Scientific report: comparison of treatment uniformity of laser assisted liposuction (LAL) and radiofrequency assisted liposuction (RFAL). Medesthetics. 2013;2 (3):39-41.
5. Blugerman G, Scvhalvezon D, Mulholland RS, et al. Gynecomastia treatment using radiofrequency-assisted liposuction (RFAL). Eur J Plast Surg. 2013;36:231-6.
6. Rohrich RJ, Gosman AA, Brown SA, et al. Mastopexy preferences: a survey of board-certified plastic surgeons. Plast Reconstr Surg. 2006;118(7):1631-8.
7. Hammond DC, Alfonso D, Khuthalia DK. Mastopexy using the short scar periareolar inferior pedicle reduction technique. Plast Reconstr Surg. 2008;121(5):1533-9.
8. Hall-Findlay EJ. Pedicles in vertical breast reduction and mastopexy. Clin Plast Surg. 2002;29(3):379-91.
9. Migliori E. "Upside-down" augmentation mastopexy. Aesthetic Plast Surg. 2011;35(4):593-600.

10. de la Plaza R, de la Cruz L, Moreno C. Mastopexy utilizing a dermoglandular hammock flap. Aesthet Surg J. 2005; 25(1):31-36.
11. Rubin JP, Gusenoff JA, Coon D. Dermal suspension and parenchymal reshaping mastopexy after massive weight loss: statistical analysis with concomitant procedures from a prospective registry. Plast Reconstr Surg. 2009;123(3):782-9.
12. Benelli L. A new periareolar mammaplasty: the "round block" technique. Aesthetic Plast Surg. 1990;14(2):93-100.
13. Lassus C. A 30-year experience with vertical mammoplasty. Plast Reconstr Surg. 1996;97(2):373-80.
14. Lejour M. Vertical mammoplasty and liposuction of the breast. Plast Reconstr Surg. 1994;94(1):100-114.
15. Rohrich RJ, Thornton JF, Jakubietz RG, et al. The limited scar mastopexy: current concepts and approaches to correct breast ptosis. Plast Reconstr Surg. 2004;114(6):1622-30.
16. Keskin M, Tosun Z, Savaci N. Seventeen years of experience with reduction mammoplasty avoiding a vertical scar. Aesthetic Plast Surg. 2008;32(4):653-9.
17. Marconi F. The dermal pursestring suture: a new technique for a short inframammary scar in reduction mammoplasty and dermal mastopexy. Ann Plast Surg. 1898:22(6):484-93.
18. Gryskiewicz JM, Hatfield AS. "Zigzag" wavy-line periareolar incision. Plast Reconstr Surg. 2002;110(7):1778-83.
19. Loustau HD, Mayer HF, Sarrabayrouse M. The owl technique combined with the inferior pedicle in mastopexy. Aesthetic Plast Surg. 2008;32(10):11-15.
20. Honig JF, Frey HP, Hasse FM, et al. Autoaugmentation mastopexy with an inferior-based pedicle. Aesthetic Plast Surg. 2009;33(3);302-7.
21. Botti G. Personal mastopexy algorithm with auto-augmentation. International Master Course on Aging Skin (IMCAS), China 2012, Shanghai, July 28–29.
22. Gonzalez R. The PAM method—periareolar augmentation mastopexy: a personal approach to treat hypoplastic breast with moderate ptosis. Aesthet Surg J. 2012;32(2):175-85.
23. Ceydeli A, Freund RM. "Tear drop augmentation mastopexy": a technique to augment superior pole hollow. Aesthetic Plast Surg. 2003;27(60:425-32.
24. Keleman N, Kannan RY, Offer G. A stacked technique of mastopexy: volume redistribution mastopexy with inferior flap and superomedially based pedicle. Aesthetic Plast Surg. 2013;37(2):349-53.
25. Pozner J. 2013. [online] Available from Web address. http://www.youtube.com/watch?v=lw9Fm4GvJM. Accessed June 7 2013.
26. Duncan D. Ulthera microfocused ultrasound for soft tissue tightening. International Master Course on Aging Skin (IMCAS) Asia 2011, Singapore, July 17-19.
27. Baxt S. The scarless breast reduction. Available from http://www.youtube.com/watch?v=MKu9V8rh30. [Accessed June 7, 2013].
28. Gray L. Available from http://www.atlanticplasticsurg.com/scarless-breast-reduction.html. [Accessed June 8, 2013].
29. Jakubietz RG, Jakubietz DF, Gruenert JG, et al. Breast reduction by liposuction in females. Aesthetic Plast Surg. 2011;35(3):402-7.
30. Trelles MA, Mordon SR, Bonanad E, et al. Laser-assisted lipolysis in the treatment of gynecomastia: a prospective study in 28 patients. Lasers Med Sci. 2013;28(2):375-82.
31. Blugerman G, Schavelzon D. Mixed gynecomastia, reduction by laser lipolysis and transmammilar adenectomy. Am J Cosm Surg. 2003;20(4):233-8.
32. Romano J. The scarless breast lift. JRomano.com/Breast-enhancement/Breast LiftScarless.html. [Accessed June 7, 2013].
33. Nikko. Breast enhancement procedures. Available from http://www.drnikko.com/breast-procedures/scarless-lift. [Accessed June 7, 2013].
34. Available from http://beckermd.com/breast/lift-boca-raton-fl/. [Accessed June 7, 2013].
35. DiBernardo BE. Randomized, blinded split abdomen study evaluating skin shrinkage and skin tightening in laser-assisted liposuction versus liposuction control. Aesthet Surg J. 2010;30(4):593-602.
36. Paul M, Blugerman G, Kreindel M, et al. Three-dimensional radiofrequency tissue tightening: a proposed mechanism and applications for body contouring. Aesthetic Plast Surg. 2010;33(5):687-94.
37. Mulholland RS. Radiofrequency energy for non-invasive and minimally invasive skin tightening. Clin Plast Surg. 2011;38:437-48.
38. Key D. Improving the clinical response of skin tightening by "targeted temperature" subdermal RF probe heating using a method of subsurface temperature monitoring combined with skin surface infrared imaging. American Society for Laser Medicine and Surgery (ASLMS), Boston, April 7, 2013.
39. Sadick N. Energy types and best applications. International Master Course on Aging Skin (IMCAS), Paris, February 3, 2013.
40. Duncan DI. Pilot study using RF assisted tissue tightening for nonexcisional breast lifting. Int Plast Reconstr Aesthetic Surg J (IPRASJ). 2012;8:76.
41. Duncan D. Nonexcisional RF-assisted breast lifting: a prospective 50 patient study with 1 year results. Presented at American Society for Laser Medicine and Surgery (ASLMS), Boston, April 6, 2013.

11 Inverted "T" Superior Pedicle Technique with Inferior-Based Dermal Adipose Flap for Reduction Mammaplasty

Paolo Persichetti, Pierfranco Simone, Carlo Carusi

INTRODUCTION

Plastic surgery textbooks abound with descriptions of reduction mammaplasty techniques, each aiming to put forward an original approach to excise breast tissue and reshape a new breast mound. The results vary according to the excision pattern and concomitant gland coning, leading to different breast shapes, nipple-areola complex position, location and extent of the scar.[1] Many articles have focused the attention on the advantages of specific techniques highlighting the short scars or outstanding aesthetic outcomes. The authors believe that it is fundamental to consider the stability of the results, in terms of shape, projection, harmony of the quadrants, with the passage of time. The technique described in this chapter was demonstrated to provide stable results in the long run, as showed in a previous study, where the stability of the reduced breast was assessed in comparison to a contralateral reconstructed breast, 5 years postoperatively.[2]

PATIENT SELECTION

The inverted "T" superior pedicle technique, with inferior-based dermal adipose flap, for reduction mammaplasty, is applicable in most cases of breast reduction. In fact, the best candidates for this procedure are patients without overstretched Cooper's ligaments, considering the limited direct gland rearrangement and the fact that the breast mound is reshaped mainly through skin reapproximation. The connections between the skin and the gland are assessed preoperatively with the "pinch test" (Fig. 11.1).

Candidates for this breast reduction technique are patients needing minor or major reduction; however, the stability offered by this technique is obviously more noteworthy in larger breasts.

Patients' eligibility for surgery is carefully assessed through medical history, preoperative laboratory tests, mammogram, and ultrasound. Special attention is devoted to the acquisition of standardized preoperative pictures. In particular, the following views are recommended:

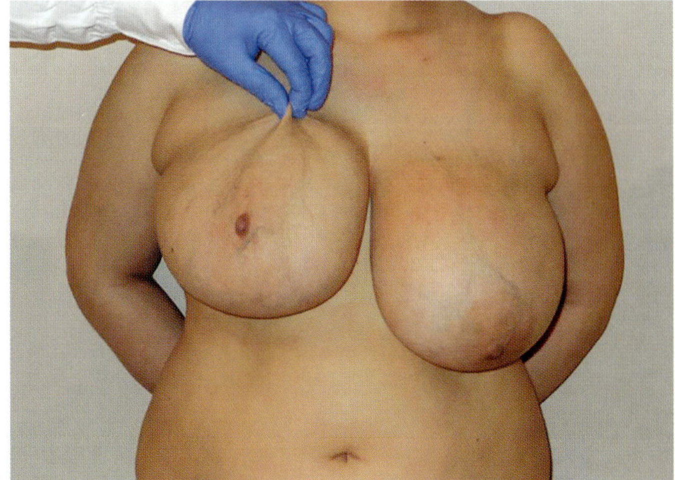

Fig. 11.1: Pinch test.

Frontal view: The upper margin is the clavicles and shoulders, and the lower margin is the line running between the anterosuperior iliac spines. The patient is in the upright position, with arms relaxed behind the back and one hand holding the contralateral wrist. This view allows for evaluation of symmetry, shape, and dimensions (Figs. 11.2A and B).

Oblique view (Figs. 11.2A and B): The patient rotates 45° from the frontal view. The upper and lower margins remain the same.

Lateral view (Figs. 11.2A and B): The patient rotates 90°. Points of reference are the same as for the oblique view (Figs. 11.2A and B).

Other views advised include the following:

Frontal view with arms raised and hands placed over the head: This view allows symmetry of inframammary folds to be assessed.

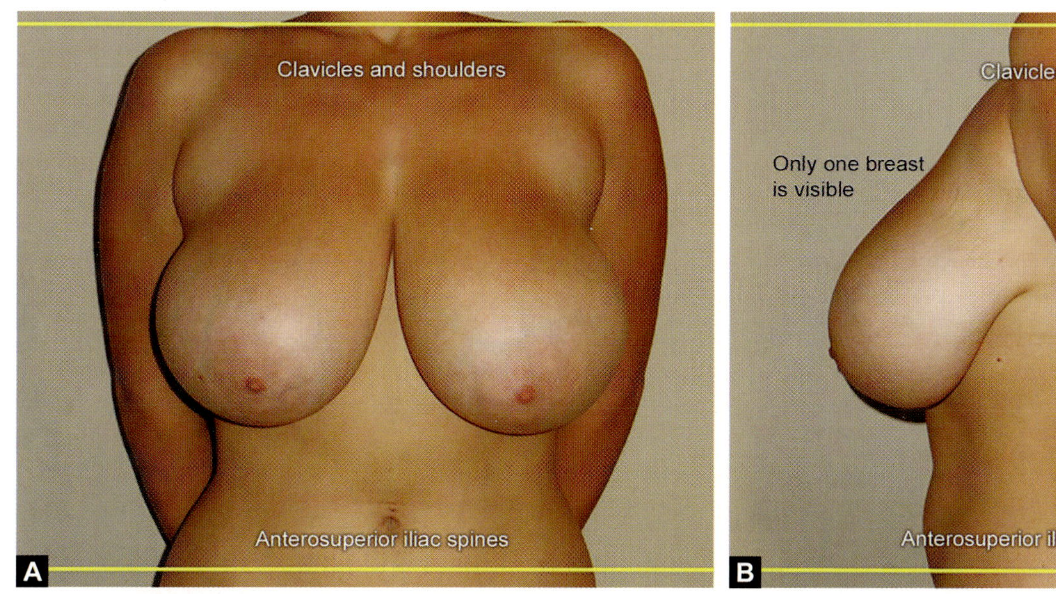

Figs. 11.2A and B: Standardized preoperative pictures. (A) Frontal view. (B) Left lateral view.

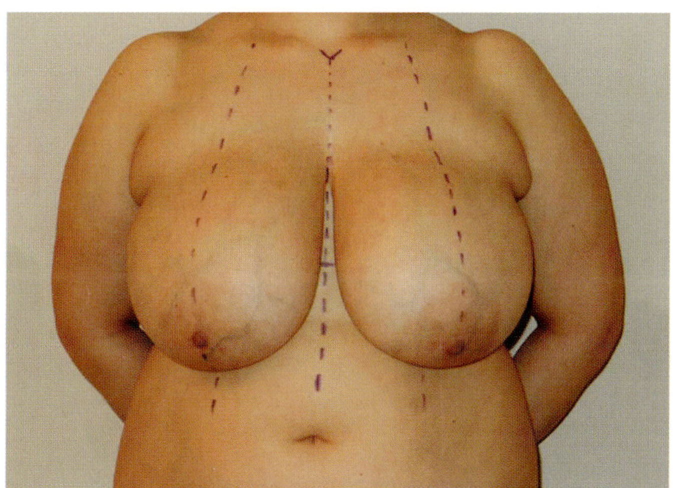

Fig. 11.3: Preoperative marking: midline, hemimammary lines, and the inframammary folds.

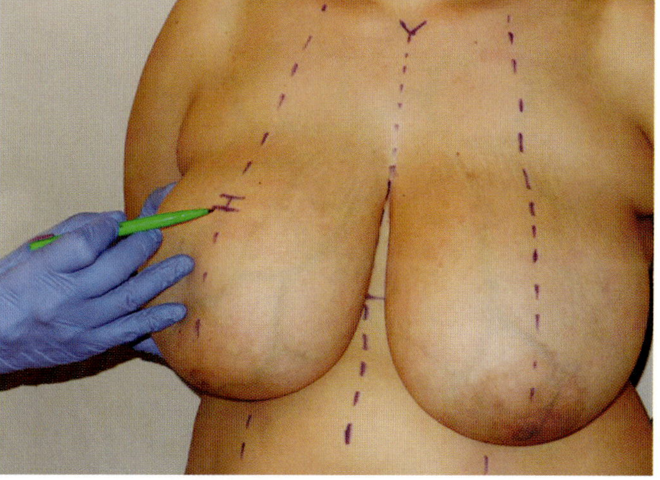

Fig. 11.4: Preoperative marking: Pitanguy's maneuver.

Frontal view with hands on flanks: Contracting pectoral muscles. The points of reference are the same as for the standard frontal view. This view permits assessment of mammary gland adherence to the underlying muscular fascia, revealing such pathologic adherences as observed in tuberous and tubular breasts.[3]

SURGICAL PROCEDURE

Marking

The preoperative drawing is made with the patient standing. The midline and hemimammary lines, and the inframammary folds, are marked (Fig. 11.3). Point A is calculated using Pitanguy's maneuver: the index finger is positioned in the inframammary fold and the palpation of this finger, on the anterior surface of the breast, allows the surgeon to establish the projection of the inframammary crease on the hemimammary line.[4] The authors prefer to mark point A, which is an approximate indication of the future site of the nipple, 1 cm lower than the actual projection of the inframammary crease (Fig. 11.4). In this way, the nipple is prevented from being too high after the lower pole of the breast has become fuller as a result of postoperative "bottoming out".[5] Points B and C are marked by moving the breasts medially and laterally in such a way that lines A–B and A–C correspond to the hemimammary line (Figs. 11.5A and B). A–B and A–C distances vary from 7 to 9 cm (longer for bigger excisions). B–C distance varies with the extent of the excision and is generally 8–12 cm. Lines from points B and C to the ends of the inframammary creases are then marked (Fig. 11.6).

A rectangular flap is marked based on the inframammary fold and centered on the hemimammary line, with the width of its base varying from 12 to 14 cm and the height from 10 to 12 cm (Fig. 11.7).

Technique

The patient is placed semi-sitting on the operating table. An areolar marker with a 4.2 cm diameter is used in all cases and the area is de-epithelialized (Figs. 11.8A and B). In particular, vertical strips are marked at the level of the lower pole flap and saline solution is infiltrated vigorously in the dermis with a 60-mL syringe and a 14-gauge needle. In this way, very tumescent and turgid tissues are obtained and the dermis is evidently expanded. Incision is made along the vertical lines, down to the dermis, and then one of the ends of the strips of skin is elevated with a knife. The strip is seized with a sturdy clip and forcefully drawn, rolling it around the clip, and de-epithelialization is carried out with the help of a blade[6] (Figs. 11.9A and B).

The dermal adipose flap is raised from the lower pole, 1 cm away from the areola. It is based at the fourth and fifth intercostal spaces, with a width that varies from 12 to 14 cm. Particular attention is paid to raising the flap so as not to

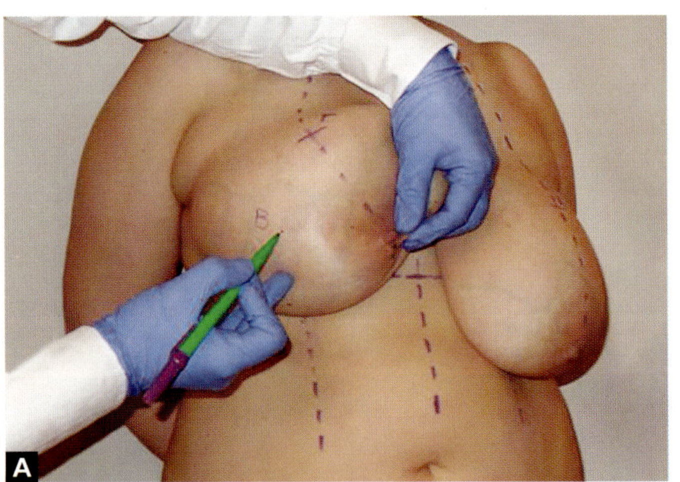

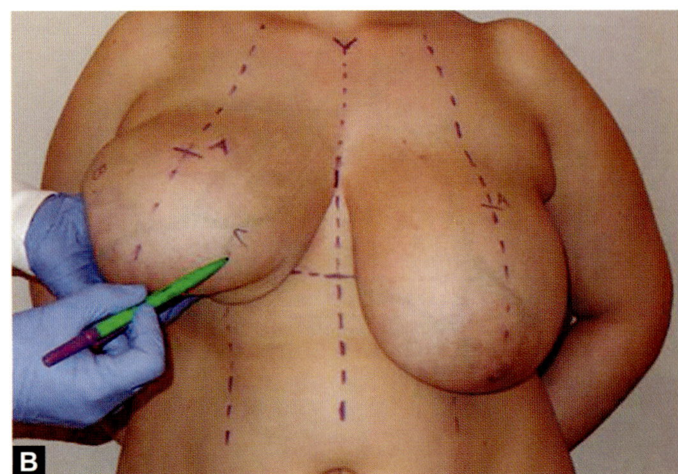

Figs. 11.5A and B: Preoperative marking: (A) Point B. (B) Point C.

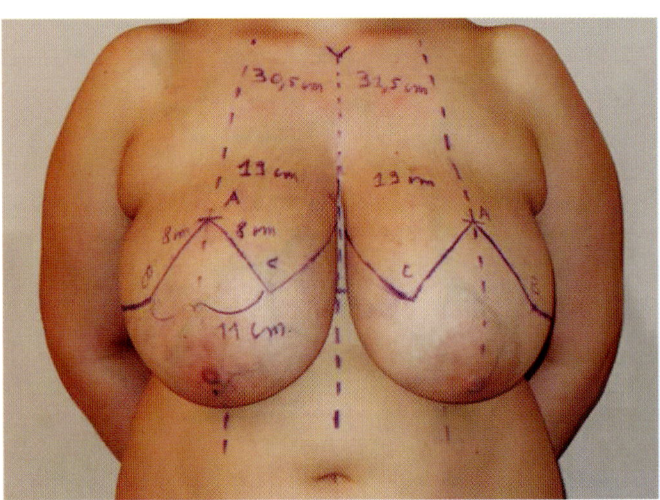

Fig. 11.6: Complete preoperative marking.

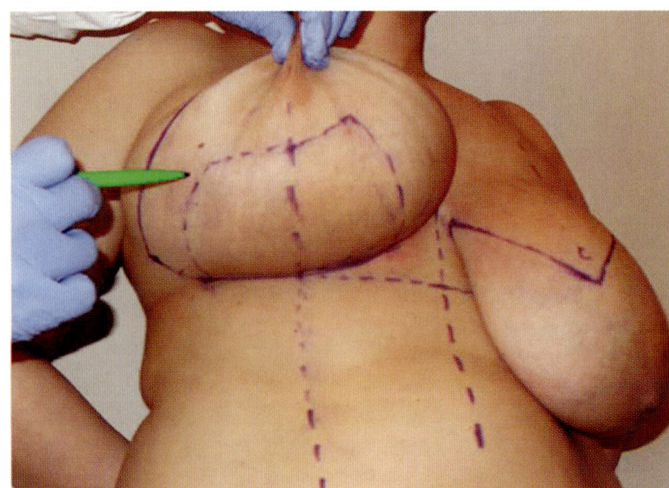

Fig. 11.7: Preoperative marking: flap.

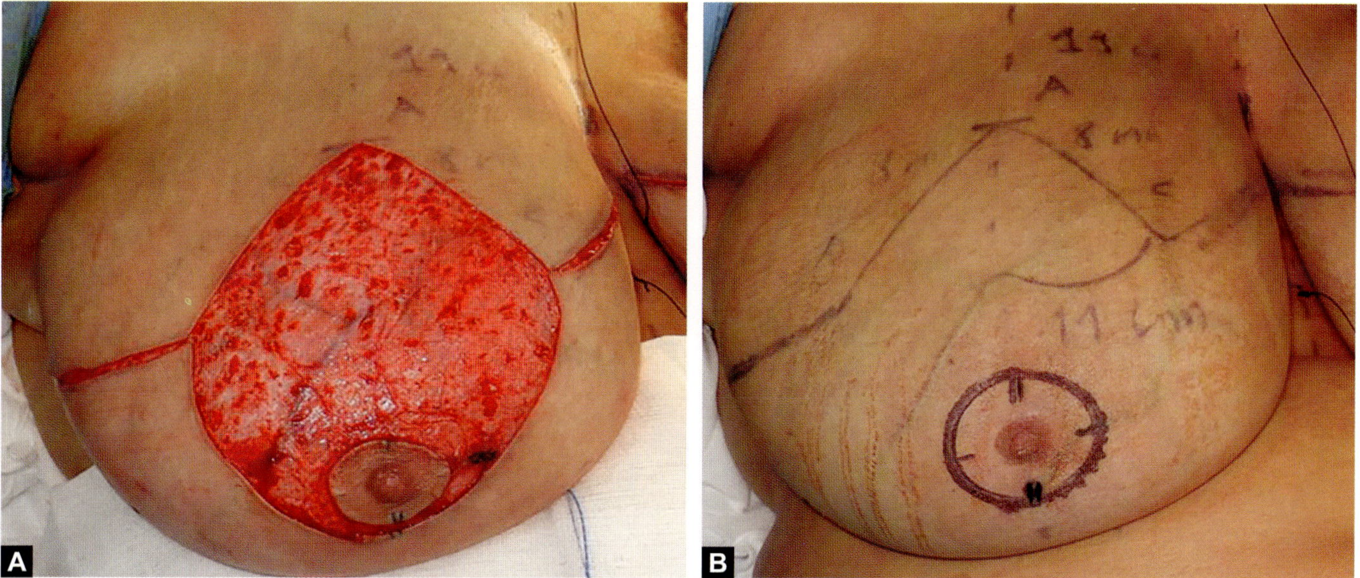

Figs. 11.8A and B: (A) Deepithelialization right breast; (B) Areolar marking right breast.

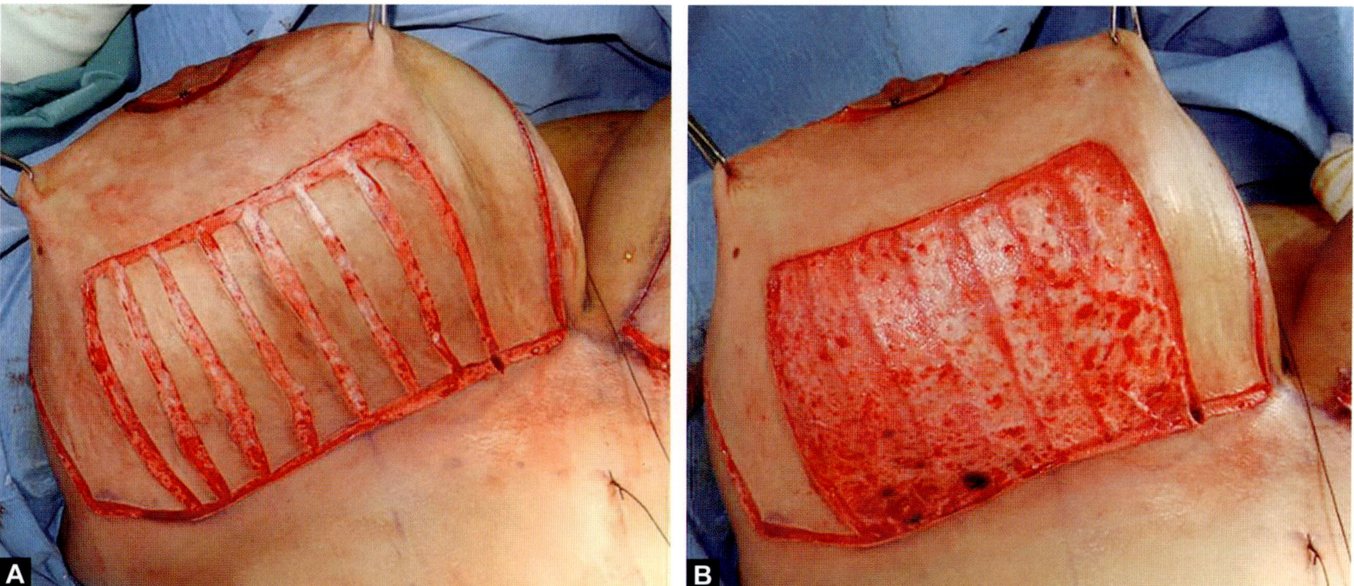

Figs. 11.9A and B: Flap de-epithelialization. (A) Skin incisions. (B) De-epithelialization.

include any of the gland in it (Fig. 11.10). Breast tissue is excised from the lateral, medial, and lower parts, and a keel resection made in the subareolar area (Fig. 11.11). Dissection on the underlying muscular fascia is prolonged cephalad, as far as the second rib. The dermal adipose flap is moved upward and when its thickness is such that it can affect the breast shape, it is adjusted medially or laterally, depending on which area needs filling. It is secured to the muscular fascia with polyglactin 910 (Vicryl) 0 sutures at the level of the second rib[7] (Fig. 11.12). The new breast is then assembled. The upper pole of the areola is lifted and sutured to point A and the new breast is coned by suturing the two lateral skin flaps above the dermal adipose flap. As a result the nipple is buried under the surrounding skin. The new areola is marked centered on point A, which is lower than the apex of the breast, and the marked area is de-epithelialized. Once exposed, the areola is sutured into its new position with single sutures of 4-0

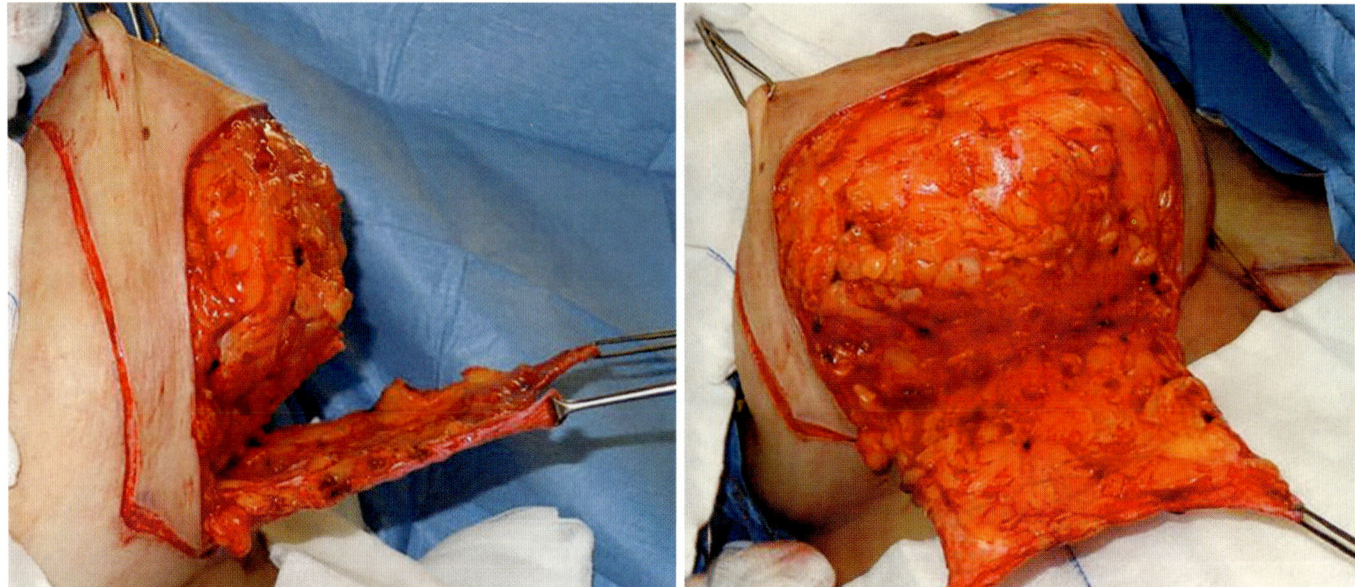

Fig. 11.10: Dermal adipose flap elevation.

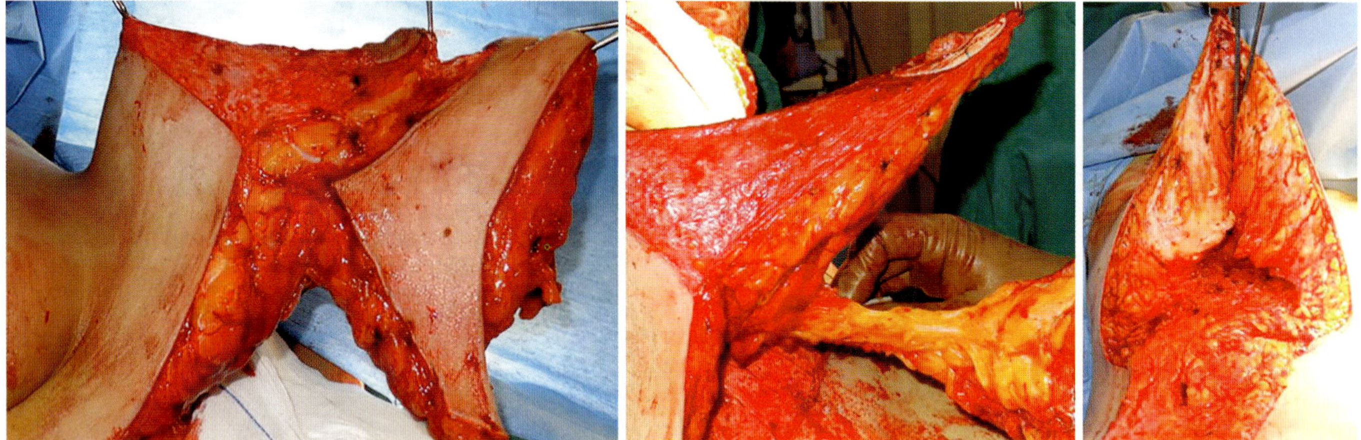

Fig. 11.11: Breast tissue resection.

nylon (Fig. 11.13). No drains are used, and a pressure dressing is applied. The average duration of the procedure is 2.5 hours.

Antibiotics are administered intravenously solely prior to the surgery.

POSTOPERATIVE CARE

Patients are discharged on the first postoperative day. Sutures around the areolas are removed after 2 weeks. A sports bra is worn day and night for at least 2 months after the operation. Paper taping of the scars for 3 months following surgery is recommended; afterward, patients are instructed to apply silicon gel.

COMPLICATIONS

Complications concerning the nipple–areola complex vascularization, observed following the inverted "T" superior pedicle technique with inferior-based dermal adipose flap, are in line with the rates reported in the medical literature for superior pedicle techniques.

Seroma was never reported, despite the authors' preference not to place drains. This is probably due to the use of the knife for dissection as opposed to the electrocautery. Another issue that may account for this finding is that the dissection performed during the inverted "T" superior pedicle technique with a dermal adipose flap does not imply a large dead space.

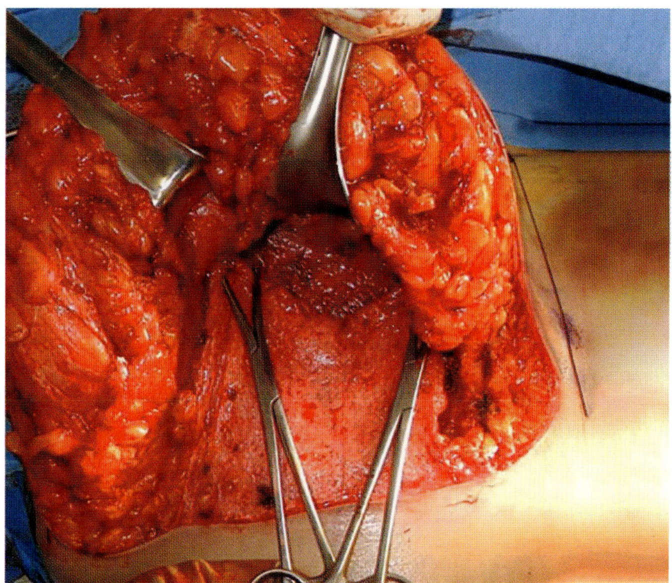

Fig. 11.12: Dermal adipose flap "in situ."

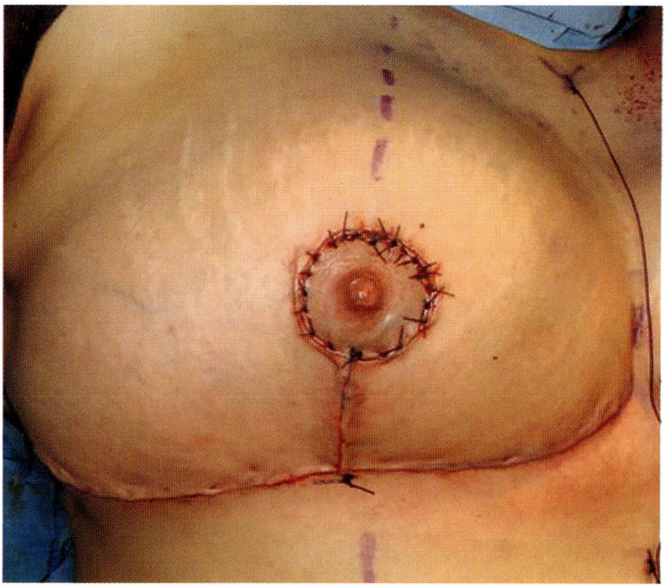

Fig. 11.13: Areola sutured in its new position.

No cases of dermal adipose flap malposition or complications related to the flap were reported.

DISCUSSION

It may sound unpopular to propose a traditional inverted "T" scar technique at a time when most surgeons are leaning toward short scars such as vertical mammaplasty to reduce residual scarring.[8-10] However, the authors are convinced that the stability of the reduced breast, in terms of shape and ptosis, is a pivotal element when selecting the appropriate technique for breast reduction.[7,11-13]

In a previous study, recurrent ptosis was assessed in reduced breasts 5 years postoperatively, considering the position of the nipple relative to the inframammary fold according to Regnault's classification. Glandular ptosis was reported in 29% and grade 1 ptosis in 25% of the cases included. The remaining patients had no ptosis, which shows remarkable stability in the long run. The best candidates are those whose Cooper's ligaments were not overstretched, as this approach relies on skin approximation to create the new breast, and patients with very lax connections between gland and skin are more prone to having early recurrence of ptosis.

The authors think that the reason for this stability is the adhesion of the gland to the raw surface of the flap, which is sutured to the underlying muscular fascia. Fixation of the gland in its new position is facilitated by a pressure garment, such as a sports bra, worn day and night for at least 2 months after the operation. It is evident that during the early postoperative period the upper pole gradually loses its initial fullness, even though it maintains its global shape.

The dermal adipose flap offers some further advantages. Especially in cases with considerable subcutaneous tissue, the flap can be positioned and adjusted to improve the shape of the breast, contributing to contour enhancement where needed. In selected cases, the flap can be elevated as a perforator flap based on perforator vessels from the fifth to seventh intercostal spaces. The resection of the dermal pedicle, isolating the perforator vessels, allows further mobility of the flap, which can contribute to upper pole fullness, similarly to the anterior intercostal artery perforator flap.[14]

Special care is taken in the flap elevation. In particular infiltration prior to de-epithelialization causes dermis hydrotomy and the traction on the skin exerted by the clip further acts in this way. The tumescent infiltration exposes the tissues, flattens concave surfaces, and facilitates countertraction. Therefore, the strip of skin comes off very rapidly and de-epithelialization is less time-consuming, even in the lower pole of the breast, where the dermis is extremely compact and difficult to dissect.

No gland tissue is included when the dermal adipose flap is raised and this separates the authors' procedure from the one described by Ribeiro and Backer.[15,16] This precaution allows avoidance of transferring gland tissue on to the muscular fascia or under it, as described in other techniques.[9,17] This is an important detail as transferring glandular tissue and juxtaposing it to the muscular fascia might have relevant consequences in case of breast cancer. In addition, the dermal adipose flap is a barrier that separates the breast from the chest wall.[18]

The inverted "T," superior pedicle technique, with an inferiorly based dermal adipose flap, is a standardized and versatile procedure, which is applicable to most patients with different breast shapes and volumes. In patients needing major reduction, with a great deal of skin in the lower quadrants, an inverted "T" technique is essential.[19] Especially in these cases, the approach allows roundness of the breasts to be obtained and limits excessive projection (Figs. 11.14A and B). This is a predictable procedure unlike other well-known techniques, which are considerably more intuitive and operator dependent.

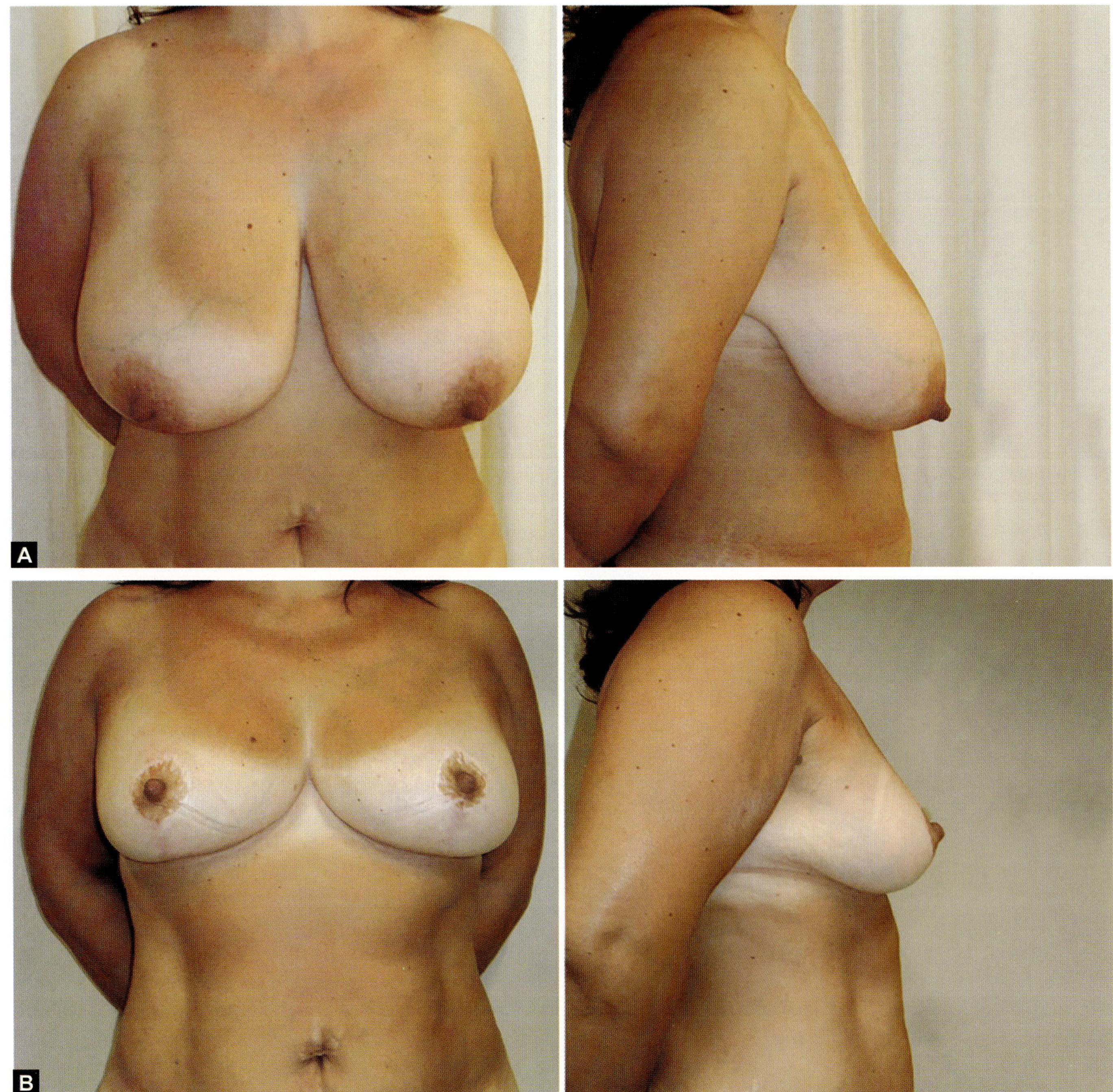

Figs. 11.14A and B: (A) Preoperative. (B) Four years postoperative.

REFERENCES

1. Shiffman MA. History of breast reduction. In: Shiffman MA, Di Giuseppe A (Eds). Body Contouring: Art, Science, and Clinical Practice. Berlin: Springer-Verlag; 2010. pp. 149-53.
2. Persichetti P, Simone P, Palazzolo D, et al. Reduction of the opposite breast in patients with a breast reconstructed with an implant: validity of the inverted "T," superior pedicle technique, with an inferiorly-based dermal adipose flap. J Plast Surg Hand Surg. 2012;46(5):339-43.
3. Persichetti P, Simone P, Langella M, et al. Digital photography in plastic surgery: how to achieve reasonable standardization outside a photographic studio. Aesthetic Plast Surg. 2007;31(2):194-200.
4. Pitanguy I, Caldeira AML, Alexandrino A, et al. Mamaplastia redutora e mastopexia. técnica Pitanguy. 25 anos de experiência (Reducing mammaplasty and mastopexy Pitanguy's technique. 25 years of experience). Rev Bras Cir. 1984;74(5): 265-88.
5. Vogt PM, Mühlberger T, Torres A, et al. Method for intraoperative positioning of the nipple-areola complex in vertical scar reduction mammaplasty. Plast Reconstr Surg. 2000;105(6):2096-9.
6. Simone P, Carusi C, Palazzolo D, et al. An extremely simple and systematic approach to deepithelialization during breast reduction and mastopexy. Ann Plast Surg. 2007;58 (3):348-9.
7. Regnault P. Breast ptosis. Definition and treatment. Clin Plast Surg. 1976;3(2):193-203.
8. Spear SL, Howard MA. Evolution of the vertical reduction mammaplasty. Plast Reconstr Surg. 2003;112(3):855-68.
9. Spector JA, Kleinerman R, Culliford AT 4th, et al. The vertical reduction mammaplasty: a prospective analysis of patient outcomes. Plast Reconstr Surg. 2006;117(2):374-81.
10. Hidalgo DA. Vertical mammaplasty. Plast Reconstr Surg. 2005;115(4):1179-2297.
11. Giovanoli P, Meuli-Simmen C, Meyer VE, et al. Which technique for which breast? A prospective study of different techniques of reduction mammaplasty. Br J Plast Surg. 1999;52(1):52-59.
12. Chalekson CP, Neumeister MW, Zook EG, et al. Outcome analysis of reduction mammaplasty using the modified Robertson technique. Plast Reconstr Surg. 2002;110(1): 71-9.
13. Abramson DL, Pap S, Shifteh S, et al. Improving long-term breast shape with the medial pedicle wise pattern breast reduction. Plast Reconstr Surg. 2005;115(7):1937-43.
14. Persichetti P, Tenna S, Brunetti B, et al. Anterior intercostal artery perforator flap autologous augmentation in bariatric mastopexy. Plast Reconstr Surg. 2012;130(4):917-25.
15. Ribeiro L, Backer E. Mastoplastia: modificaciòn personal de la técnica. Prensa Med Argent. 1973;60:944-5.
16. Ribeiro L. A new technique for reduction mammaplasty. Plast Reconstr Surg. 1975;55(3):330-4.
17. Graf R, Biggs TM. In search of better shape in mastopexy and reduction mammaplasty. Plast Reconstr Surg. 2002;110(1):309-17.
18. Jones SA, Bain JR. Review of data describing outcomes that are used to assess changes in quality of life after reduction mammaplasty. Plast Reconstr Surg. 2001;108(1):62-7.
19. Hidalgo DA. Improving safety and aesthetic results in inverted T scar breast reduction. Plast Reconstr Surg. 1999; 103(3):874-86.

12 A Novel Approach in Male Breast Contouring after Massive Weight Loss: The Central Pedicled Breast Reduction Technique

Alexander Stoff, Fernando Velasco-Laguardia, Dirk F Richter

INTRODUCTION

Male patients after mild-to-massive weight loss often suffer from excess skin and excess fat tissue in the area of the anterior and lateral chest wall, presenting as pseudogynecomastia or gynecomastia. Pseudogynecomastia is characterized by increased retroareolar fat without enlargement of the mammary gland. In contrast, gynecomastia is a morphostructural impairment of the mammary region in men caused by parenchymal hypertrophy or a cutaneous distortion of breast skin covering or both.[1] Up to date, several schemes have been devised for the classification of gynecomastia.[2,3] Treatment of gynecomastia is dependent on the extent of mammary hypertrophy and the amount of skin excess, resulting in multiple methods such as combined liposuction with subcutaneous mastectomy, with or without excessive skin removal, in severe cases with free-nipple-areola grafting. In cases of gynecomastia with mild-to-moderate mammary hypertrophy and most cases of pseudogynecomastia, treatment options include free-nipple-areola grafting versus superiorly or inferiorly based pedicle techniques for nipple–areola preservation.[4,5] The more time-consuming pedicled transposition of the nipple–areola complex (NAC) allows for preservation of the neurovascular system with a more natural appearance without the risk of depigmentation.[5] Various excision patterns are available for removal of chest tissue excess in patients after mild-to-massive weight loss.[6,7] As a modification of the superiorly and inferiorly based pedicle in an horizontal elliptical chest wall excision pattern we have established a novel technique, based on a central pedicled NAC preservation, with simultaneous extensive liposuction of the pedicle and a wide elliptical excision pattern for anterior and lateral chest reshaping.[8]

PREOPERATIVE MANAGEMENT

Patients have to be informed prior to the operation regarding the technique in detail, the specific risks and complications, the resulting scar line, the possible postoperative variations of the scar line, and about all alternatives that could be performed. All patients have to sign an informed consent form with the indication of an optional free NAC grafting in case of an insufficient blood supply. All patients should be photo-documented preoperatively and 3 months postoperatively in a standard manner. Smokers have to be advised to refrain from smoking 6 latest 2 weeks prior to the procedure. Further the authors advise all patients to perform intensive training of the chest and shoulder muscles with main focus on the pectoralis major muscle for minimum 8 weeks preoperatively and starting earliest at 4 weeks postoperatively. Differential diagnosis of gynecomastia has to be excluded through preoperative palpation and mammography. Patient mobilization has to be forced at day one postoperatively and standard heparin is applied for thrombosis prophylaxis. Compression garments are fitted immediately postoperative with reduced compression during the initial 48 hours and worn for 8 weeks day and night.[8]

PREOPERATIVE MARKING

The patients' marking is performed while the patient is standing upright. During this phase, the patient can be actively involved in the planning of the resulting scar line and new NAC position, ideally faced to a mirror. First, the chest midline and a line from the mid-clavicular point down through the center of the NAC are marked. The resulting line should be located slightly lateral to the breast meridian. The submammary fold and upper breast margin are marked next. The submammary line has then to be continued laterally as an upward curve to the axillary crease at the posterior axillary line while the patient elevates his arm. The extent of redundant lateral chest tissue is estimated by manual pinching, which allows an optimal planning of the scar positioning. In cases of redundant skin and fat tissue in the upper abdomen, we advise to mark additional lower breast incision lines further inferiorly at the upper abdominal region for sufficient upper abdominal tissue tightening, again estimated through precise pinching (Fig. 12.1). This maneuver simulates best possible the expected tissue dynamics, which enables an optimal scar positioning at the lower pectoralis muscle margin. Supportingly at this timepoint, we ask the patient to constrict his pectoralis major muscle. The precise marking of a line running from the clavicular center inferior through the nipple–areola center and continuing inferiorly beyond the inferior incision line allows an optimal repositioning of the NAC, while the breast is pulled upward in standing position or while the patient lying down in supine position.[8]

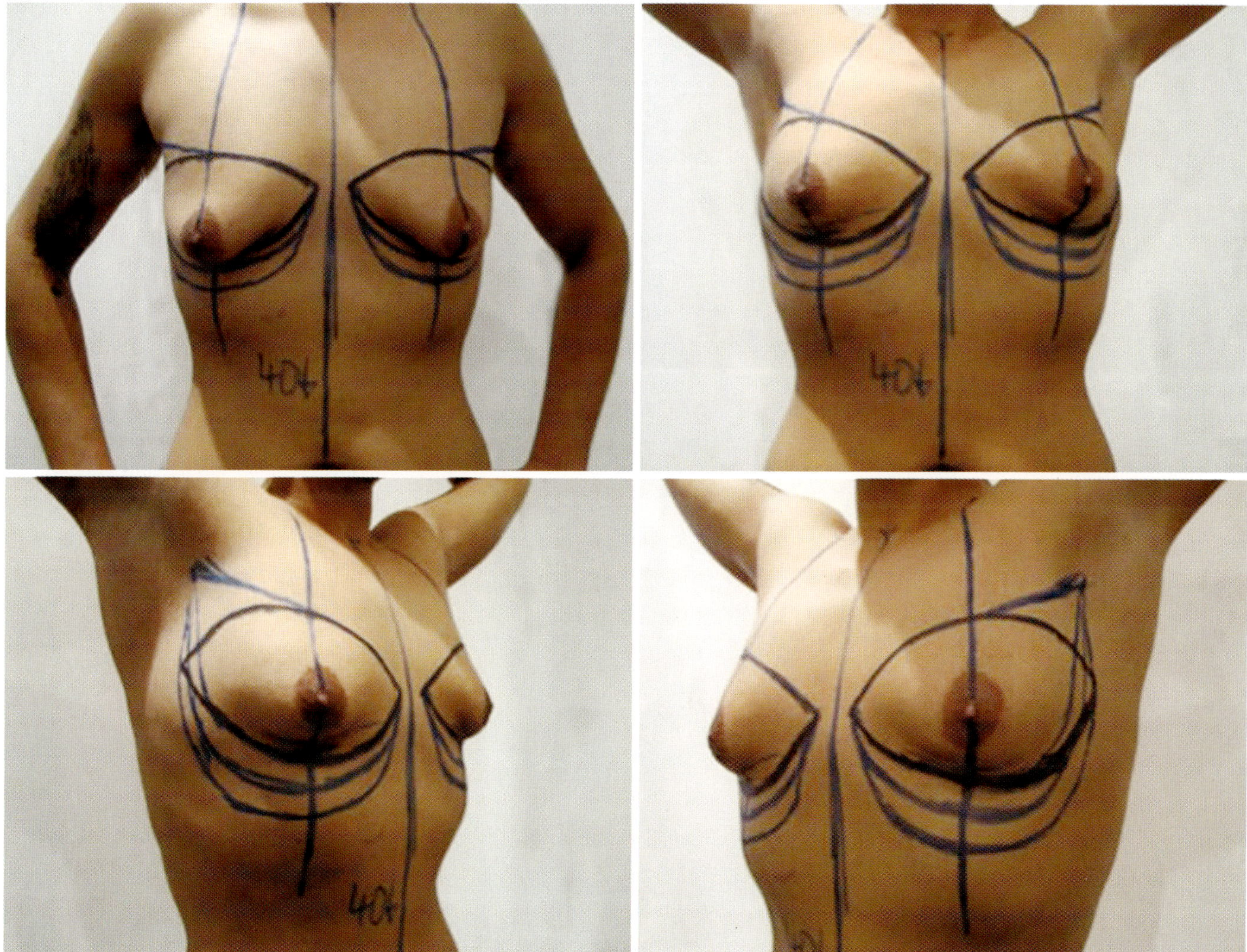

Fig. 12.1: Preoperative marking with the most important marking line running from the midclavicular point down through the existing nipple–areola complex (NAC) line and extending further caudally. This line allows a precise positioning of the new NAC in the vertical axis. In cases of NAC medialization, it should be raised cranially during marking to its original position. The black lines indicate the margins of the breast tissue, the blue lines demonstrate the upper and lower incision line for a full chest lift, including the breast, upper abdomen, and lateral thorax. The upper line position should be checked through downward movement to the submammary fold, the inferior line may vary for more or less reduction of the upper abdomen tissue, recognizing a caudal distraction of the resulting scar line. *Source*: Stoff A, Velasco-Laguardia FJ, Richter DF. Central pedicled breast reduction technique in male patients after massive weight loss. Obes Surg. 2012;22(3):445-51. Printed with kind permission from Springer.

SURGICAL TECHNIQUE (FIGS. 12.2 TO 12.11)

The operation is generally performed under general anesthesia, the patient lying in supine position and receiving a single-shot antibiotic therapy. For the marking of the central pedicle, it is advised to respect a pedicle diameter of 8–10 cm. The entire central pedicle and the entire marked excision pattern is then infiltrated with tumescence solution and consequently thinned out by extensive liposuction

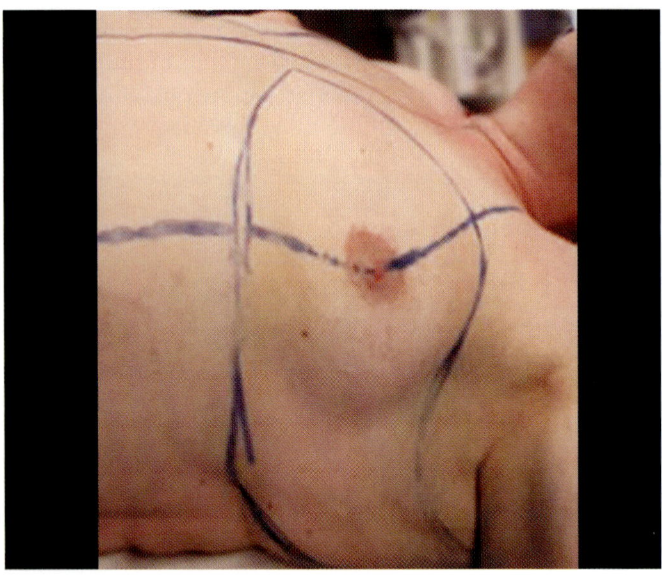

Fig. 12.2: Anterior and lateral chest lift.

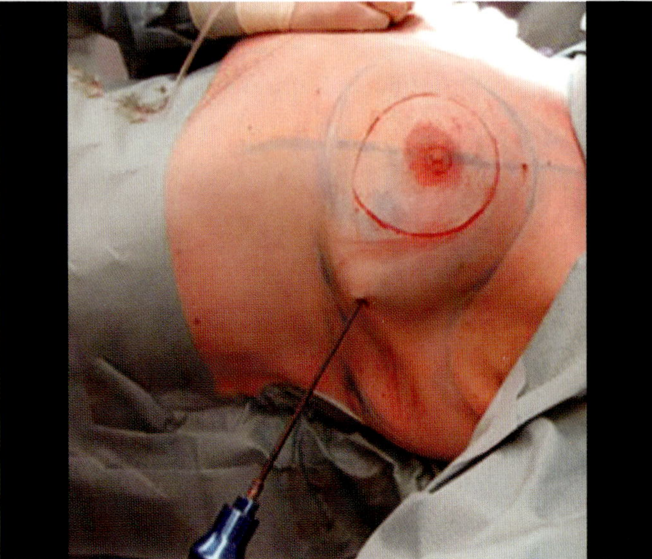

Fig. 12.3: Central breast reduction procedure. Infiltration of tumescence solution in the entire area of the excision pattern and the pedicle have already been performed. Vibration-assisted liposuction of the pedicle and entire excision area. The pedicle has been incised circularly with 8–10 cm in diameter.

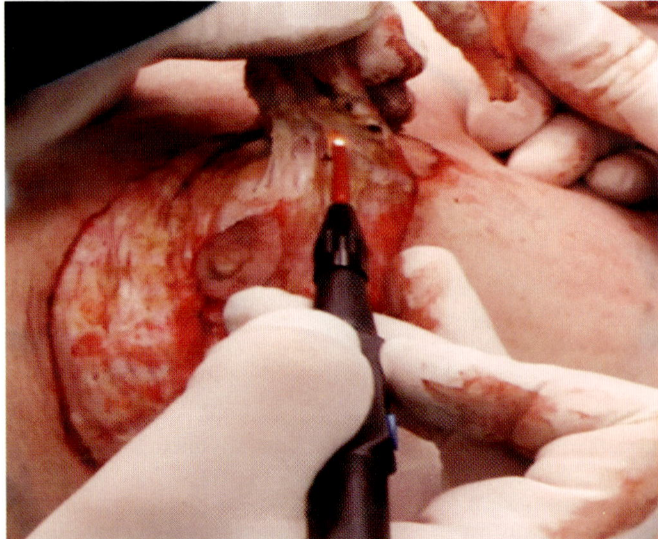

Fig. 12.4: The entire skin and adipose tissue preparation can easily be performed utilizing the Colorado microdissection. It has shown to be a perfect tool for de-epithelialization of the skin, since preparation time and dermal bleeding can be obviously reduced.

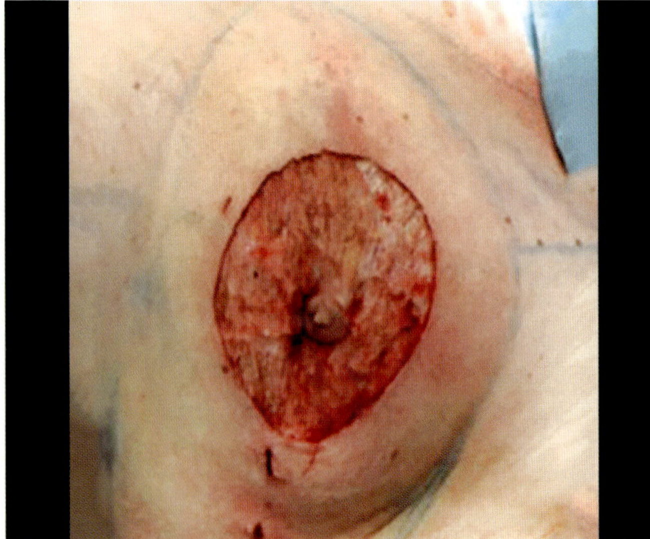

Fig. 12.5: De-epithelialization of the pedicle has been performed.

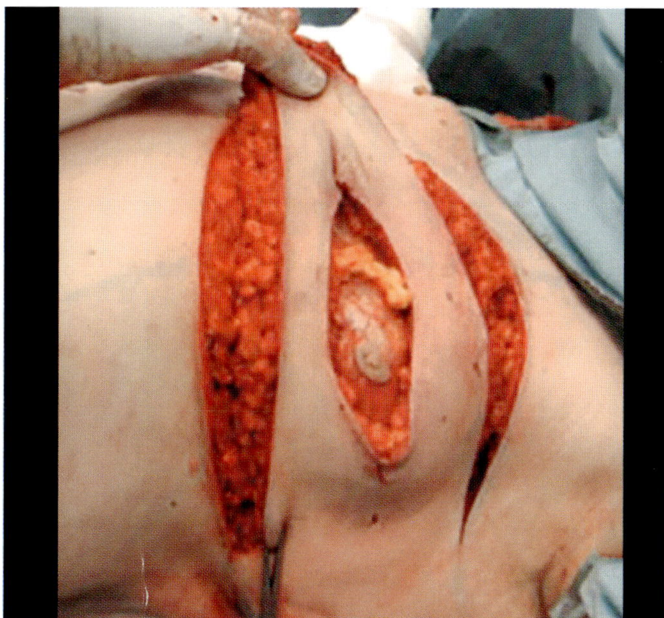

Fig. 12.6: The central pedicle has been prepared en bloc and mobilized from the redundant breast tissue.

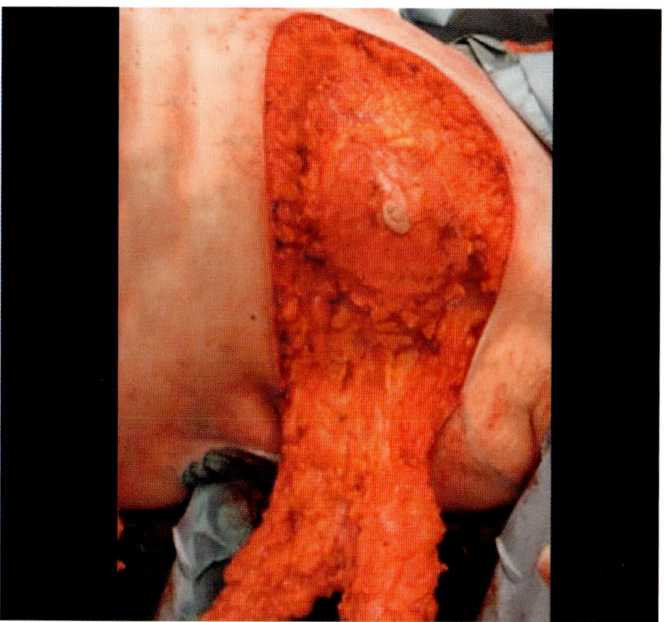

Fig. 12.7: The redundant tissue has been excised from medial to lateral, always ensuring a complete attachment of the central pedicle.

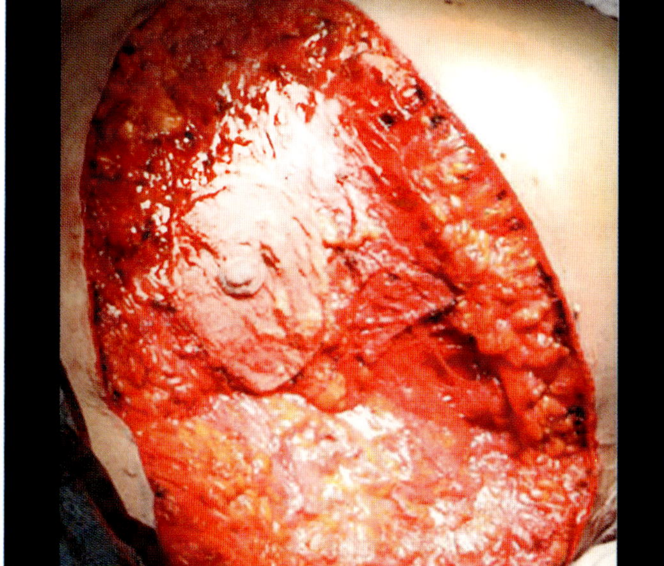

Fig. 12.8: The central pedicle is restored after total tissue resection. Fascial attachment has proved to be unnecessary.

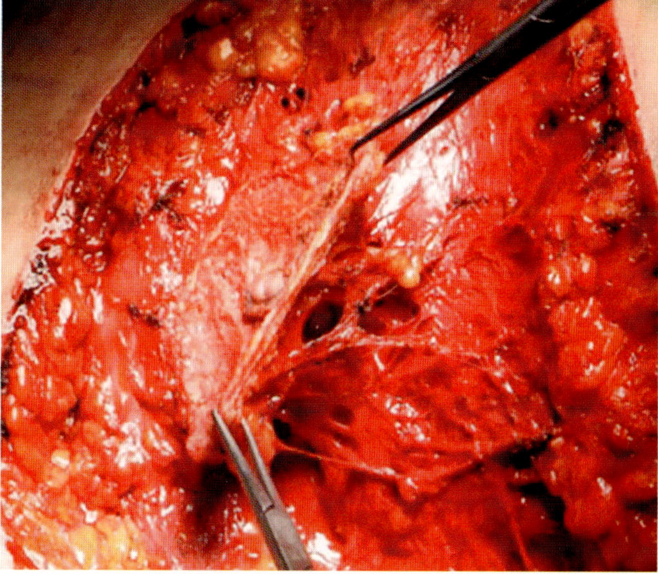

Fig. 12.9: An extensive, maximal possible liposuction of the entire pedicle has been performed without impairment of the blood perfusion. The remaining fibrous and vascular structures are obviously preserved.

(5 mm cannula), allowing a maximum reduction of the subcutaneous tissue with sole preservation of the dermal layer. In cases of glandular hypertrophy, thorough retromamillary liposuction is performed, utilizing a thinner cannula (3–4 mm). An adequate glandular reduction can be generally achieved. Next, the NAC is incised with a diameter of 2 cm (e.g. the stamp of a 20-mL syringe plunger top) and the entire pedicle is de-epithelialized, utilizing the Colorado microdissection needle. The pedicle is entirely mobilized down to the pectoralis major fascia.

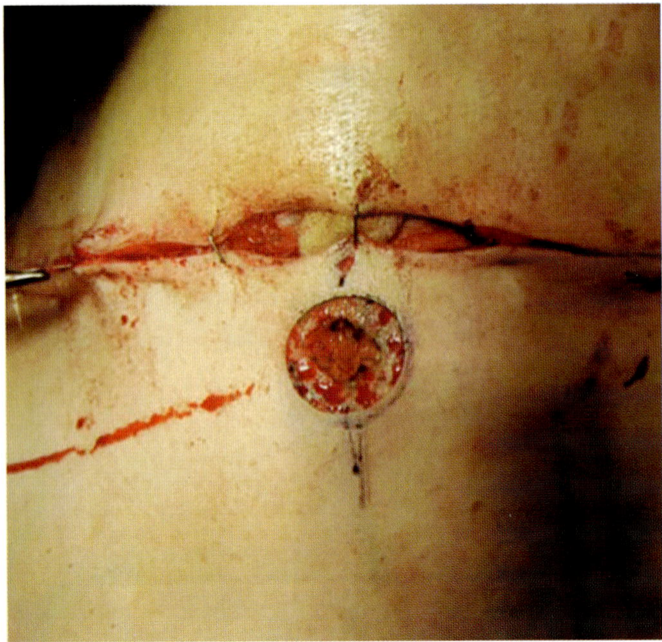

Fig. 12.10: After assessment of the new nipple–areola complex (NAC) position, the skin is de-epithelialized and an X-shaped dermal incision for integration of the nipple–areola complex is performed to avoid a distension of the NAC.

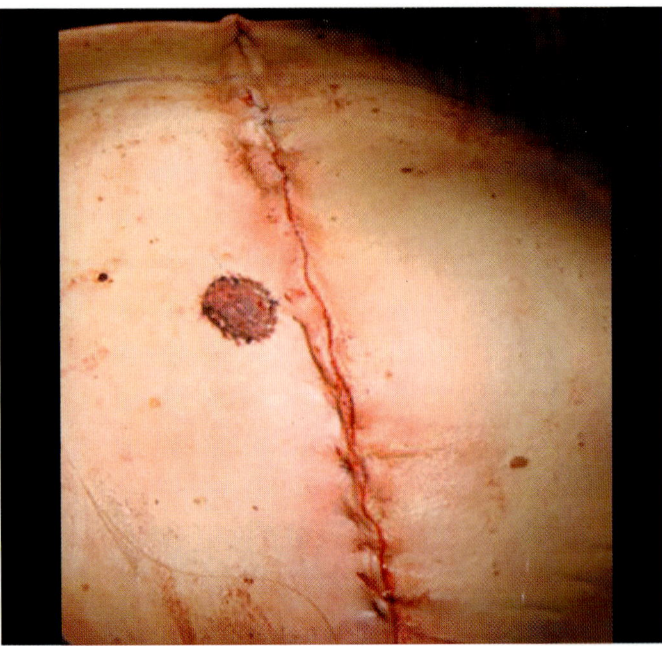

Fig. 12.11: Final wound closure is performed, including the insertion of the nipple–areola complex after an adequate perfusion is ensured. A blue discoloration can generally be observed at this stage of the procedure.

During this step, it is essential to respect the borderline of the pedicle, meaning to refrain from accidently mobilizing pedicle tissue. At this step of the procedure, an adequate perfusion of the pedicle lacks due to the persisting vascular constriction from tumescence solution. Continuing, the entire excision pattern is incised and mobilized from the underlying connective tissue, preserving the lymphatic structures in the lateral chest region. Intermittently, an adequate wound closure can be ensured by repetitive pinching.

Resection of the subfascial adipose layer above the latissimus dorsi is not done, since seroma formation due to the damage of lymphatic vessels may be more frequent. As an important step the fixation of the superficial fascia of the inferior skin flap to the pectoralis and serratus anterior fascia is then accomplished at the height of the lower pectoralis major muscle boundary. This maneuver will allow a secure positioning of the scar at the lower pectoralis muscle margin. The superior skin flap has to be mobilized cranially about 4–5 finger wide to allow an overlying on the central pedicle. During temporary wound closure utilizing staples, it is crucial to adapt wound edges accurately, connecting the central vertical line from the superior and the inferior skin flap. Next, the wound closure is performed from lateral and medial using absorbable 2–0 sutures for subcutaneous single knots, hereby sparing the central region.

At this time, blood perfusion of the NAC has to be checked. In case of insufficiency, a free nipple–areola transpositioning can now be achieved safely. The new NAC position is rechecked and marked on the vertical breast line, maintaining a diameter of maximal 2 cm (e.g. the stamp of a 20-mL syringe plunger top) and, as far as the patient agreed, a distance of approximately 2 cm from the lower NAC pole to the resulting scar line. De-epithelization is performed with the Colorado microdissection needle and the dermis is incised in a cross pattern to avoid maximal spreading when the nipple is inset and the tissue under maximal tension. Subcutaneous tissue in then excised in a cylindrical manner and the NAC is passed through the upper flap and sutured in place with nonresorbable 5–0 single knot and running sutures. Further wound closure is continued after drain insertion with subcutaneous resorbable 2–0 sutures in single knot and 3 × 0 intracuticular in running manner. A dark blue and sometimes white discoloration of the NAC at this step of the procedure may be observed, appearing not to be a reason for wariness.

DISCUSSION

Up to date, multiple classifications with treatment recommendations have been published for the treatment of gynecomastia and pseudogynecomastia including the lateral thoracic wall.[2,3,9-13]

The male chest deformity in patients after weight loss often presents a combination of excess skin and excess adipose tissue in the breast and lateral thoracic region. The deformities vary considerably in terms of shape, volume, and consistency of the excess tissue.

The ideal male breast consists of a trained and hypertrophic pectoralis major muscle and a NAC that is situated close above the submammary fold, which corresponds to the inferior border of the pectoralis major muscle. The course of the submammary fold in men is usually a curved line, starting lateral to the midline and descending on the way to the breast median, before ascending to the anterior axillary line. The position of the NAC in relation to the submammary fold has not received adequate consideration when determining the new location of the male NAC on the chest wall.[14-16]

Gusenoff et al.[5] have evaluated a poor aesthetic score of enlarged and ptotic NAC deformities in male breast deformities after massive weight loss and recommend a distance of 4–5 cm from the submammary fold or resulting scar, which should follow the silhouette of the pectoralis muscle.

In every individual case the extent of the surgical procedure has to be revealed to the patient. The resulting scar line has to be visualized by marking the expected scar line and the alternative procedures have to be discussed. Since most of these patients usually do not present a glandular hypertrophy, a subcutaneous mastectomy is not required. However, in cases of glandular hypertrophy an extensive liposuction of the glandular tissue can be safely performed.

The correction of gynecomastia and pseudogynecomastia after massive weight loss with elliptical tissue excision in the breast and lateral chest region can easily be performed with free NAC transfer, which excludes the need for pedicled transfers and minimizes the risk of tissue flap and NAC necrosis. A major disadvantage of free NAC grafting is the postoperative discoloration, unnatural stuck-on appearance and numbness of the transferred NAC.[17] Gusenoff et al. modified this technique utilizing an inferior pedicled dermoglandular nipple–areola transfer, evaluating a higher postoperative acceptance of pedicled NAC versus the free graft.[5] The scar course with this horizontal ellipse technique is placed at the level of the submammary fold without any additional vertical scars and can be combined with a lateral chest enhancement through an upper lateral thoracic lift (ULTL).[18,19] The technique with inferior pedicle can be performed in almost all cases, accept for patients with large distances between the NAC and the inferior incision, since the extended pedicle length may result in flap necrosis. In such cases, when the distance between the NAC and the upper incision is smaller than the distance between the NAC and the inferior incision, a superior pedicle for NAC transfer may be performed, nevertheless, precluding the ability of NAC positioning superior to the resulting scar.[4]

As a modified procedure of the horizontal ellipse technique, an NAC transfer on a central pedicle is established, which allows the implementation on almost every case, regardless of the degree of NAC ptosis and its position related to the superior and inferior incision line. Since a simultaneous extensive liposuction of the central pedicle is performed for significant volume reduction, a postoperative bulginess is excluded. In cases of associated glandular hypertrophy, the glandular tissue can be adequately eliminated, although liposuction of glandular tissue requires abundance of patience. In these cases, the authors emphasize the requirement of a preoperative mammography. For an optimal reinsertion of the NAC superior to the resulting scar and optimal wound closure, the authors recommend the preparation of a subcutaneous pocket for embedding of the pedicle by limited mobilization of the superior skin flap. A fixation of the pedicle dermis to the anterior pectoralis fascia has proven to be unnecessary, since the NAC reinsertion should correspond to the former position on the chest wall. For an adequate NAC positioning slightly above the inframammary fold, a distance of 2 cm from the lower pole caudal to the final horizontal scar line is measured. The adequate horizontal position refers to the preoperatively marked vertical NAC line, which varies in distance to the chest meridian and considers the ptosis process with possible NAC medialization (see Fig. 12.1). Conclusively, the ability of controlling the NAC perfusion during tissue excision and partial wound closure allows a safe insertion. Up to date, the authors have not experienced any partial or complete NAC loss. Further, a high postoperative patient satisfaction may allow us to recommend this modification of the horizontal ellipse technique as an effective and safe alternative in male breast and chest reconstruction procedures after mild-to-massive weight loss (Figs. 12.12 and 12.13).[8]

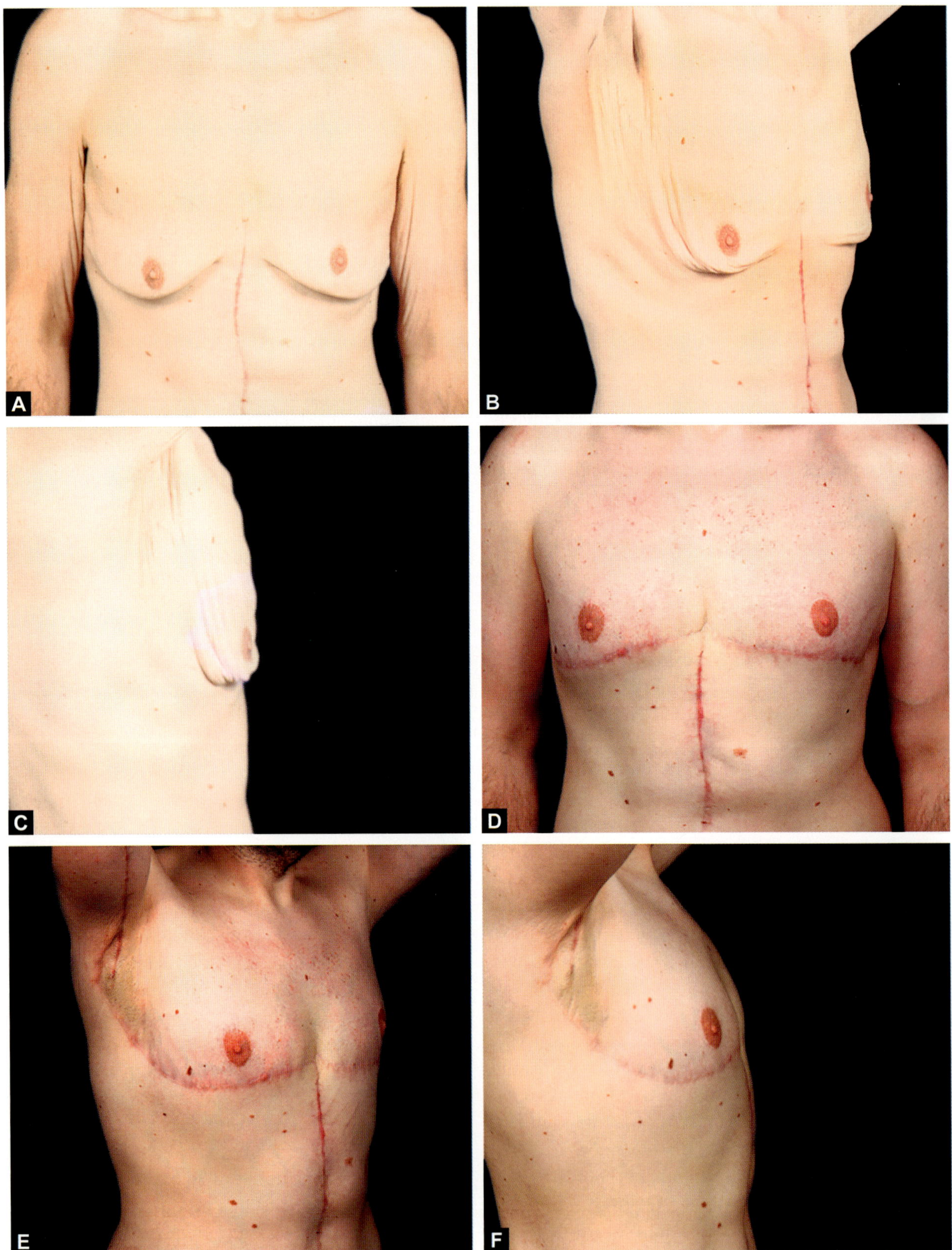

Figs. 12.12A to F: (A to C) Preoperative 40-year-old patient after 110 kg diet induced weight loss. (D to F) Twelve months postoperative.

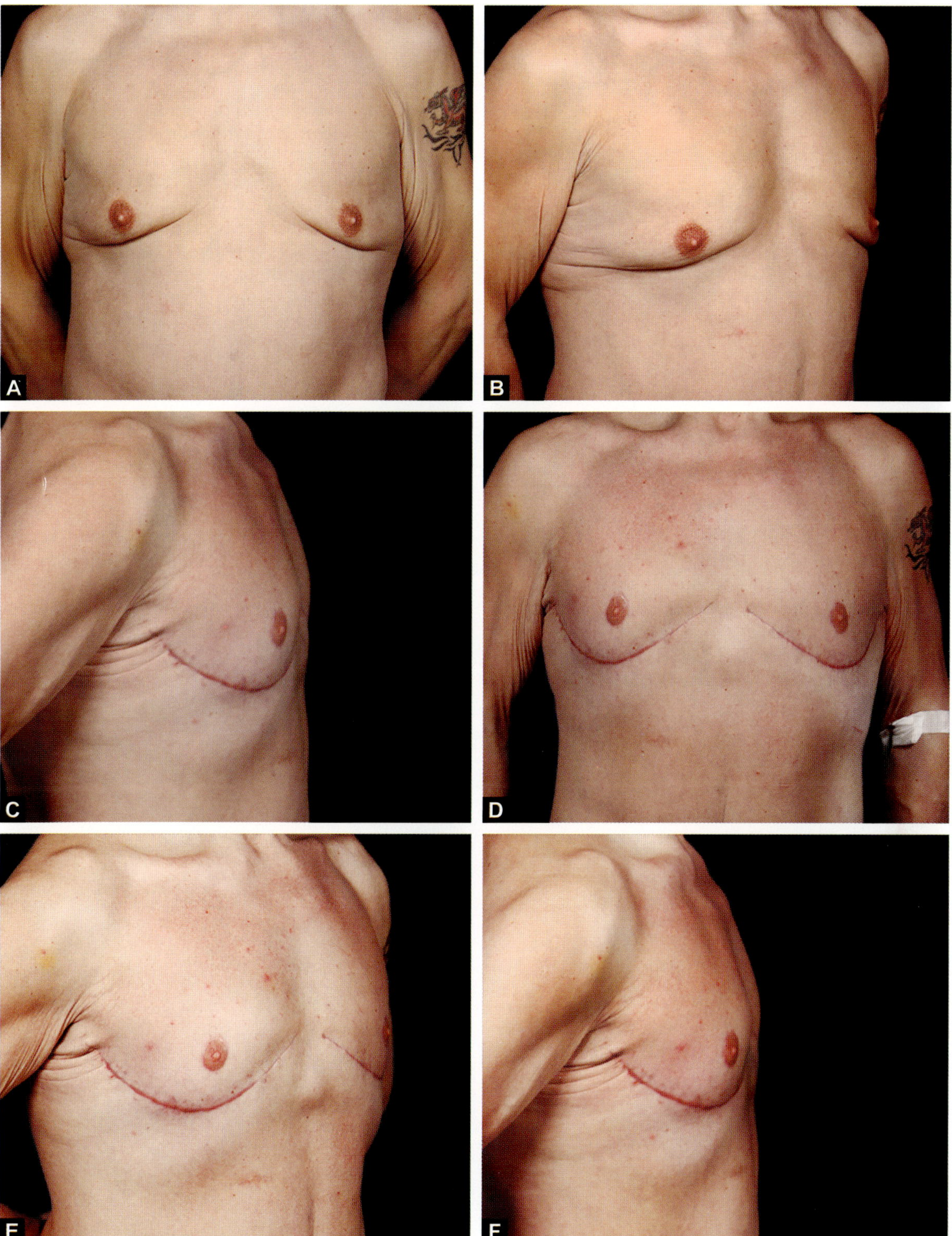

Figs. 12.13A to F: (A to C) Preoperative 49-year-old patient with gastric sleeve after 83 kg weight loss. (D to F) Four months post-operative. In this specific case, the patient refused a simultaneous extended lateral chest lift, since the skin excess in the lateral axillary region did not impair his daily life. Further, he preoperatively asked for a nipple–areola complex settled >2 cm above the resulting scar line.

REFERENCES

1. Braunstein GD. Cinical practice. Gynecomastia. N Engl J Med. 2007;357(12):1229-37.
2. Simon BE, Hoffman S, Kahn S. Classification of gynecomastia. Plast Reconstr Surg. 1973;51(1):48-52.
3. Rohrich R, Ha R, Kenkel J, Adams WP Jr. Classifications and management of gynecomastia: defining the role of ultrasound-assisted liposuction. Plast Reconstr Surg. 2003;111 (2):909-23.
4. Gheita A. Gynecomastia: the horizontal ellipse method for its correction. Aesthetic Plast Surg. 2008;32(5):795-801.
5. Gusenoff JA, Coon D, Rubin JP. Pseudogynecomastia after massive weight loss: detectability of technique, patient satisfaction, and classification. Plast Reconstr Surg. 2008; 122(5):1301-11.
6. Aly AS. Body Contouring after massive weight loss. St Louis, MO: Quality Medical Publishing; 2006.
7. Stoff A, Reichenberger MA, Richter DF. Male breast contouring after massive weight loss. Handchir Mikrochir Plast Chir. 2006;38(4):209-16.
8. Stoff A, Velasco-Laguardia FJ, Richter DF. Central pedicled breast reduction technique in male patients after massive weight loss. Obes Surg. 2012;22(3):445-51.
9. Hodgson EL, Fruhstorfer BH, Malata CM. Ultrasonic liposuction in the treatment of gynecomastia. Plast Reconstr Surg. 2005;116(2):646-53.
10. Tashkandi M, Al-Qattan MM, Hassanain JM, et al. The surgical management of high grade gynecomastia. Ann Plast Surg. 2004;53(1):17-20.
11. Kornstein AN, Cinelli PB. Inferior pedicle reduction technique for larger forms of gynecomastia. Aesthetic Plast Surg. 1992;16(4):331-5.
12. Persichetti P, Berloco M, Casadei RM, et al. Gynecomastia and the complete circumareolar approach in the surgical management of skin redundancy. Plast Reconstr Surg. 2001;107(4):948-54.
13. Song AY, Jean RD, Hurwitz DJ, et al. A classification of contour deformities after bariatric weight loss: the Pittsburgh rating scale. Plast Reconstr Surg. 2005;116(5):1535-44.
14. Beckenstein MS, Windle BH, Stroup RT Jr. Anatomical parameters for nipple position and areolar diameter in males. Ann Plast Surg. 1996;36(1):33-6.
15. Beer GM, Budi S, Seifert B, et al. Configuration and localization of the nipple-areola complex in men. Plast Reconstr Surg. 2001;108(7):1947-52.
16. Shulman O, Badani E, Wolf Y, et al. Appropriate location of the nipple-areola complex in males. Plast Reconstr Surg. 2001;108(2):348-51.
17. Mladick RA, Hunstad JP, Pitman GH, et al. Practice forum: male body contouring. Aesthetic Surg J. 2006;26(3):307-3136.
18. Richter DF, Wynands JF, Stoff A. The upper lateral thoracic lift (ULTL). Plastic Surgery Pulse News. September 2010;2(1):1-3. Available from http://www.plasticsurgerypulsenews.com/2/article_dtl.php?QnCategoryID=18&QnArticleID=42&QnCurPage=2. Accessed May 30, 2013.
19. Richter DF, Stoff A. Back and lateral fold contouring. In: Nahai F (Ed). The Art of Aesthetic Surgery: Principles and Techniques, 2nd edition. St Louis, MO: Quality Medical Publishing; 2010.

Section 5

Body

Chapter Outline

- Perforator Flaps for Pressure Sore Treatment
- Gluteal Perforator Flaps for Coverage of Pressure Sores
- Using Radiofrequency Energy for Heat-Mediated Tissue Tightening: Minimally Invasive and Noninvasive Modalities

13 Perforator Flaps for Pressure Sore Treatment

Luca Grassetti, Matteo Torresetti, Matteo Gioacchini, Manuela Bottoni, Alessandro Scalise, Giovanni Di Benedetto

INTRODUCTION

Several strategies for closure have been attempted in the past in pressure sores surgery. The temptation to perform a primary closure should be resisted. By definition, a pressure sore has an absolute tissue deficiency and simply pulling tissue together over a bony prominence will almost surely lead to tension and dehiscence. Skin grafting has been attempted with limited success because of the lack of bulk and poor durability in the face of the pressure and shearing forces. More successful strategies include the use of a variety of local flaps, such as musculocutaneous and fasciocutaneous flaps, each of them having its advantages. Most flap coverage strategies use pedicled flaps. Alternatively, a number of surgeons have advocated the use of free tissue transfer to address multiply recurrent pressure sores (common donors are the latissimus dorsi and serratus anterior muscles).

Muscle flaps have significant bulk and excellent blood supply. They therefore can be useful where a significant soft tissue defect is present and also where a history of infection is a consideration. On the downside, muscle is susceptible to ischemic injury. Fasciocutaneous flaps are durable, maintain good blood supply, are less susceptible to ischemia, and are closer to the normal anatomical tissue arrangement.[1] Indeed, all pressure points in the human body are covered by fasciocutaneous tissue alone, not by muscle.[2] Thus, they are especially useful in wounds of limited depth, as are many in the sacral area. However, they become less useful if significant filling of dead space is required.[1]

The clinical data described by the literature demonstrate that the use of myocutaneous flaps for reconstruction of a complicated pressure sore has greatly reduced the incidence of early postoperative complications.[3–5] However, good long-term results with muscle-flap coverage of pressure sores cannot be expected because the muscle portion in the transferred myocutaneous or muscle flaps shows remarkable atrophic changes clinically, and a high incidence of muscle necrosis in response to pressure without cutaneous necrosis was significantly noted in the animal studies.[6,7] Furthermore, muscle flaps leave the donor area exposed to new ulcer occurrences because of the absence of a sort of "pillow" effect on the loading surface created by the vascularized myocutaneous unit.[1] Recent reports show no differences in outcome between the use of fasciocutaneous and muscle flap,[8,9] and one study reported even better results for fasciocutaneous flaps likely due to the less susceptibility to ischemia of this type of flaps.[10] Yamamoto et al. in 1997[11] concluded that because early wound closure and absence of recurrence over long periods should be required in the surgical management of pressure ulcers, the use of myocutaneous or muscle flaps is inadequate over the long term because of the recurrence rate of 63% compared to the 27.8% recurrence rate for fasciocutaneous flaps.

Available local flap options are limited in number and must be cautiously preserved as long as possible for these patients who are destined to have a lifelong vulnerability for recurrence.

In the last decades, perforator flaps have been introduced for the treatment of sacral, ischial, and trochanteric pressure ulcers. Since their introduction, perforator flaps have occasionally been used as an alternative option for achieving reliable wound coverage without sacrificing muscle tissue.[12] After the initial enthusiasm for their use, a lot of concerns were raised regarding their reliability for pressure ulcers, particularly for their ability to provide adequate soft tissue bulk and lengthening of the operatory time. These flaps limit donor site morbidity and better achieve flap mobility and viability when compared to a pedicled fasciocutaneous flap.

The most common perforator flaps performed in the authors' practice were the inferior gluteal artery perforator (IGAP) flap, followed by the superior gluteal artery perforator (SGAP) flap, first or second perforator of the profunda femoris artery flap (PFAP-1, PFAP-2), and first medial perforator of the profunda femoris artery perforator (PFAP-am) flap.

PREOPERATIVE AND POSTOPERATIVE MANAGEMENT

All patients are examined preoperatively, and the perforating vessels are marked on the skin with the assistance of a handheld 8 MHz Doppler ultrasound scanner. When a perforator could not be found, you have to use a traditional flap. In very few cases, a reliable perforator pedicle could not be identified intraoperatively when a Doppler signal was present preoperatively. In such cases, you have to convert the design to a salvage traditional pedicled flap.

All flaps are raised in the subfascial layer because the procedure is quicker and very straightforward in patients with tissues of poor quality and to allow a flap-raising time comparable to that of local pedicled flaps. As standard procedure, after injecting methylene blue into the pressure sore bursa, the sore is accurately removed and the bony base accurately debrided by high-pressure water with VersaJet (Smith & Nephew Medical Limited, Hull HU3 2BN, England). A bone biopsy is carried out with a sterile osteotome and sent for a bone culture to guide the appropriate antibiotic therapy. The area is disinfected again before proceeding to immediate reconstruction.

After an initial exploratory incision to locate the perforators, the closest free scar and granulation tissue is chosen and the flap design is rechecked and eventually slightly moved. The flap is elevated and the pedicle skeletonized by dissecting all its fascial strands and muscle arborizations from its origin from the source vessel up to the point where it pierced the deep fascia to enter the flap. The flap is then completed and papaverine is applied and left in place for 10 minutes around the pedicle to avoid vasospasm and to allow adequate perfusion. When the flap perfusion is satisfactory, the flap could be advanced or rotated into the defect. The use of a flap in which the design allowed the donor-site primary closure without tension is recommended. Two big caliber suction drains are usually inserted underneath the flap and secured far from the pedicle.

All patients should always receive the same preoperative and postoperative protocol management: the same outpatient care team provides an adequate wound bed preparation; a urologist is consulted to assess bladder status and urinary catheter management; a plain pelvic radiogram is obtained to assess osteomyelitis and bone fractures; the same in-patient nursing team and physician team under the guidance of the same physical medicine and rehabilitation team took care of the patients. Both passive and active ranging of the uninvolved extremities and upper body strengthening exercises are initiated in the immediate postoperative setting and are performed regularly during the immobilization period. For 2–3 weeks after operation, air-fluidized-bed rest (KCI International, 8023 Vantage Drive, San Antonio, TX, USA) is used in all patients. Only patients with positive bone culture receive an antibiogram-guided antimicrobial therapy during their hospital stay. All patients have a consultation with a nutritionist team to determine the appropriate nutritional program, and the same outpatient team followed up all the patients after hospital discharge.

Supervised by Physical Medicine and Rehabilitation Services, the patient's progress through a graduated 7- to 10-day sitting regimen at home until they achieved an upright seated posture on properly padded wheelchairs for a 3-hour period per day. Wound status should be repeatedly assessed throughout the progressive mobilization period. Pressure-release maneuvers are taught and then performed at 15-minute intervals by the patients while seated.

SUPERIOR GLUTEAL ARTERY PERFORATOR FLAP

Allen and Tucker, in 1995,[13] described an alternative technique of skin/fat flap transfer from the buttock with a long vascular pedicle without gluteus maximus muscle sacrifice. The flap is based on the superior gluteal artery perforators and accordingly is called the SGAP flap or superior gluteal artery perforator flap. The SGAP flap differs from both previously described myocutaneous flap by eliminating the muscle component and by providing a much longer vascular pedicle. Gluteus maximus muscle function and bulk were preserved with a muscle-splitting approach (this is particularly important in nonparalyzed patients). It was also recognized that as dissection of the vascular structures proceeded through the muscle, the length of the pedicle increased significantly.

Koshima et al.[14] first described the pedicled SGAP flap for use in pressure sore treatment. Use of the superior gluteal artery perforator flap preserves the entire contralateral side as a future donor site. On the ipsilateral side, the gluteal muscle itself is preserved and all flaps based on the inferior gluteal artery are still possible. This flap is recommended in an area where reconstructive possibilities are limited, as it preserves other reconstructive flap options, both on the ipsilateral and contralateral sides.[15] This flap can be used in sacral reconstruction.

Since the advent of perforator flaps, harvesting flaps from the gluteal region without inclusion of Gluteus Maximus muscle has supplanted Gluteus Maximus muscle flaps in most reconstructions because the gluteal perforator flaps have the following advantages:

1. Better intraoperative exposure, less blood loss, and a longer vascular pedicle compared to its myocutaneous predecessor. The length of the pedicle gives the flap an appropriate arch of rotation and allows for easy tissue transposition without tension.
2. *Satisfactory quality of the tissues*: In the case of a pedicled flap, the tissues used in the gluteal perforator flap come from a further distance from the ulcer or wound and, as such, they are less inflamed, less edematous, and less prone to dehiscence. The inset of the flap is always tension free and the donor site can always be closed primarily.
3. *Reduced donor site morbidity*: This itself will lead to a shorter hospital stay and therefore reduced costs.
4. *The potential for a neurosensory flap*: The possibility of including a sensate branch of the nervi clunium superiores within a gluteal perforator flap provides better quality and quantity of sensation to the flap in nonparalyzed patients.[16]

Vascular Anatomy

The superior gluteal artery is a terminal branch of the internal iliac artery and exits the pelvis through the greater sciatic foramen. Its length ranges from 2 to 3 cm and its diameter ranges from 2 to 3 mm. Veins usually accompany the arteries. The superior gluteal vein receives multiple tributaries from other pelvic veins at the level of entering the pelvis. After its exit, the superior gluteal artery divides into superficial and deep branch. The superficial branch continues above the pyriformis muscle into the gluteus maximus muscle. As it travels toward the skin surface, the artery divides into multiple branches (average of four) that perforate the muscle and go on to supply the overlying angiosome.

The perforating vessels travel in superior and lateral directions. The intramuscular length for these vessels is 4–5 cm, depending on thickness of the gluteus muscle mass. The perforating vessels that supply the medial portions of the skin paddle travel in a strictly superior direction toward the skin surface. Perforators that supply the lateral portions of the skin paddle travel through the muscle substance in a more horizontal manner for 4–6 cm before turning upward toward the skin surface. The perforating vessels can be separated from the gluteus maximus muscle and the fascia and traced down to the parent vessel, forming the basis for the superior gluteal artery perforator flap. The length of the superior gluteal artery perforator and the resultant pedicle length for the overlying SGAP flap range from 5 to 7 cm.

Flap Design

Markings are placed on the patient in the prone position. The posterior superior iliac spine and the great trochanter are palpated and marked; a line connecting these two points is drawn. Perforator pedicles are located adjacent to the medial two thirds of these lines.

Common surgical practice is to harvest the superior gluteal artery perforator flap as an ellipse, as this geometry lends itself more easily to primary closure.[17] The skin paddle is marked in an oblique pattern from inferior medial to superior lateral to include these perforators (Figs. 13.1A and B). However, its orientation can vary from being angled upward or downward along the previously marked line to a more horizontal orientation. The outline of the flap may be modified to almost any orientation, as long as it contains the perforating vessels. The flap can be designed 7–12 cm wide (average width of 10 cm) and 20–30 cm long (average length of 24 cm).

Flap Harvesting

In the case of a perforator flap, a fusiform skin island is drawn over the perforators, ideally centered on selected perforators. The position of the gluteal vessels can be identified using a handheld 5–8 MHz Doppler. The main perforators for SGAP flap are localized in an area above the pyriform muscle. Choice of the perforator depends on the strength of the Doppler signal but also on the location of the perforator. Choosing the most remotely located perforator from the SGA exit will provide a longer pedicle to reach the defect easily.

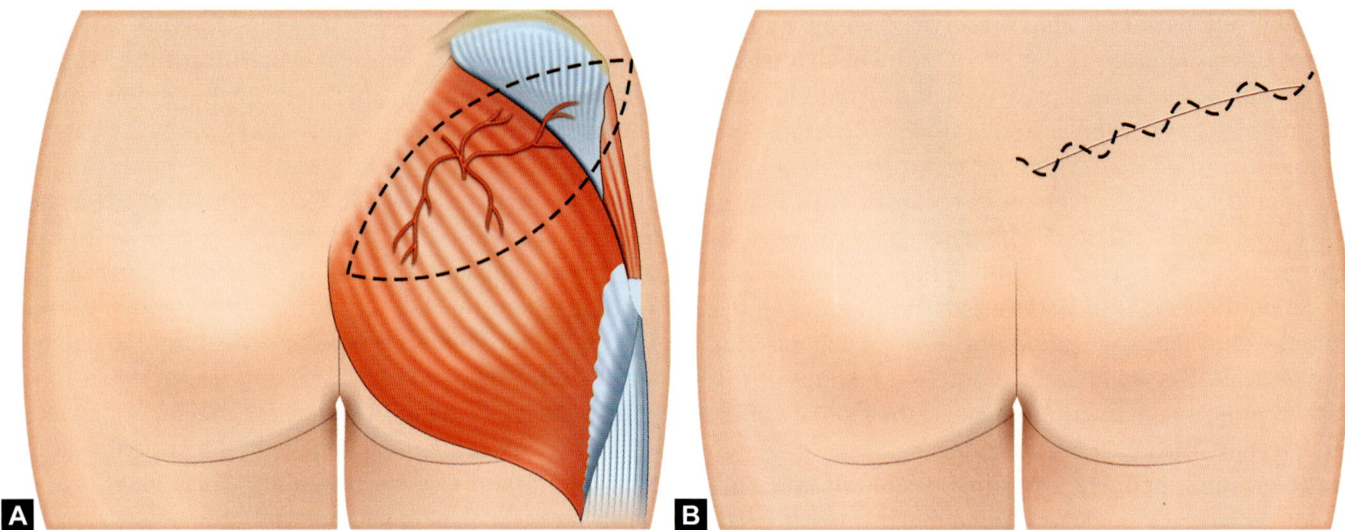

Figs. 13.1A and B: SGA-P flap design and closure of donor site.
Source: From Wei FC, Mardini S (Eds). Flaps and Reconstructive Microsurgery. Philadelphia, PA: Saunders Elsevier Inc; 2009.

The flap is dissected and transferred as a transposition flap but it is designed in such a way that it can be converted to a rotation flap if no perforators are found. The flap is then advanced or rotated 90° to cover the defect and the donor site is closed primarily.[16]

Case Report

This tetraplegic 61-year-old male patient had a sacral third stage pressure sore, without spontaneous healing despite advanced dressings (Figs. 13.2A to F). The patient underwent to three cycles of VAC therapy to clean the bottom of the lesion and afterward to surgical excision of the lesion after marking of the pressure sore bursa with methylene blue. Surgical debridement was completed with high-pressure water. The patient underwent to immediate reconstruction by using a superior gluteal artery perforator flap with a rotation of 90°. Primary closure of the donor site was performed. No recurrence at 2 years.

INFERIOR GLUTEAL ARTERY PERFORATOR FLAP

Le-Quang[18] was the first to describe the use of an inferior gluteal musculocutaneous free flap in 1979 and published his work in 1992. To circumvent some of the drawbacks of myocutaneous flaps, an alternative method for harvesting gluteal tissue was performed by Allen and Tucker in 1993.[13] The same technique initially applied to the SGAP flap was then applied in 2002 by Higgins et al.[19] with equal success, to the inferior gluteal vasculature for the realization of the IGAP flap.

This flap has the same advantages of the SGAP flap. Furthermore, it has other important characteristics: uses excess lower buttock tissue with a cosmetic location of the scar (leaves the scar in the natural depression of the inferior gluteal crease), reliable anatomy, ubiquitous donor site with good volume, firm consistency of the fat for extra padding. Pedicled IGAP flaps could be used for ischial pressure sores.

Vascular Anatomy

The inferior gluteal artery is a terminal branch of the anterior division of the internal iliac artery and exits the pelvis through the greater sciatic foramen. Landmarks can also be used to identify the location of the emergence of the inferior gluteal artery outside the pelvis. A line is drawn from the posterior superior iliac spine to the outer part of the ischial tuberosity; the junction of its lower third with its middle third marks the point of emergence of the inferior gluteal and its surrounding vessels from the lower part of the greater sciatic foramen. The inferior gluteal vasculature continues toward the surface by perforating the sacral fascia. It exits the pelvis caudal to the pyriformis muscle. Once under the inferior portion of the gluteus maximus, perforating vessels are seen branching out through the substance of the muscle to feed the overlying skin and fat. The course of the inferior gluteal artery perforating vessels is more oblique through the substance of the gluteus

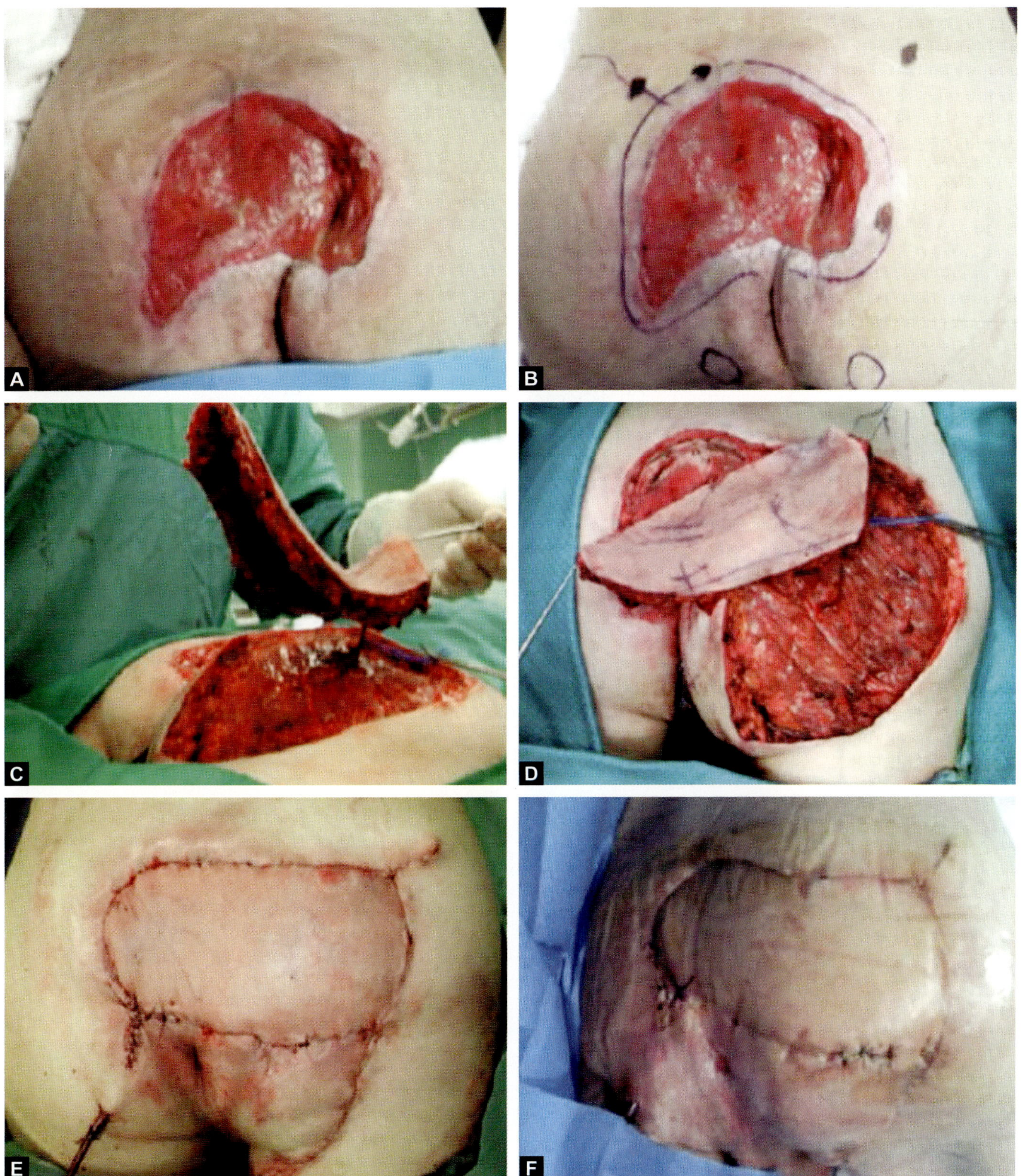

Figs. 13.2A to F: A 61-year-old man with a sacral third stage pressure sore. (A) Sacral pressure sore after wound bed preparation by using advanced dressings and VAC therapy. (B) Marking of perforators of superior gluteal artery. (C) SGAP flap raised on a single muscle perforator. (D) Flap coverage of the sacral defect. (E) Immediate postoperative. (F) Two-week postsurgery.

maximus muscle than the course of the superior gluteal artery perforators, which tend to travel more directly to the superficial tissue up through the muscle. Thus, the length of the inferior gluteal artery perforator and the resultant pedicle length for the overlying IGAP flap (7–10 cm) are greater than found with an SGAP flap (5–7 cm). Between two and four perforating vessels originating from the inferior gluteal artery will be located in the lower half of the gluteus maximus. After giving off perforators in the buttocks, the inferior gluteal artery then descends into the thigh.[16] Ninety-nine percent of the inferior gluteal artery perforators are musculocutaneous and all perforators pass through the gluteus maximus muscle.

The average cutaneous vascular territory of the inferior gluteal artery in the gluteal region is about 177 ± 38 cm^2 (69 ± 56 cm^2 for the superior gluteal artery). Each perforator of the inferior gluteal artery supplies an area (perforator zone) of 24 ± 13 cm^2 (21 ± 8 cm^2 for the superior gluteal artery). The inferior gluteal artery perforators are mostly located in the horizontal middle third of the gluteal region parallel to the gluteal crease. Inferior gluteal artery perforators can be also found at approximately 5 cm superior to the lateral third of the gluteal crease.[20]

Flap Design

A line is drawn from the greater trochanter to the middle of the distance between the posterior superior iliac spine and the medial border of the gluteal crease. Perforators are located on the marked areas. The flap is designed as a horizontal ellipse with the axis centered above the gluteal crease (Figs. 13.3A and B). The inferior incision is then drawn parallel to the crease and 2–4 cm inferior to it.

The superior aspect of the skin island ellipse is then marked to capture these perforators. The orientation of the skin paddle usually parallels the inferior gluteal crease. The flap can be designed 7–12 cm wide and 20–26 cm long. Depending on the amount of skin needed and the amount of excess buttock tissue available, the design of each flap varies accordingly.[16]

Flap Harvesting

A line is drawn from the greater trochanter to the middle of the distance between the posterior superior iliac spine and the medial border of the gluteal crease. Perforators are located on the marked areas. With the patient in the lateral decubitus position, a handheld Doppler probe is used to locate perforating vessels to the skin. Choice of the perforator depends not only on the strength of the Doppler signal but also on the location of the perforator. An elliptic skin paddle is drawn to include the desirable perforators with the final shape having a longer length of the superior limb than the inferior limb and dissection proceeds as for a standard perforator flap.[16,20]

Case Reports

1. This paraplegic 53-year-old male patient had a sacral fourth stage pressure sore, without spontaneous healing despite advanced dressings (Figs. 13.4A to H). The patient underwent surgical excision of the lesion after marking of the pressure sore bursa with methylene

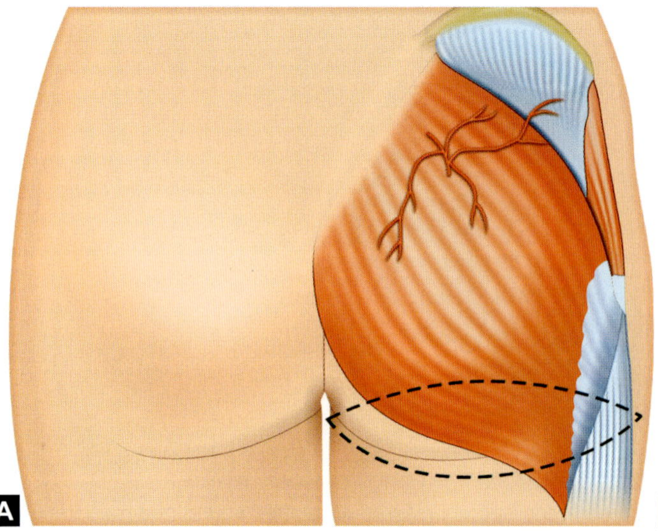

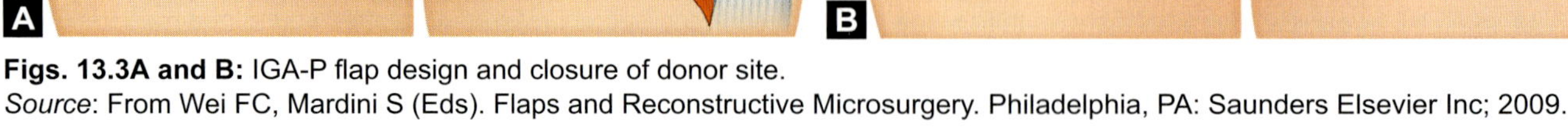

Figs. 13.3A and B: IGA-P flap design and closure of donor site.
Source: From Wei FC, Mardini S (Eds). Flaps and Reconstructive Microsurgery. Philadelphia, PA: Saunders Elsevier Inc; 2009.

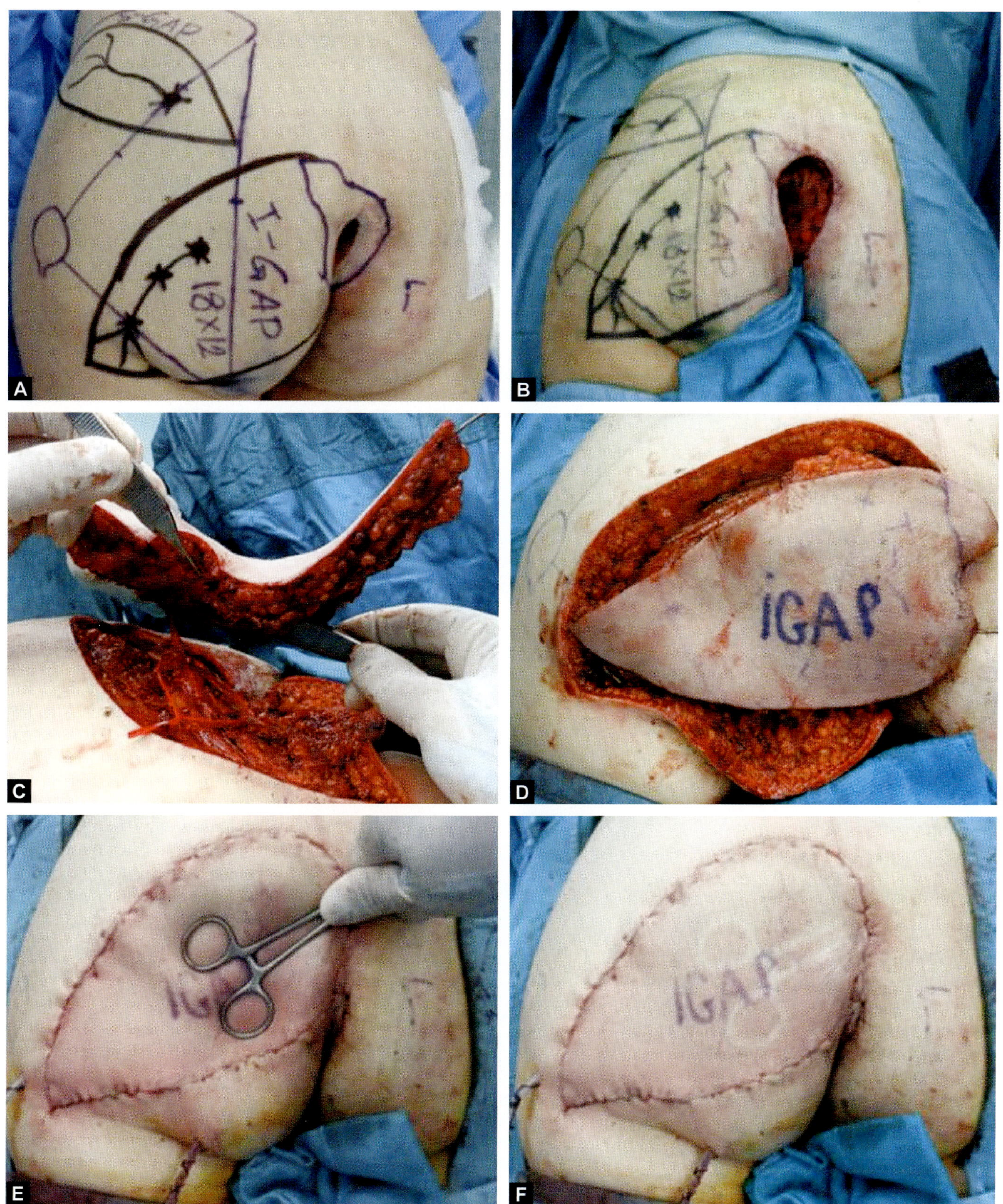

Figs. 13.4A to F

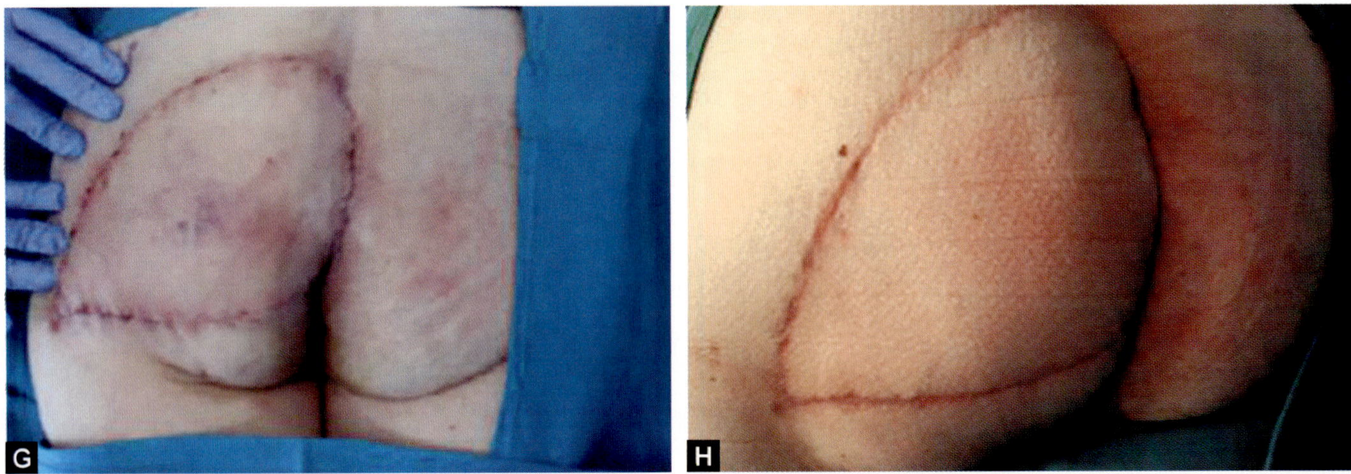

Figs. 13.4A to H: A 52-year-old female with late-stage sacral pressure sore. (A) Marking of typical SGAP and IGAP flaps. (B) The lesion has been resected. (C) IGAP flap raised on a single muscle perforator. (D) Flap coverage of the sacral defect. (E and F) Capillary refill sign, with two drains in place. (G) Two-week follow-up showing excellent color texture match. (H) Four-week follow-up.

blue. Surgical debridement was completed with high-pressure water. Immediate reconstruction by using an IGAP flap with V-Y advancement was performed. Primary closure of the donor site was possible. No recurrence at 1 year.

2. This paraplegic 48-year-old male patient had an ischial fourth stage pressure sore, without spontaneous healing despite advanced dressings (Figs. 13.5A to D). The patient underwent surgical excision of the lesion after marking of the pressure sore bursa with methylene blue. Surgical debridement was completed with high-pressure water. Immediate reconstruction by using an IGAP flap. Primary closure of the donor site was possible. No recurrence at 1 year.

POSTERIOR THIGH PERFORATOR FLAPS

The posterior thigh region is loosely defined as a region bordered by the inferior gluteal fold superiorly, the iliotibial tract laterally, the thigh adductors medially, and the popliteal fossa inferiorly. The thigh donor site has been used extensively for microsurgical tissue transfer; however, the posterior thigh has been somewhat neglected as a potential donor site.

The posterior thigh flap was first described in 1980 by Hurwitz.[21] It was transferred as a free flap by Song et al.[22] in 1984, and it has been used as a pedicled flap, a pedicled island flap and a free flap. Cadaver studies have shown that the dominant blood supply to the posterior thigh is from the profunda femoris artery perforators (PFAPs).[23]

The profunda femoris branches off the lateral side of the femoral artery and passes posteriorly between the adductor longus and pectineus muscles to enter the posterior compartment of the thigh. It runs distally and gives medial and lateral branches. The medial branches enter the adductor compartment. The lateral branches, or perforating arteries, are usually three and enter the lateral compartment of the thigh by piercing the adductor magnus muscle insertion; the profunda femoris artery ends as the fourth perforating artery. The first perforating artery gives branches to the adductor muscles and the gracilis. The second and third perforating arteries supply the semimembranosus, biceps femoris, and vastus lateralis muscles. All of these perforating arteries give rise to musculocutaneous and/or septocutaneous perforators. Cadaver studies have shown that most perforators could be found on a line extending from the ischium to the lateral femoral condyle. The most proximal perforators were located at the inferior gluteal fold, and the most distal perforators were found on average 10 cm proximal to the lateral femoral condyle (Fig. 13.6). These perforators could be readily used for perforator skin flap harvest.

FIRST AND SECOND PERFORATOR OF THE PROFUNDA FEMORIS ARTERY PERFORATOR FLAP

Vascular Anatomy

The first perforator of the profunda femoris artery arises superior to the adductor brevis muscle and pierces the

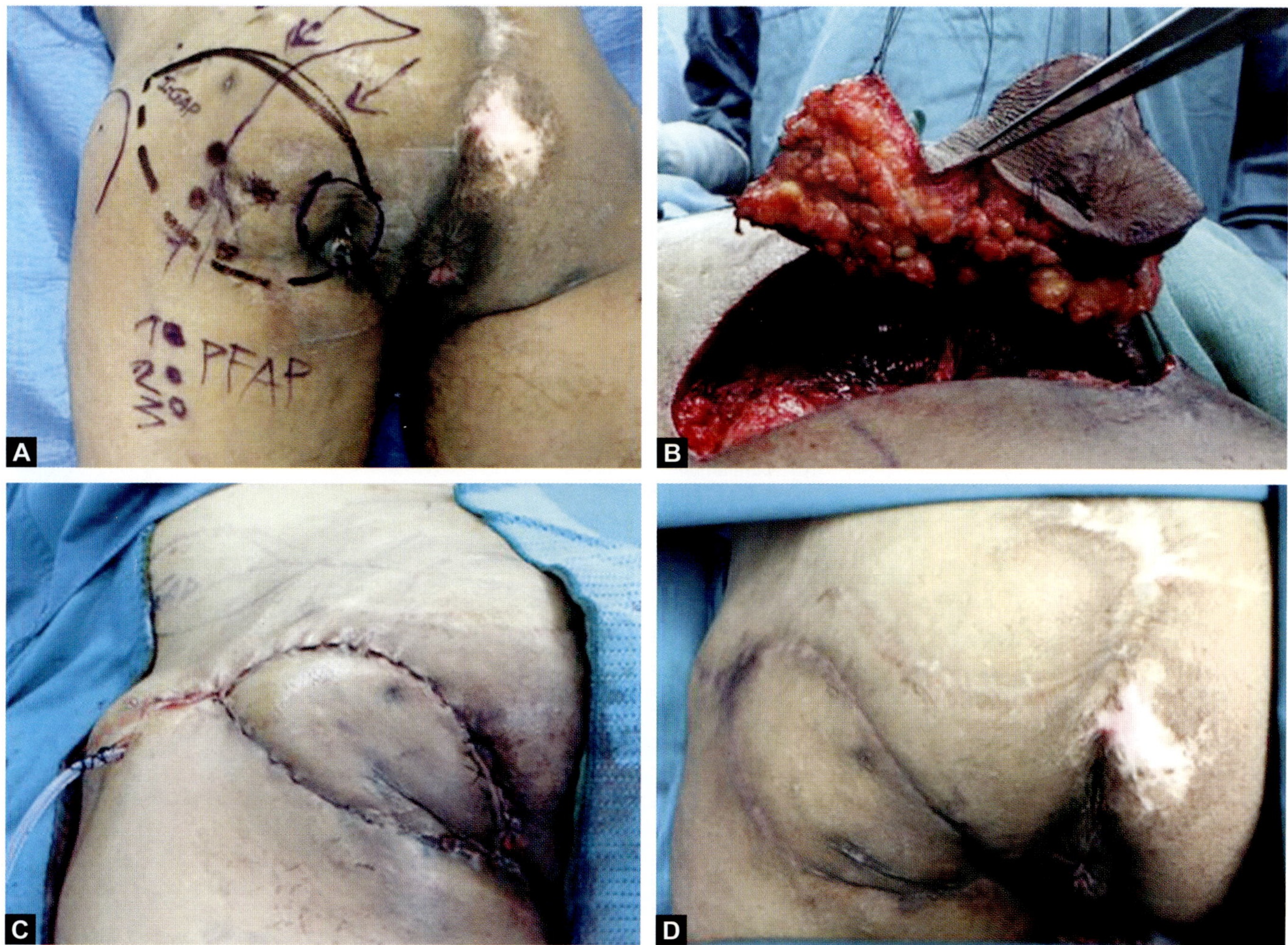

Figs. 13.5A to D: A 48-year-old male with late-stage ischial pressure sore. (A) Marking of IGAP flap and its perforators. (B) IGAP flap raised on a single muscle perforator and flap coverage of the ischial defect. (C) Immediate postoperative with one drain in place. (D) Six-week follow-up.

adductor magnus muscle 2–4 cm inferior to the ischial tuberosity. A large muscular branch ascends superolaterally to supply the lower part of the gluteus maximus and adductor muscles. A fasciocutaneous branch (1–2 mm in diameter) supplies the upper posterolateral thigh skin. After piercing the fascia, a lateral branch proceeds to supply the skin overlying the iliotibial tract and great trochanter. A posteriorly directed branch supplies the posterolateral aspect of the thigh. This branch is located near the junction of the gluteus maximus muscle's insertion into the iliotibial tract and the biceps femoris muscle.

The second perforator of the profunda femoris artery enters the posterior thigh after piercing the insertion of the adductor brevis and the adductor magnus muscle, 4–6 cm inferior to the ischial tuberosity. Branches pierce the fascia overlying the lateral intermuscular septum to supply the mid posterior thigh.[24]

Flap Design

With the patient in the prone position, a line is drawn from the ischium to the lateral femoral condyle. Several anatomic studies demonstrate that most perforators could be found on this line. A handheld Doppler probe is used to locate the PFAPs. On average, five perforators are located on the previously marked line between the inferior gluteal fold and 10 cm proximal to the condyles. A skin paddle is centered over the most suitable (size and position considered) perforator and dissection proceeds as with a standard perforator flap. These flaps are particularly useful for ischiatic pressure sores coverage.

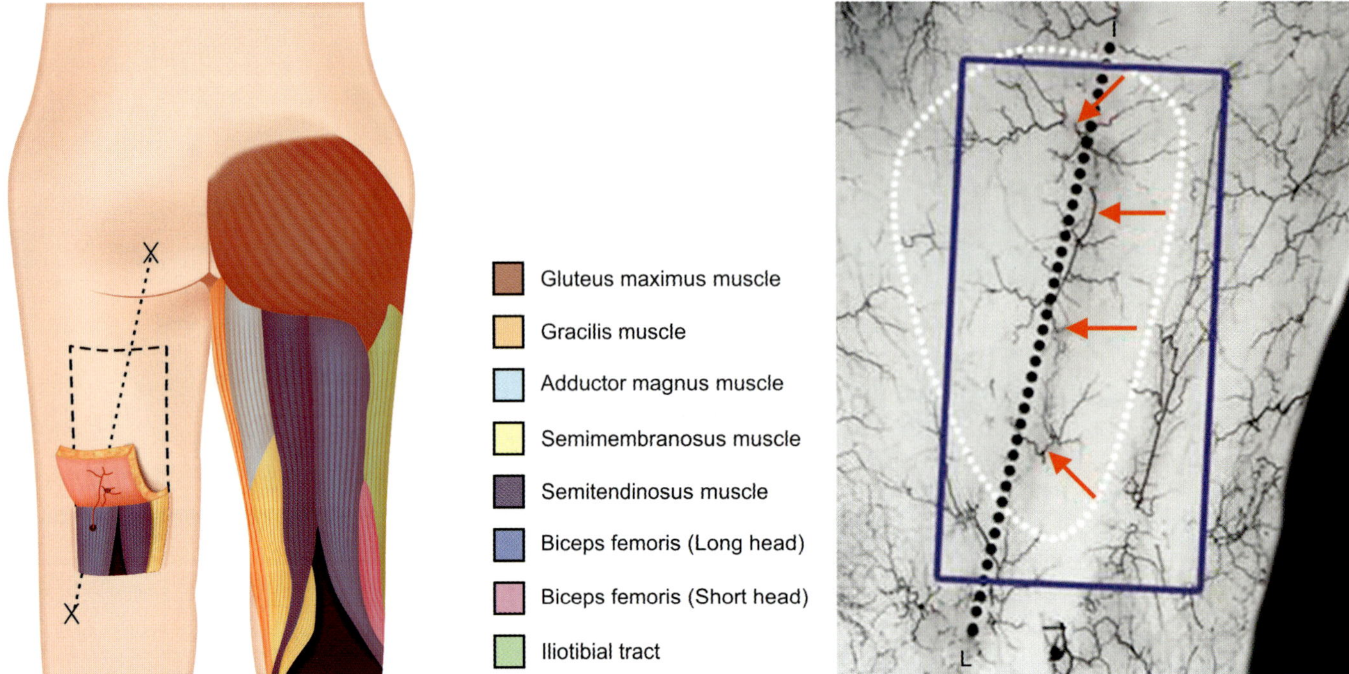

Fig. 13.6: Profunda femoris perforators (arrows) are located along a line extending from the ischium to the lateral femoral condyle. The posterior thigh region is outlined by the rectangle. The profunda femoris vascular territory is shown by the white dotted line. (I: Ischium; L: Lateral femoral condyle).
Source: From Ahmadzadeh R, Bergeron L, Tang M, et al. The superior and inferior gluteal artery perforator flaps. Plast Reconstr Surg. 2007;120(6):1551-6.

Case Reports

1. Paraplegic 58-year-old man with an ischiatic fourth stage pressure sore (15 × 12 cm), without spontaneous healing despite advanced dressings (Figs. 13.7A to F). The onset of the ulcer was 28 months earlier, with bone exposure and high risk of osteomyelitis. According with the preoperative planning, we have located the perforators of the PFA by using a handheld Doppler probe. After 7 days from admission the patient underwent to surgical excision of the lesion after marking of the pressure sore bursa with methylene blue. Surgical debridement was completed with high-pressure water. Immediate reconstruction by using a propeller flap based on the PFAP-1. No recurrence at 1 year.
2. Paraplegic 37-year-old male with an ischiatic fourth stage pressure sore, without spontaneous healing despite advanced dressings (Figs. 13.8A to F). Patient underwent to surgical excision of the lesion after marking of the pressure sore bursa with methylene blue. Surgical debridement was completed with high-pressure water. Immediate reconstruction by using a perforator flap based on the second perforator of the profunda femoris artery (PFAP-2). No recurrence at 1 year.

FIRST MEDIAL PERFORATOR OF THE PROFUNDA FEMORIS ARTERY PERFORATOR FLAP OR ADDUCTOR FLAP

The medial and posterior portions of the thigh are useful donor site areas to harvest soft-tissue flaps for a variety of difficult defects coverage with minimal donor-site morbidity because of the abundant tissue in those regions.

The use of the medial thigh for pressure sores coverage was first described by Conway et al. in 1947.[25] McCraw et al. in 1976[26] described the gracilis flap, a musculocutaneous flap from the medial aspect of the thigh that has traditionally been used before the introduction of perforator flaps to the reconstructive surgeon's choice of techniques. However, one of the known drawbacks of the gracilis myocutaneous flap is inconsistent skin paddle size, which results in moderate to high rates of partial distal skin necrosis.

Since the advent of perforator flaps, their popularity and use have increased dramatically due to their reliable cutaneous territories and minimal donor-site morbidity. Angrigiani et al. in 2001[27] were the first to describe the

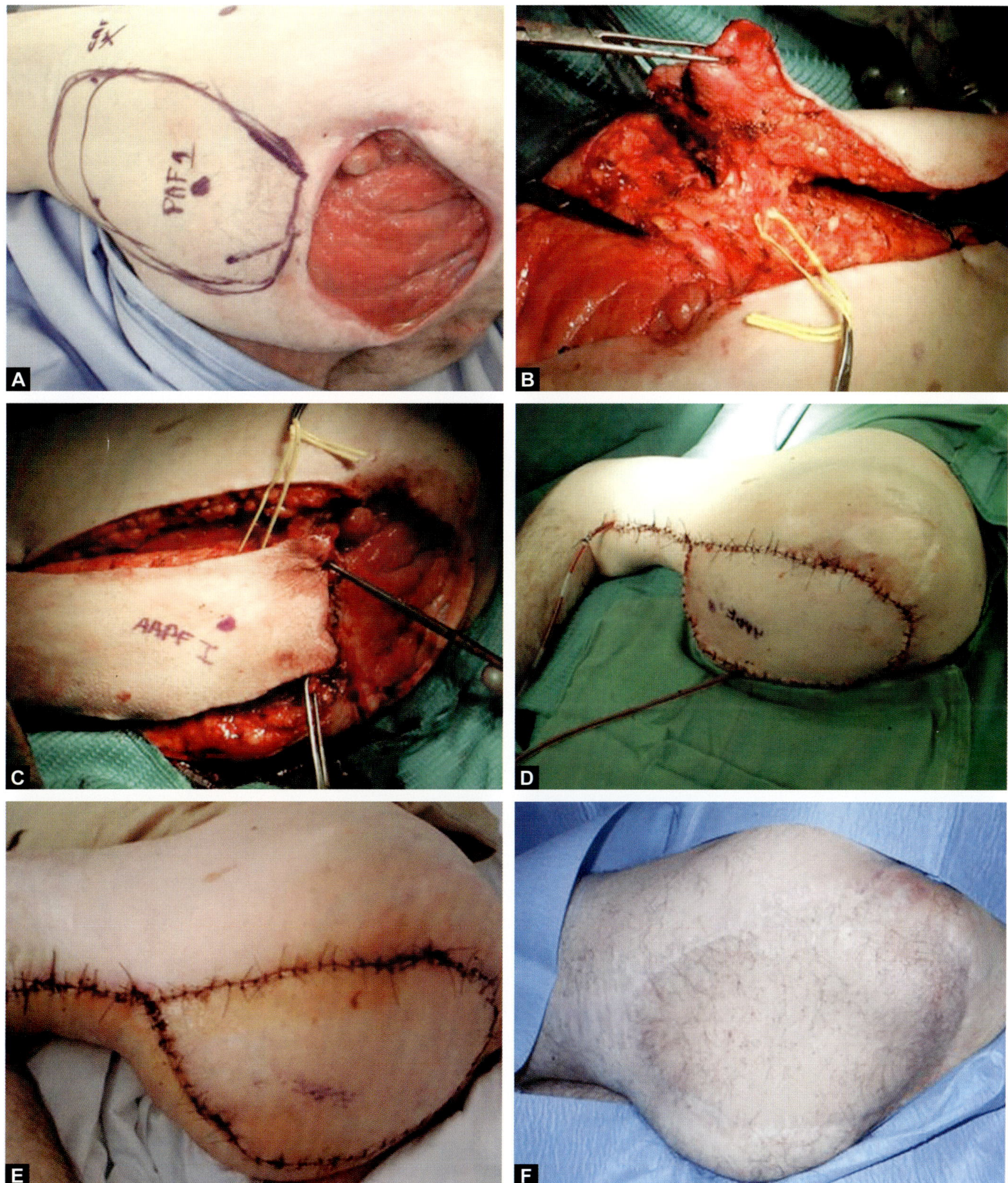

Figs. 13.7A to F: A 58-year-old male with late-stage ischial pressure sore. (A) Marking of PFAP-1 flap and its perforators. (B and C) PFAP-1 flap raised on a single muscle perforator before the propeller rotation. (D) Immediately postoperative with two drains in place. (E) Two-week follow-up. (F) One-year follow-up.

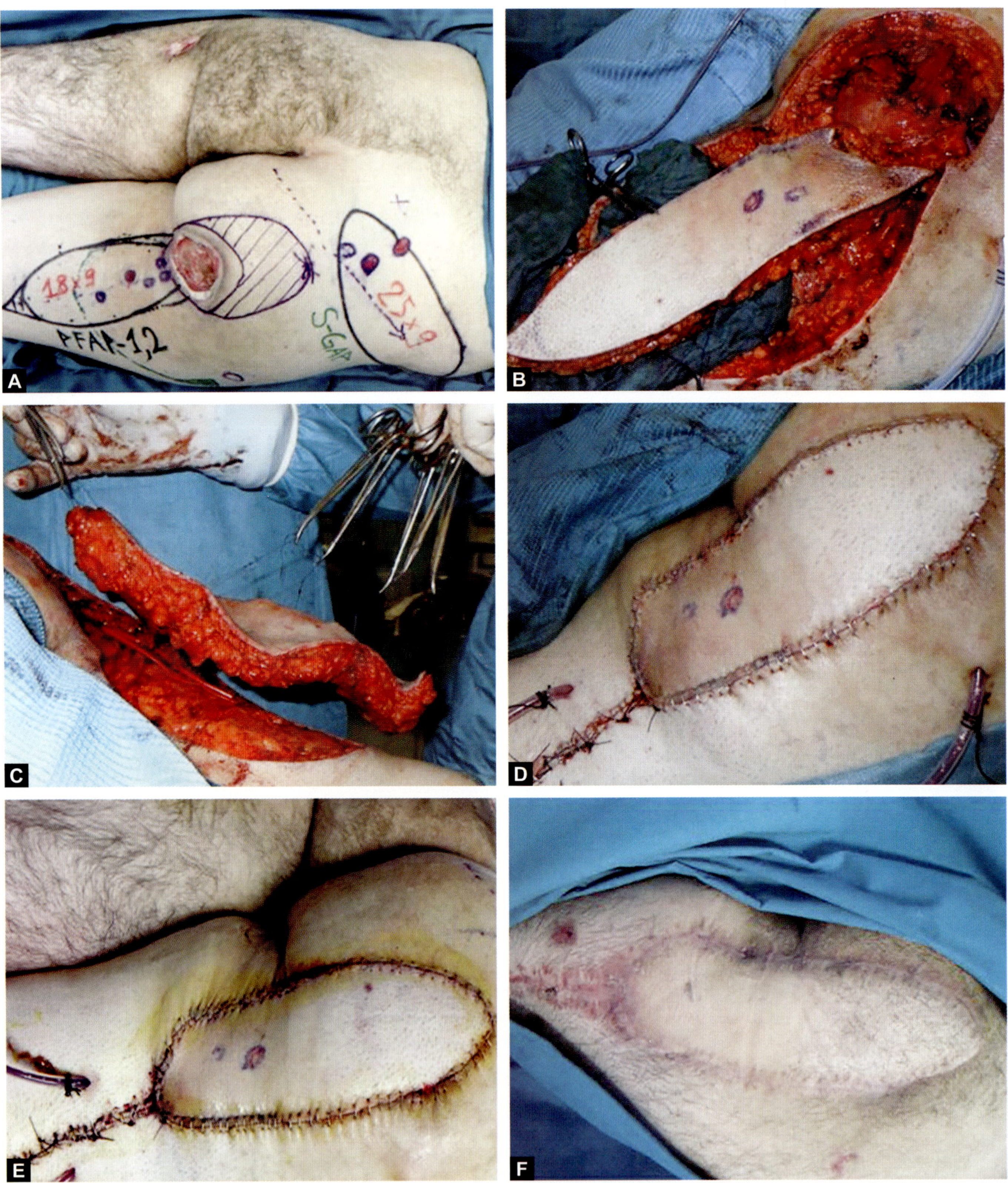

Figs. 13.8A to F: A 37-year-old man with late-stage ischial pressure sore. (A) Marking of PFAP-2 flap and its perforators. (B and C) PFAP-1 flap raised on a single muscle perforator after surgical debridement of the pressure sore and flap coverage of the ischial defect. (D) Immediately postoperative with two drains in place. (E) One-week follow-up. (F) Two-month follow-up.

adductor magnus perforator (AMP) flap and has been shown to have a very reliable skin paddle as well as a reproducible pedicle.

Vascular Anatomy

Reviewing the regional anatomy, the profunda femoris artery enters the posterior compartment of the thigh and divides into medial and lateral branches. The lateral branches pierce the adductor magnus muscle insertion achieving the lateral compartment of the thigh. The medial branches enter the adductor compartment. The first medial branch originates from the profunda femoris at approximately 8 cm below the groin crease and runs medially and posteriorly between the adductor major and brevis muscles posteriorly and the adductor longus muscle anteriorly. The vessel enters the adductor magnus muscle, giving off several branches to this muscle and to the adductor brevis. The vessel reaches the superficial surface of the muscle and pierces the fascia, where it emerges as a large caliber cutaneous artery and arborizes profusely in the subcutaneous tissue. That perforator is reliably found approximately 8 cm distal to the groin crease and 2 cm posterior to the posterior border of the gracilis muscle. The First Medial Perforator of the Profunda Femoris Artery Perforator (PFAP-AM) flap or Adductor flap is based on this pedicle.[27]

Hurwitz et al. in 2011[28] with several anatomic studies described that a second perforator consistently accompanies the first perforator described by Angrigiani located approximately 2 cm distally. Dissection approximately 1–2 cm into the adductor magnus muscle revealed a Y-configuration of these two perforators (Figs. 13.9A and B). This configuration was confirmed in 100% of the cadaveric dissections and was supplied by the first medial branch of the profunda femoris artery.

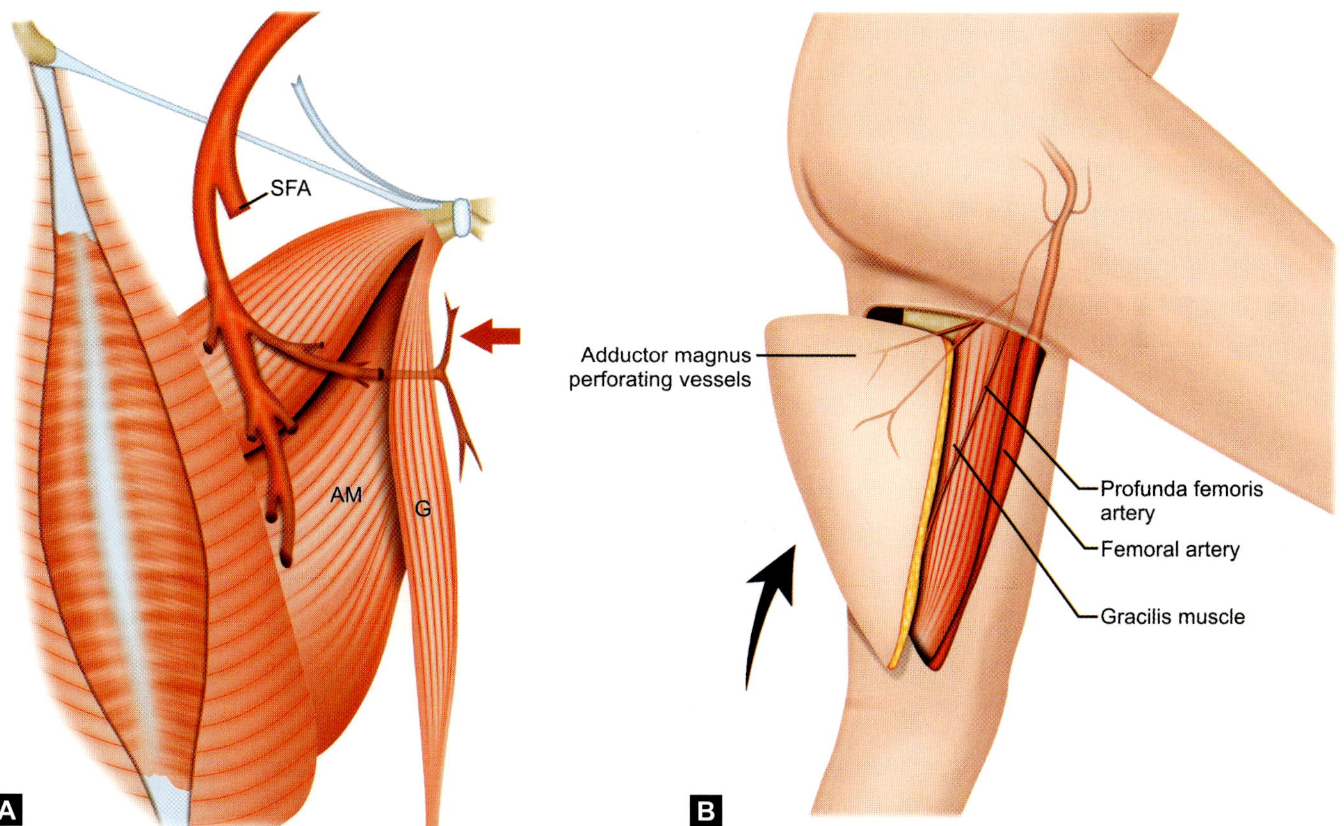

Figs. 13.9A and B: : Adductor magnus perforator flap. (A) The first medial branch of the profunda femoris artery entering the adductor magnus (AM), coursing posterior to the gracilis (G) muscle, and emerging in the posteromedial thigh. The adductor artery (the arterial pedicle for the adductor flap) is indicated by the red arrow. SFA, superficial femoral artery. *Source*: From Angrigiani C, Grilli D, Thorne CH. The adductor flap: a new method for transferring posterior and medial thigh skin. Plast Reconstr Surg. 2001;107:1725-31.
(B) AMP flap designed as a V–Y advancement with the Y-configuration supplying a large cutaneous territory. *Source*: From Hurwitz ZM, Montilla R, Dunn RM, et al. Adductor magnus perforator flap revisited. Ann Plast Surg. 2011;66:438-443.

Flap Design

The prone position allows simultaneous access to an ischial pressure sore and the posterior thigh donor site. A line along the inguinal crease is extended from its medial side onto the posterior thigh. The posterior border of the gracilis muscle as palpated is marked. The AMP is near a point 8 cm inferior to the extended line of the inguinal crease and 2 cm posterior to the gracilis muscle. An audible Doppler probe is used to verify its location. The flap is drawn around this point and should have a width equal to that of the debrided pressure sore.

The flap can be designed 12–23 cm wide and 16–30 cm long.

Flap Harvesting

The flap is elevated from distal to proximal in a plane superficial to the deep fascia, from anterior to posterior until the posterior border of the gracilis muscle. The adductor flap could be transferred as pedicled flaps for coverage of ischial pressure sores as V-Y advancement flap. In this case skin grafting of the donor site is usually required.

Hallock in 2006[29] proposed the propeller flap version of the adductor muscle perforator flap for coverage of ischial or trochanteric pressure sores. If designed as a propeller flap, this version after rotation will cover the defect and simultaneously allow direct donor-site closure to avoid the need for a skin graft. The flap is carefully turned 180° about the hub so that its distal portion fills the defect. The distal thigh usually has enough elasticity to allow some direct closure, while the rest of the donor site can be closed by insetting what was originally the proximal part of the flap.

Case Reports

This paraplegic 56-year-old man had an ischiatic fourth stage pressure sore, without spontaneous healing despite advanced dressings (Figs. 13.10A to H). Patient underwent to surgical excision of the lesion after marking of the pressure sore bursa with methylene blue. Surgical debridement was completed with high-pressure water. Immediate reconstruction by using an AMP flap (18 × 8 cm). The donor area was skin grafted. Patient had complete flap failure due to a technical error in which the pedicle was incompletely skeletonized during flap elevation. Four days later patient underwent to surgical debridement of the necrotic flap and after 8 days of VAC therapy underwent to second reconstruction by using a gluteal myocutaneous flap.

This paraplegic 44-year-old man had an ischiatic fourth stage pressure sore, without spontaneous healing despite advanced dressings (Figs. 13.11A to F). Patient underwent to surgical excision of the lesion after marking of the pressure sore bursa with methylene blue. Surgical debridement was completed with high-pressure water. Immediate reconstruction by using an AMP flap designed as a propeller flap. Only the first perforator was kept to facilitate the rotation about the hub of the propeller.

AUTHORS' PROCEDURE TECHNIQUE AND RESULTS

Pressure sores have been a significant problem for the reconstructive surgeon. Despite various flap alternatives, the rate of recurrence is high. Muscle and musculocutaneous flaps have extensively been used in the past.

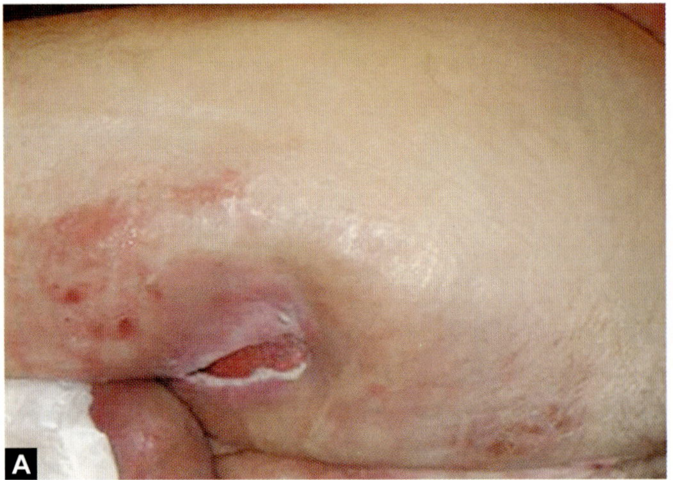

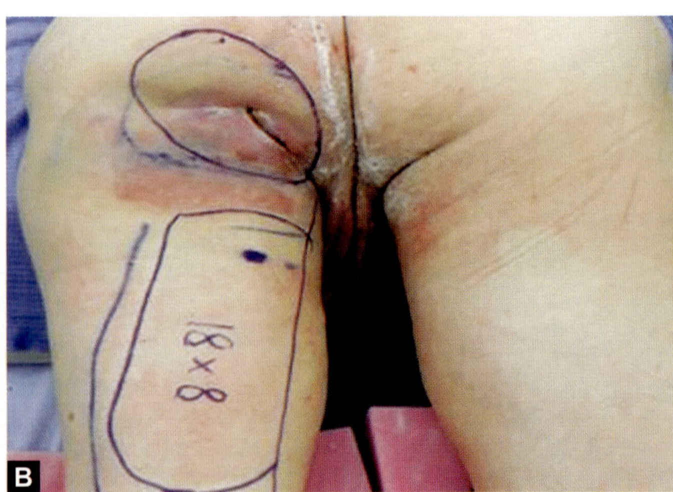

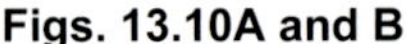
Figs. 13.10A and B

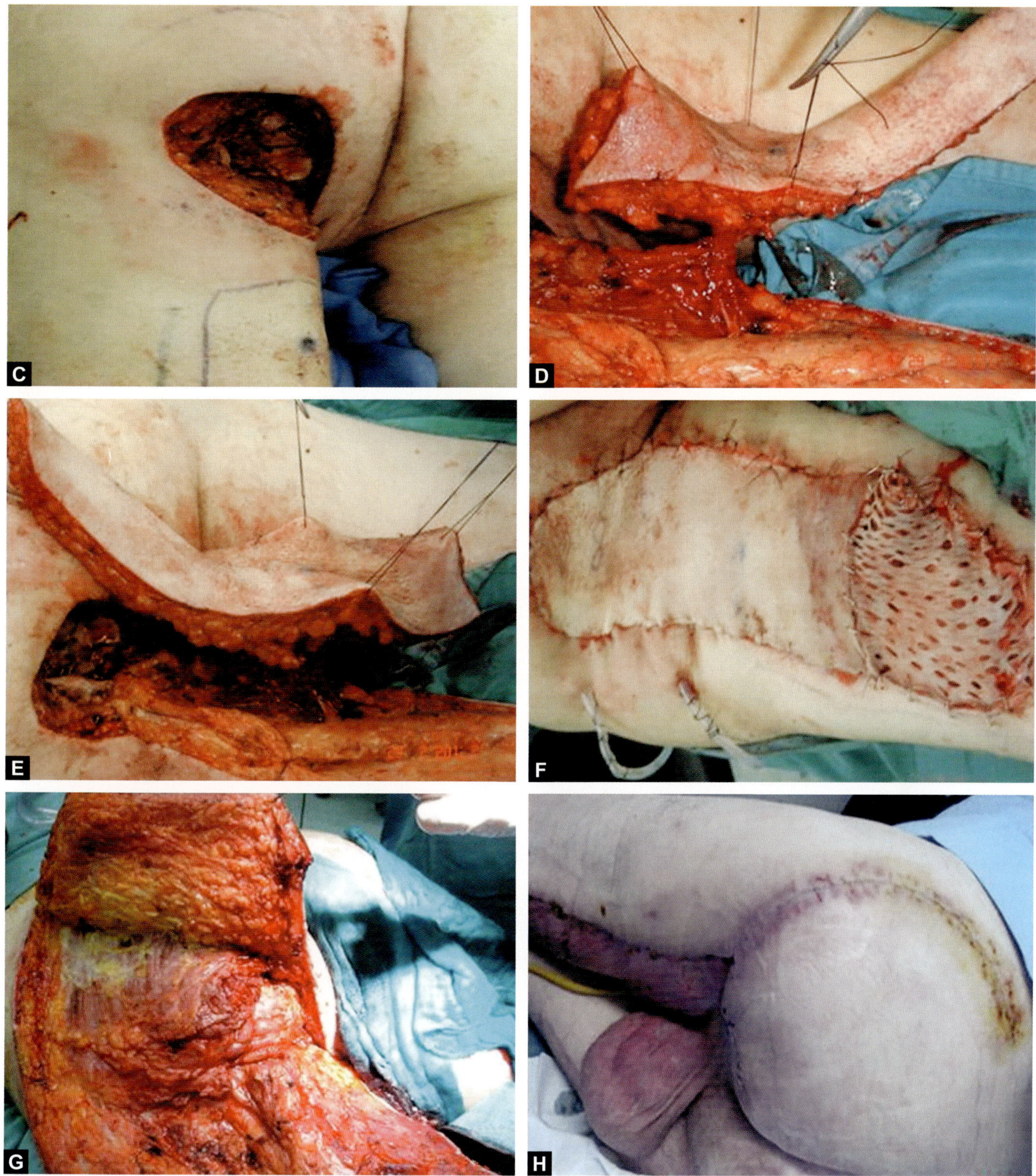

Figs. 13.10A to H: A 56-year-old male with late-stage ischial pressure sore. (A) Preoperative. (B) Marking of PFAP-am flap. (C) Pressure sore after surgical debridement. (D and E) PFAP-am flap raised on a single muscle perforator and flap coverage of the ischial defect. (F) Immediately postoperative with two drains in place. (G) Second reconstruction by using a gluteal myocutaneous flap. (H) Four-week follow-up.

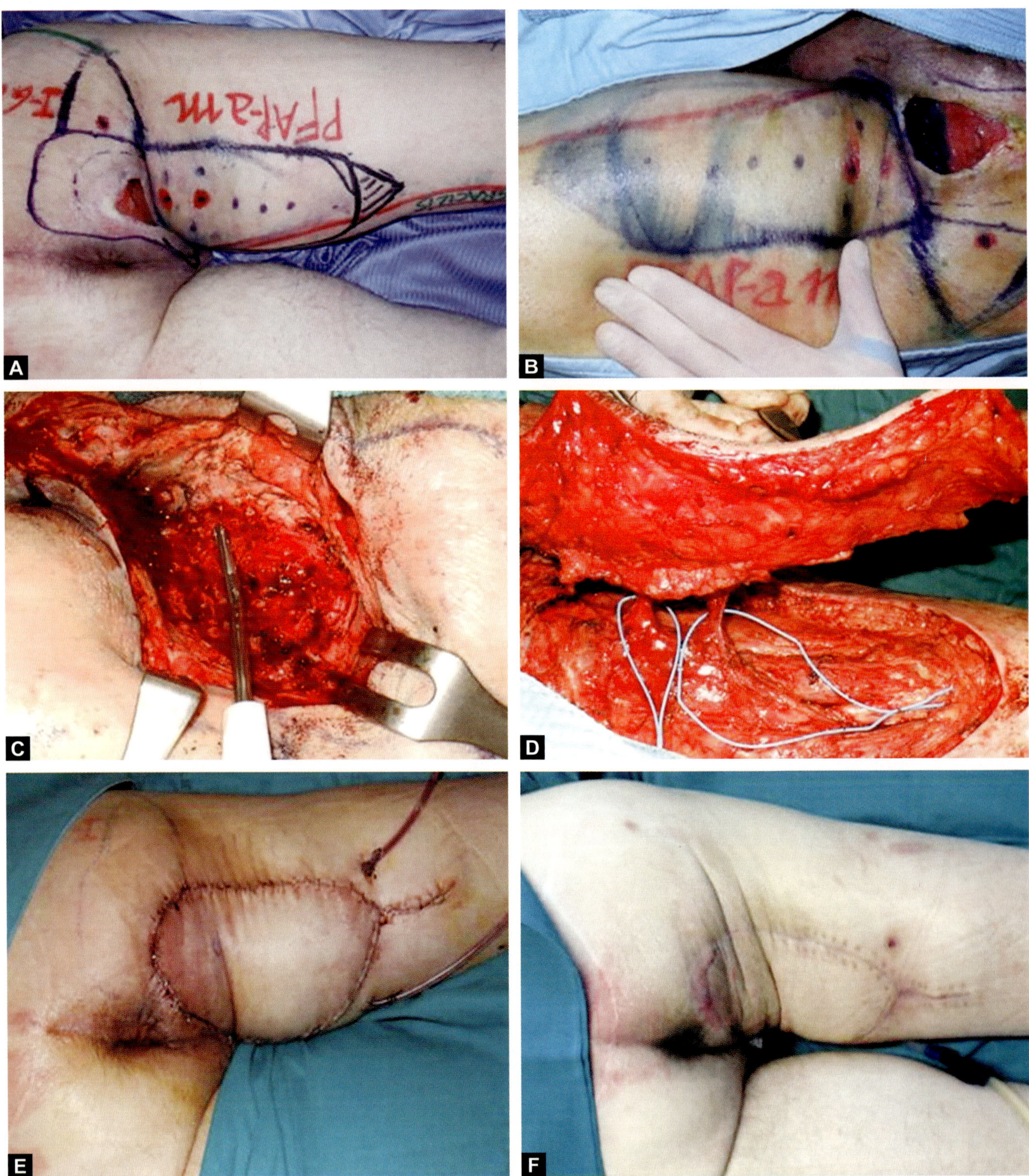

Figs. 13.11A to F: A 44-year-old male with late-stage ischial pressure sore. (A) Marking of PFAP-am flap. (B) Surgical excision of the lesion after marking of the pressure sore bursa with methylene blue. (C) Surgical debridement was completed with high-pressure water. (D) PFAP-am flap raised; only the first perforator was kept to facilitate the propeller rotation. (E) One-week follow-up with two drains in place. (F) Five-week follow-up.

However, introduction of perforator flaps to the reconstructive surgeon's choice of techniques has improved the reconstructive strategy during the past decade.

Between April 1999 and April 2010, the authors had 143 patients undergo surgical treatment with perforators flaps for late-stage pressure sores. Only ulcers graded as stage 4 according to the National Pressure Ulcer Advisory Panel staging system that underwent immediate reconstruction with perforator flaps were included in the study. Inclusion criteria were independent of sex, ethnicity, mental or physical condition, kind of flap movement to allow the defect coverage and number of perforators included in each flap. All the patients were examined preoperatively, and the perforating vessels were marked on the skin with the assistance of a handheld 8 MHz Doppler ultrasound scanner. When a perforator could not be found, a traditional flap was used. In very few cases, a reliable perforator pedicle could not be identified intraoperatively when a Doppler signal was present preoperatively. In such cases, the design was converted into a salvage traditional pedicled flap and did not include the patient in the study.

Surgical Procedure

All flaps were raised in the subfascial layer because we found the procedure quicker and very straightforward in patients with tissues of poor quality and to allow a flap-raising time comparable to that of local pedicled flaps. As standard procedure, after injecting methylene blue into the pressure sore bursa, the sore was accurately removed and the bony base accurately debrided by high-pressure water with VersaJet (Smith & Nephew Medical Limited, Hull HU3 2BN England). A bone biopsy was carried out with a sterile osteotome and sent for a bone culture to guide the appropriate antibiotic therapy. The area was disinfected again before proceeding to immediate reconstruction.

After an initial exploratory incision to locate the perforators, the closest vessel free of scar and granulation tissue was chosen and the flap design was rechecked and eventually slightly moved. The flap was then elevated and the pedicle skeletonized by dissecting all its fascial strands and muscle arborizations from its origin from the source vessel up to the point where it pierced the deep fascia to enter the flap. The flap was then completed islanded and papaverine was applied and left in place for 10 minutes around the pedicle to avoid vasospasm and to allow adequate perfusion. When the flap perfusion was satisfactory, the flap could be advanced or rotated onto the defect. We always used a flap in which the design allowed the donor-site primary closure without tension. Two big caliber suction drains were inserted underneath the flap and secured far from the pedicle.

The data were stored in the electronic database of the Regional Hospital. The evaluated outcomes were as follows: new ulcer occurrence, defined as a new pressure sore in a location different from the original; ulcer recurrence, defined as an ulcer occurring >3 months after a previously treated pressure sore at the same location. Complications were classified as major, requiring a re-operation, or minor. Minor complications included dehiscence, distal flap necrosis, and infection. Suture-line dehiscence was defined as any recorded break in the skin, excluding the donor site, which occurred at any point before or during the mobilization protocol. The occurrence of a significant dehiscence necessitating a return to the operating room for flap revision was noted as distinct from suture-line dehiscence that healed without intervention.

Statistical Analysis

Clinical characteristics of patients and sore's features were summarized according to recurrence using absolute and relative frequencies for categorical variables and quartiles (median, and first and third quartiles) for quantitative variables. Comparisons between groups were performed using Fisher exact test for qualitative variables and Wilcoxon test for the quantitative ones. Cumulative probability of developing recurrence according to patients' sores features and subjects' clinical characteristics were estimated by Kaplan–Meier curves, and comparisons between strata were evaluated using log-rank test. Cox regression analysis was used to evaluate the prognostic role of the considered variables to have clinical relevance and to estimate the hazard ratio of developing ulcer recurrence. The statistical significance was assessed using a P value < 0.05, and confidence intervals were calculated with a probability of 95% (95% CI); all the analysis was performed using R package.

RESULTS

Ninety-three percent of 143 patients were white Caucasian, and 61% were men, with median age of 51 years (first to third quartile: 35–65 years). No significant differences resulted in terms of age, in-hospital period, smoking habits, and comorbidity, except for coronary disease that was significantly more frequent in patients with recurrence.

The most common cause of pressure sores was traumatic paraplegia/tetraplegia (74.9%); no significant difference was found in initial diagnosis distribution between patients who developed recurrence and those who did not. Nontraumatic diagnoses included spinal cord tumors, spina bifida, transverse myelitis, multiple sclerosis, and one case of postintensive care unit ulcer. Of the 143 pressure sores included, 46.2% were ischial, 42.7% were sacral, and 11.2% were trochanteric. The most common perforator flap performed was the IGAP flap, followed by the SGAP flap, the first perforator of the profunda femoris artery flap (PFAP-1), and the profunda femoris artery adductor magnus flap (PFAP-AM). No significant differences were found in ulcer location and perforator flap used between the two groups at bivariate analysis. Only 8 patients (5.6%) had major complications requiring a reoperation. In such cases, we performed a further dissection of the perforator pedicle to free it some more, allowing the flap to advance without perfusion problems. In case of flap failure, we used a near traditional myocutaneous flap advancement. Moreover, 4.2% of patients developed a new occurrence. The overall complication percentage was 22.4% and included suture dehiscence (14%) and distal flap necrosis (6.3%), which were managed by accurately debriding them with blade or collagenase ointment and eventually suturing the margins at the patient bed whenever necessary. Complication resulted in average of 5.8 additional days of bed rest. The median postoperative hospitalization time was 16 days with no more draining liquid after an average of 15 days. Thirty-two patients (22.4%) developed a recurrence. Recurrent and nonrecurrent subjects did not show significant differences in the distribution of complication, reoperation percentage, and in-hospital period (Table 13.1).

Figures 13.12A to J show the results of Kaplan-Meier survival analysis. The overall cumulative probability of recurrence at 2 years was 22.4% (95% CI, 15.2–28.9%). Patients who suffered from coronary artery disease had a significant higher probability of developing recurrence. No significant differences resulted between strata when the other factors were evaluated. Six patients developed a new occurrence with a probability at 2 years of 4.2% (95% CI, 0.9–7.4%).

The final and best model of risk estimation of developing recurrence according to clinical and sore's characteristics is shown in Table 13.2. The type of perforator flap used and the comorbidities played a significant effect on recurrence; subjects for whom PFAP flap (PFAP-1 + PFAP-AM) was used had a significant higher risk of developing recurrence than subjects treated with IGAP flap; no significant difference resulted between SGAP and IGAP flaps. The recurrence risk was significantly higher for subjects suffering from coronary artery disease, while a significant protective role of renal disease was found. No significant effect resulted when the role of diagnosis was investigated. Nevertheless, this variable was included in the model because it contributed to a better model's goodness of fit.

DISCUSSION

In the last decades, perforator flaps have been introduced for the treatment of sacral, ischial, and trochanteric pressure ulcers. The authors have used these flaps since 1999 because they limit donor site morbidity and better achieve flap mobility and viability when compared to a pedicled fasciocutaneous flap. The patients in the study were evaluated for complications, recurrence, and occurrence rates in comparison with current literature data. The patients underwent debridement and immediate reconstruction with fasciocutaneous perforator flaps. All the patients underwent the same pre-, intra- and postoperative treatments performed by the same teams. Different types of perforators were used according to the ulcer location and the preoperative Doppler signs. The results showed an overall recurrence rate of 22.4% at the 24-month follow-up, which is quite low when compared with the previously published rates of 16.8–82%.[11,30] The 24-month follow-up was used to evaluate recurrence because the literature suggests that the recurrence curve tends to flatten at 18 months, with the most critical time period being between 15 and 22 months.[11,31]

Within the last 10 years, reported dehiscence rates have ranged between 9% and 45%.[32,33] Again, the rate depends on the definition of dehiscence used by the authors. The dehiscence rate in our population was 14%, using a very conservative definition.

The 5.6% requiring operative revision is slightly lower than the 17% reported by Foster et al.[34] and the 19% of Larson et al.[32] Conversely, the occurrence of distal flap necrosis is higher (6.3%) than the 0.6% of Larson et al. who used myocutaneous flaps. This could be explained by the increased risk rate of a perforator flap when compared to a "traditional" flap.

Our overall complication rates and infection rates are consistent with other already published rates.[30,32] When examining our new-occurrence rate, we found 4.2% which

Table 13.1: Patient's clinical characteristics and sore's features according to recurrence (bivariate analysis)

		Recurrence		
Median (first to third quartiles)	*No (n = 111)*	*Yes (n = 32)*	*Total (n = 143)*	*P*
Age (years)	50 (38–65)	52 (40–63)	51 (38–65)	0.725[a]
In-hospital period (days)	16 (14–17)	16 (15–19)	16 (14–17)	0.299[a]
n (%)				
Diabetes	12 (10.8)	7 (21.9)	19 (13.3)	0.137
Smoking	37 (33.3)	13 (40.6)	50 (35)	0.529
Renal disease	13 (11.7)	3 (9.4)	16 (11.2)	1.000
COPD	29 (26.1)	10 (31.3)	39 (27.3)	0.653
Coronary disease	19 (17.1)	12 (37.5)	31 (21.7)	0.026
Diagnosis				
Nontraumatic paraplegic	16 (14.4)	5 (15.6)	21 (14.7)	0.832
Nontraumatic tetraplegic	12 (10.8)	2 (6.3)	14 (9.8)	
Traumatic paraplegic	43 (38.7)	15 (46.9)	58 (40.6)	
Traumatic tetraplegic	39 (35.1)	10 (31.3)	49 (34.3)	
Ulcer location				
Ischial	48 (43.2)	18 (56.3)	66 (46.2)	0.357
Sacral	51 (45.9)	10 (31.3)	61 (42.7)	
Trochanteric	12 (10.8)	4 (12.5)	16 (11.2)	
Perforator flap used				
I-GAP	63 (56.8)	15 (46.9)	78 (54.5)	0.438
S-GAP	34 (30.6)	10 (31.3)	44 (30.8)	
PFAP-1	12 (10.8)	6 (18.8)	18 (12.6)	
PFAP-am	2 (1.8)	1 (3.1)	3 (2.1)	
Reoperation	6 (5.4)	2 (6.3)	8 (5.6)	1.000
Complications				
No	89 (80.2)	22 (68.8)	111 (77.6)	0.189
Suture dehiscence	14 (12.6)	6 (18.8)	20 (14.0)	
Distal flap necrosis	7 (6.3)	2 (6.3)	9 (6.3)	
Infections	1 (0.9)	2 (6.3)	3 (2.1)	

Wilcoxon test
Fisher exact test.

was much lower than Larson et al. and Foster et al. who used myocutaneous flaps. Muscle flaps leave the donor site exposed to new ulcer occurrences because a "pillow" effect no longer exists on a loading surface created by the vascularized myocutaneous unit. This is also consistent also with our hospitalization time of 16.2 days with no more draining liquid after an average of 14.8 days. Comparatively, periods of 20 days[32,34] up to 45–70 days[35,36] have

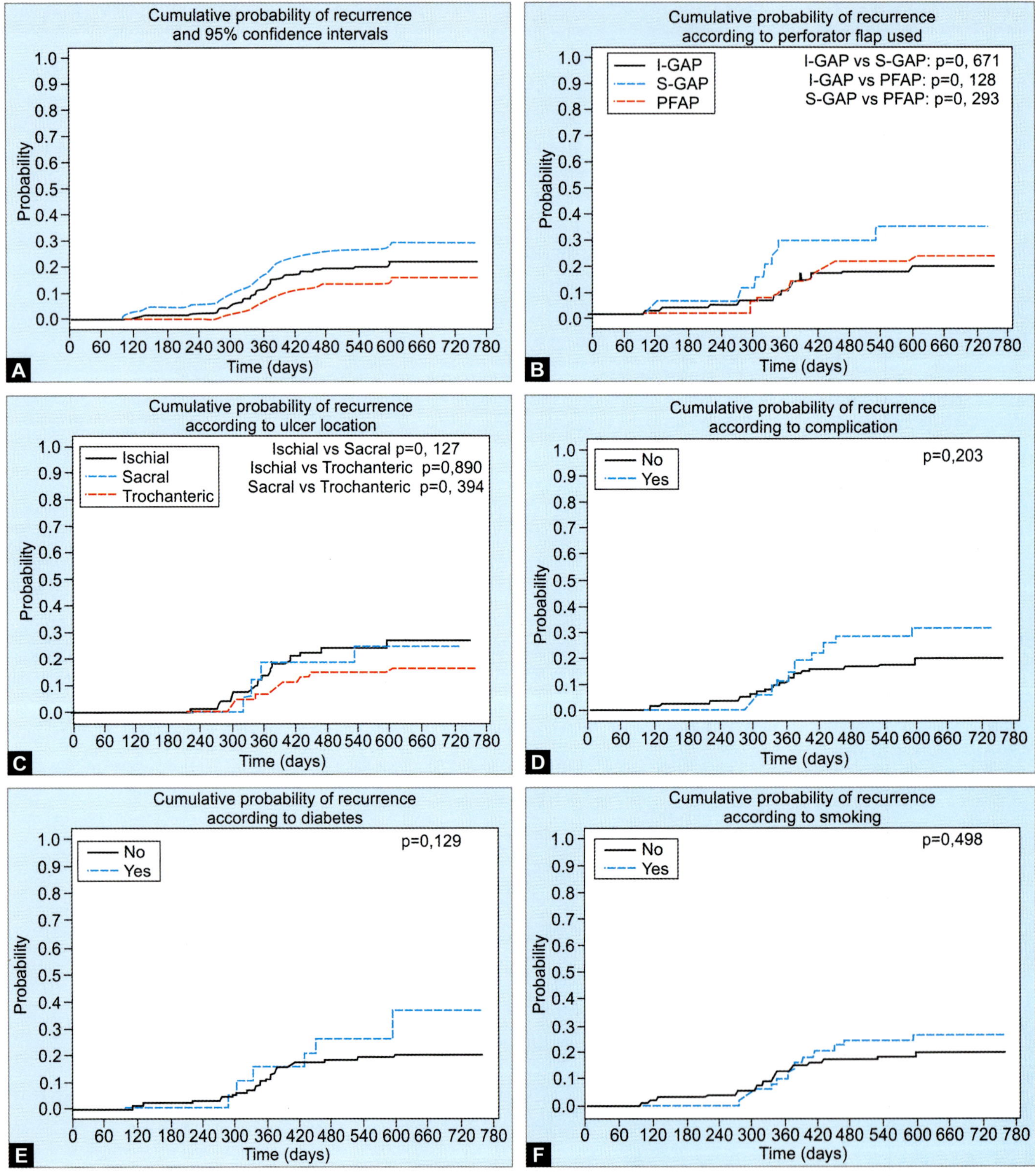

Figs. 13.12A to F

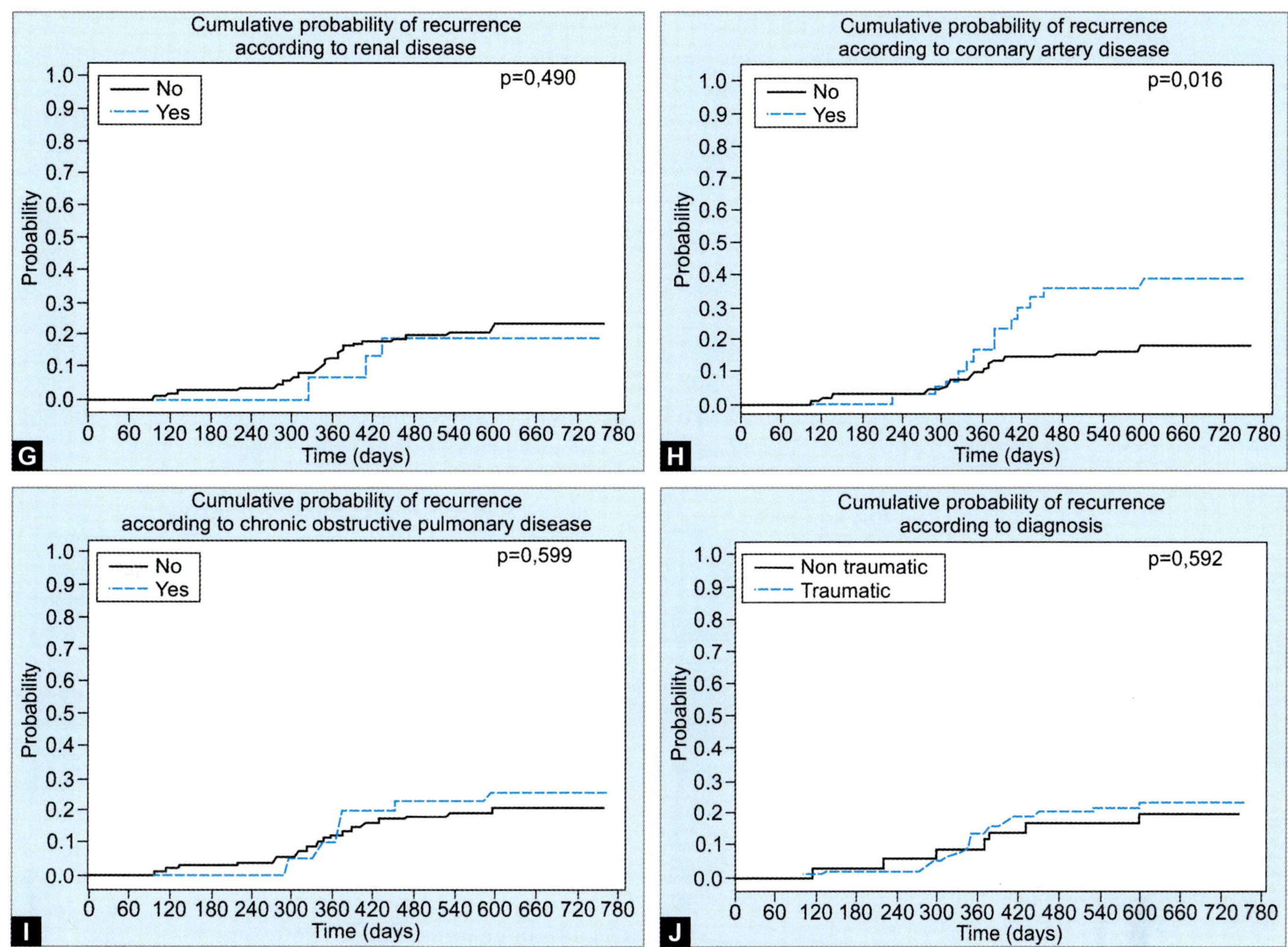

Figs. 13.12A to J: Cumulative probability of recurrence according to selected variables.

Table 13.2: Estimation of hazard ratios according to selected variable (cox regression analysis)

Prognostic factors	*Hazard Ratio*	*95% CI LL*	*95% CI UL*	*P*
P-FAP vs. I-GAP	2.75	1.07	7.04	0.035
S-GAP vs. I-GAP	1.11	0.49	2.52	0.806
Renal disease	0.17	0.04	0.73	0.017
Coronary disease	5.27	2.27	12.21	<0.001
Nontraumatic tetraplegic vs. nontraumatic paraplegic	0.18	0.03	1.13	0.068
Traumatic paraplegic vs. nontraumatic paraplegic	0.66	0.21	2.03	0.469
Traumatic tetraplegic vs. nontraumatic paraplegic	0.56	0.17	1.83	0.337

been described for muscle flaps. It is possible that the extent of edema was reduced using the perforator flap because one more unit of muscle was allowed to move.

CONCLUSION

When compared to previously published data, perforator flaps showed the same recurrence and complication rates as myocutaneous flaps, with a slightly higher distal flap necrosis rate (6.3%, with the best reported being 0.6%), but they significantly reduced the postoperative hospital stay (by an average of nearly 1 week), new occurrence rates, reoperation procedures, and donor-site morbidity. Coronary artery disease was the only feature significantly associated with a significant higher probability of recurrence at 2 years in both the bivariate and multiple analyses.

REFERENCES

1. Bauer J, Phillips LG. MOC-PSSM CME article: pressure sores. Plast Reconstr Surg. 2008;121(1 Suppl):1-10.
2. Daniel RK, Faibisoff B. Muscle coverage of pressure points: the role of myocutaneous flaps. Plast Reconstr Surg. 1982; 8(6):446-52.
3. Vasconez LO, Bostwick JIII, McCraw J. Coverage of exposed bone by muscle transposition and skin grafting. Plast Reconstr Surg. 1974;53(5):526-30.
4. Ger R, Levine SA. The management of decubitus ulcers by muscle transposition: an 8-year review. Plast Reconstr Surg. 1976;58(4):419-28.
5. Minami RT, Mills R, Pardoe R. Gluteus maximus myocutaneous flaps for repair of pressure sores. Plast Reconstr Surg. 1977;60(2):242-9.
6. Nola GT, Vistnes LM. Differential response of skin and muscle in the experimental production of pressure sores. Plast Reconstr Surg. 1980;66(5):728-33.
7. Daniel RK, Wheatley D, Priest D. Pressure sores and paraplegia: an experimental model. Ann Plast Surg. 1985; 15(1):41-9.
8. Salgado CJ, Mardini S, Jamali AA, et al. Muscle versus nonmuscle flaps in the reconstruction of chronic osteomyelitis defects. Plast Reconstr Surg. 2006;118(6):1401-11.
9. Thiessen FE, Andrades P, Blondeel PN, et al. Flap surgery for pressure sores: should the underlying muscle be transferred or not? J Plast Reconstr Aesthet Surg. 2011;64(1): 84-90.
10. Lee JT, Hsiao HT, Tung KY, et al. Gluteal perforator flaps for coverage of pressure sores at various locations. Plast Reconstr Surg. 2006;117(7):2507-8.
11. Yamamoto Y, Tsutsumida A, Murazumi M, et al. Long-term outcome of pressure sores treated with flap coverage. Plast Reconstr Surg. 1997;100(5):1212-17.
12. Hallock GG. The propeller flap version of the adductor muscle perforator flap for coverage of ischial or trochanteric pressure sores. Ann Plast Surg. 2006;56(5):540-42.
13. Allen RJ, Tucker C Jr. Superior gluteal artery perforator free flap for breast reconstruction. Plast Reconstr Surg. 1995;95(7):1207-12.
14. Koshima I, Moriguchi T, Soeda S, et al. The gluteal perforator-based flap for repair of sacral pressure sores. Plast Reconstr Surg. 1993;91(4):678-83.
15. Verpaele AM, Blondeel PN, Van Landuyt K, et al. The superior gluteal artery perforator flap: an additional tool in the treatment of sacral pressure sores. Br J Plast Surg. 1999;52(5):385-91.
16. Wei FC, Mardini S. Flaps and Reconstructive Microsurgery. Philadelphia, PA: Saunders, Elsevier Inc; 2009.
17. Nojima K, Brown SA, Acikel C, et al. Defining vascular supply and territory of thinned perforator flaps: Part II. Superior gluteal artery perforator flap. Plast Reconstr Surg. 2006;118(6):1338-48.
18. Le-Quang C. Secondary microsurgical reconstruction of the breast and free inferior gluteal flap. Ann Chir Plast Esthet. 1992;37(6):723-41.
19. Higgins JP, Orlando GS, Blondeel PN. Ischial pressure sore reconstruction using an inferior gluteal artery perforator (IGAP) flap. Br J Plast Surg. 2002;55(1):83-85.
20. Ahmadzadeh R, Bergeron L, Tang M, et al. The superior and inferior gluteal artery perforator flaps. Plast Reconstr Surg. 2007;120(6):1551-6.
21. Hurwitz DJ. Closure of a large defect of the pelvic cavity by an extended compound myocutaneous flap based on the inferior gluteal artery. Br J Plast Surg. 1980;33(2):256-61.
22. Song YG, Chen GZ, Song YL. The free thigh flap: a new free flap concept based on the septocutaneous artery. Br J Plast Surg. 1984;37(2):149-59.
23. Ahmadzadeh R, Bergeron L, Tang M, et al. The posterior thigh perforator flap or profunda femoris artery perforator flap. Plast Reconstr Surg. 2007;119(1):194-200.
24. Blondeel P, Morris SF, Hallock GG, et al. Perforator Flaps: Anatomy, Technique & Clinical Applications. St Louis, MO: QMP Publishing; 2006.
25. Conway H, Kraissl CJ, Clifford RH. The plastic surgical closure of decubitus ulcers in patients with paraplegia. Surg Gynecol Obstet. 1947;85(3):321-32.
26. McCraw JB, Massey FM, Shanklin KD, et al. Vaginal reconstruction with gracilis myocutaneous flaps. Plast Reconstr Surg. 1976;58:176-83.
27. Angrigiani C, Grilli D, Thorne CH. The adductor flap: a new method for transferring posterior and medial thigh skin. Plast Reconstr Surg. 2001;107(7):1725-31.
28. Hurwitz ZM, Montilla R, Dunn RM, et al. Adductor magnus perforator flap revisited. Ann Plast Surg. 2011;66: 438-43.

29. Hallock GG. The propeller flap version of the adductor muscle perforator flap for coverage of ischial or trochanteric pressure sores. Ann Plast Surg. 2006;56(5):540-42.
30. Keys KA, Daniali LN, Warner KJ, et al. Multivariate predictors of failure after flap coverage of pressure ulcers. Plast Reconstr Surg. 2010;125(6):1725-34.
31. Evans GR, Dufresne CR, Manson PN. Surgical correction of pressure ulcers in an urban center: is it efficacious? Adv Wound Care. 1994;7(1):40-46.
32. Larson DL, Hudak KA, Waring WP, et al. Protocol management of late-stage pressure ulcers: a 5-year retrospective study of 101 consecutive patients with 179 ulcers. Plast Reconstr Surg. 2012;129(4):897-904.
33. Dansereau JG, Conway H. Closure of decubiti in paraplegics. Report of 2000 cases. Plast Reconstr Surg. 1964;33:474-80.
34. Foster RD, Anthony JP, Mathes SJ, et al. Flap selection as a determinant of success in pressure sore coverage. Arch Surg. 1997;132(8):868-73.
35. Isik FF, Engrav LH, Rand RP, et al. Reducing the period of immobilization following pressure sore surgery: a prospective, randomized trial. Plast Reconstr Surg. 1997;100(2): 350-54.
36. Marriott R, Rubayi S. Successful truncated osteomyelitis treatment for chronic osteomyelitis secondary to pressure ulcers in spinal cord injury patients. Ann Plast Surg. 2008; 61(4):425-29.

14 Gluteal Perforator Flaps for Coverage of Pressure Sores

O Koray Coskunfirat, Anı Cinpolat

INTRODUCTION

Managing pressure sores is a common problem for reconstructive surgeons owing to the high recurrence of the sores after flap coverage and limited flap alternatives. Pressure sores constitute an important problem not only in plegic but also in ambulatory patients. Untreated sores may cause serious complications, including death. The best treatment option is to prevent such sores before occurrence; however, despite every effort, pressure sores may occur. Surgery is the best treatment option in the vast majority of the patients and must be performed early because, when it is delayed, the ulcer and necrosis spread widely, and this limits surgical alternatives. Despite various flap options, recurrence is still a significant problem after pressure sore surgery.

Every step of the reconstructive ladder has been tried for the coverage of pressure sores.

Skin grafts and simple random pattern skin flaps have limited roles in reconstruction, but only in the early stages with small ulcers. When the pressure sore extends down to the soft tissue and includes muscles, tendons, and other structures, more robust flaps are necessary.

Flap selection differs according to the location of the defect, but muscle and musculocutaneous flaps were the most preferred and reliable options in the past. The concept of perforator flaps has progressed with improvement in understanding of flap perfusion and perforator anatomy.[1] The evolution of perforator flaps during the past decade has extended the flap options and limited the use of muscle and musculocutaneous flaps. The pedicles of the perforator flaps are musculocutaneous perforators, so they should pierce the muscle to reach the skin for the flap to be called a perforator flap.[2] In these types of flaps, there is no need to carry the muscle to provide the blood supply to the overlying skin and subcutaneous tissue.

Table 14.1: Evolution of the perforator flaps in pressure sores

Indications	*Perforator flap type*	*First time user*
	Gluteal perforator based	Koshima et al.[3]
	SGAP	Verpaele et al.[4]
	IGAP	Higgins et al.[5]
	TFL PF	Ishida et al.[6]
	Add. magnus PF	PF Hallock[7]
	Infragluteal PF	Scheufler et al.[8]

(SGAP: Superior gluteal perforator flap; IGAP: Inferior gluteal perforator flap).

Some perforator or perforator-based flaps provide various pedicled flap options for pressure sore management (Table 14.1).[3-10]

In 1993, Koshima et al.[3] used gluteal perforator flaps for sacral pressure sores. They freely designed their flap based on parasacral perforators without depending on strict anatomic landmarks. Subsequently, the superior gluteal perforator flap (SGAP)[4] and the inferior gluteal perforator flap (IGAP)[5] and their anatomic landmarks have been described in the gluteal region. Minimal donor-site morbidity and freedom in flap design overcome the major disadvantages of traditional muscle and musculocutaneous flaps, and gluteal perforator flaps became first choice for pressure sore coverage at various sites. Gluteal perforator flaps were pedicled on the musculocutaneous perforators arising from the superior gluteal artery, the inferior gluteal artery, the lateral sacral artery, and the internal pudendal artery. All of these arteries send musculocutaneous perforators to the gluteal region by penetrating the gluteal muscles. These perforators were dissected in a plane between the gluteus maximus and the overlying skin, and even one perforator can supply a large skin flap. The versatility of the flap design over the gluteus maximus muscle allowed us to use these flaps with great freedom. Gluteal perforator flaps provide sufficient endurance to resist pressure, so these flaps can be preferred for almost every type of pressure sore located at lumbosacral, trochanteric, and ischial areas. Fasciocutaneous flaps seem to be suitable to cover pressure sore defects with a similar outcome to that of muscle flaps. However, if the cavity is too extensive and large, musculocutaneous flaps are indicated to fill the cavities with adequate bulk.

Advantages of the gluteal perforator flap:[9-11]

1. Various flap designs are possible (e.g. advancement and transposition); these flaps are safe; no muscle is sacrificed; various flaps can be elevated from one donor site if designed properly; and other flap options are not restricted.
2. Donor morbidity after raising gluteal perforator flaps is the lowest, this itself will lead to a shorter hospital stay and therefore reduced costs.
3. A better intraoperative exposure, less blood loss, and a longer vascular pedicle compared to its myocutaneous counterpart. The length of the pedicle gives the flap an impressive mobility and allows for easy tissue transposition without tension.
4. The tissues used in the gluteal perforator flap come from a further distance from the ulcer or wound and, as such, they are less inflamed, less edematous, and less prone to dehiscence. The inset of the flap is always tension free and the donor defect can almost always be closed directly.

GLUTEAL VASCULAR ANATOMY

The gluteal skin is nourished mainly by perforators from the internal iliac artery branches including the superior gluteal artery, the inferior gluteal artery, the lateral sacral artery, and the internal pudendal artery. The superior parasacral region contains lateral sacral artery perforators, and the inferior parasacral region contains perforators coming from the internal pudendal artery. Also, the fourth lumbar artery terminates in the superomedial gluteal region. The gluteal perforator or perforator-based flaps can be planned based on the any of these perforators.

SUPERIOR GLUTEAL ARTERY PERFORATOR

To facilitate identification of superior gluteal artery perforators, a line is drawn from the posterior inferior iliac spine to the coccyx, and from the posterior inferior iliac spine to the apex of the greater trochanter. At the midpoint of the line from posterior inferior iliac spine to the coccyx, another line is drawn to the superior edge of the greater trochanter (GT). This corresponds to the course of the piriformis muscle. A point then marked at the proximal third of the line from the posterior inferior iliac spine to the greater trochanter (GT) coincides to where the superior gluteal artery exits the pelvis through the suprapiriform foramen. The major superior gluteal artery perforators will thus be found lateral and distal to this point of exit and above the piriformis muscle (Fig. 14.1). The more recent cadaver studies showed that the majority of perforators they found were concentrated along the medial two-thirds of the line drawn from the posterior inferior iliac spine to the greater trochanter.[12,13]

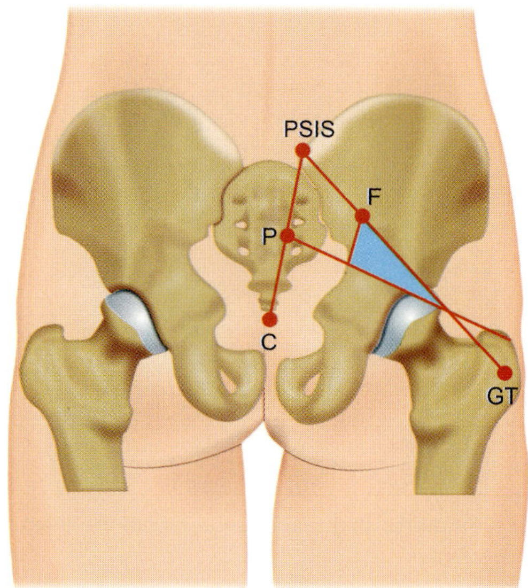

Fig. 14.1: Landmarks and markings to locate the superior gluteal artery perforators.

INFERIOR GLUTEAL ARTERY PERFORATOR

The course of the piriformis muscle is drawn from the midpoint of the line from the posterior inferior iliac spine to the coccyx to the superior edge of the greater trochanter. A vertical line is drawn from the posterior inferior iliac spine to the ischial tuberosity. Along this line, the inferior border of the piriformis marks the point of exit of the inferior gluteal artery. Preferable perforators will be found lateral to this line in the buttock region extending from the piriformis muscle to the inferior gluteal crease (Fig. 14.2).

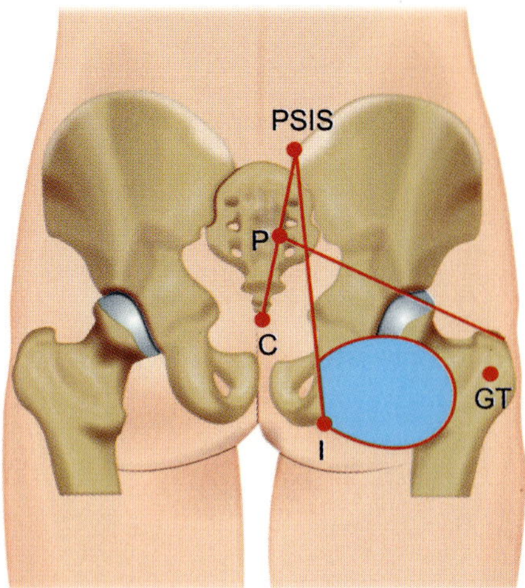

Fig. 14.2: Landmarks and markings to locate the inferior gluteal artery perforators.

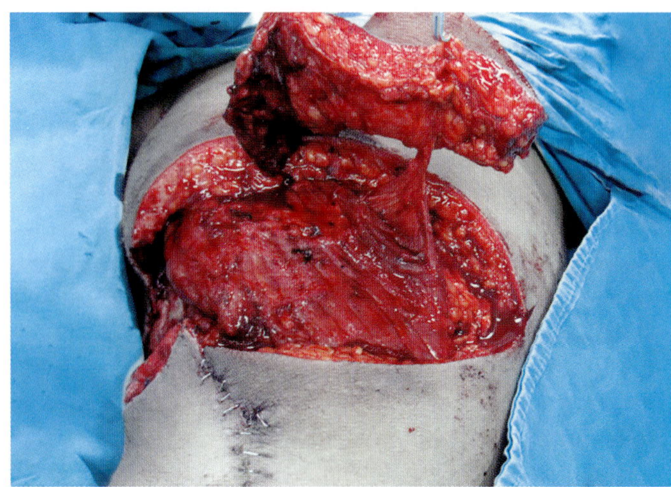

Fig. 14.3: Perforator after dissection. The perforator can be dissected inside the muscle to gain extra length.

Again in recent cadaver studies, it was determined that the majority of these perforators will be in the middle third of this region.[12,13]

PREOPERATIVE PREPARATION

Temporary or permanent intestinal stoma may be required to avoid wound contamination in complicated cases of large sacral defects. Wound culture and bone biopsy are necessary for chronic cases with signs of osteomyelitis. Spasticity contractures and vascular disease that can compromise the flap or wound healing and nutritional factors must first be managed. Intrinsic factors in bedsore physiopathology include sensory loss, diminished muscle strength or mobility, incontinence, infection, anemia, protein malnutrition, and advanced age. Obviously, if possible, these factors must be considered and corrected before surgery.

Antibiotic therapy is given at the beginning of surgery and continued at least for 24 hours postoperatively. Depending on perioperative wound culture, antibiotics should be adjusted if necessary.

SURGICAL TECHNIQUE

Preoperatively, patients were positioned according to the location of the defect. Pressure sores were excised totally and bony prominences were flattened. Doppler investigation is a useful tool for finding the musculocutaneous perforators at the gluteal region, nevertheless it is also easy to find a sizeable perforator during dissection without preoperative mapping. Currently, some authors are using a new method for perforator mapping with a 64-slice spiral computed tomography (CT) scan. This provides more accurate information concerning the vascular network and perforators. The gluteal area is very rich with musculocutaneous perforators; thus, it is always possible to find sizable perforators that can be used as a pedicle. We could easily find musculocutaneous perforators all over the gluteal muscles; however, they were more intensely located at the parasacral area, as noted previously. Flaps were planned close to the defect and shaped as rectangular, elliptical, or triangular (either transposition or V–Y advancement). Flap shape and dimensions varied according to the defect. Another important point in flap design is to consider the donor-site closure; the donor site can be closed directly even after large flap transpositions. There is no specific area of the gluteal region at which to locate the flap because we have easily found the musculocutaneous perforators at every location over the gluteus maximus muscle; however, they were located more intensely at the parasacral region. Flap elevation started with the incision of the distal site of the flap according to the defect. The incision was advanced down to the gluteus maximus muscle and the flap was elevated with the muscle fascia as a fasciocutaneous flap.

During elevation, extreme care was taken to not injure the musculocutaneous perforators.

The authors recommend use of loupe magnification for dissection of the perforators. Marginal perforators thought to restrict the transposition or advancement were ligated and cut. After finding the ideal perforators, they were skeletonized by blunt dissection, and if additional pedicle length was desired, they were dissected down into the muscle (Fig. 14.3). The maximum number of perforators were isolated and preserved, but the perforators that hindered the transposition or advancement were ligated and cut. Generally, we preserved three to five perforators for the pedicle. Nevertheless, when the number of perforators was reduced, the flap could move more easily and farther, but if the mobility of the flap was sufficient, there was no need to reduce the number of perforators. After the perforators were isolated, all boundaries of the flap were incised and the flap was prepared as an island flap supplied by the perforators arising from the gluteal muscles. The elevated flap was transposed or advanced to the defect and sutured in two layers and the donor site was closed directly in the vast majority of the cases (Figs. 14.4 and 14.5).

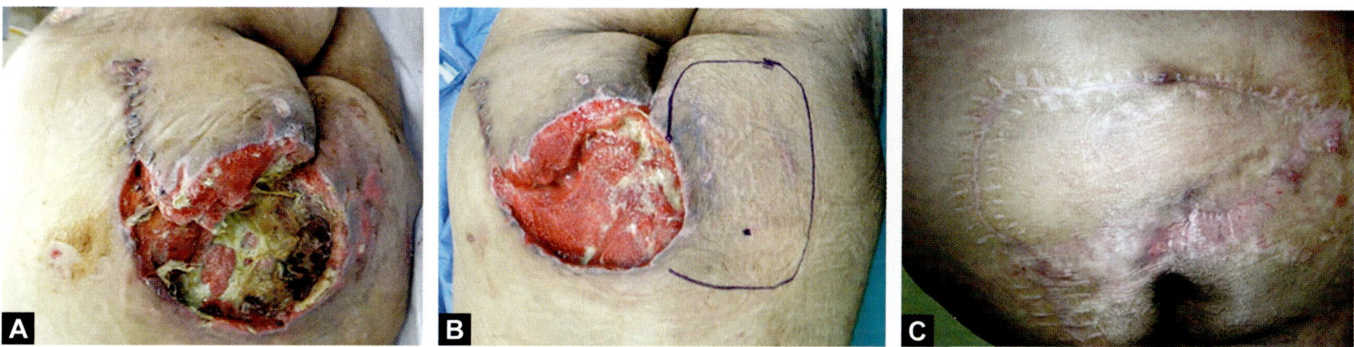

Figs. 14.4A to C: (A) Preoperative sacral pressure sore. (B) Gluteal perforator flap planning close to the defect. (C) Postoperative after transposition of the island perforator flap.

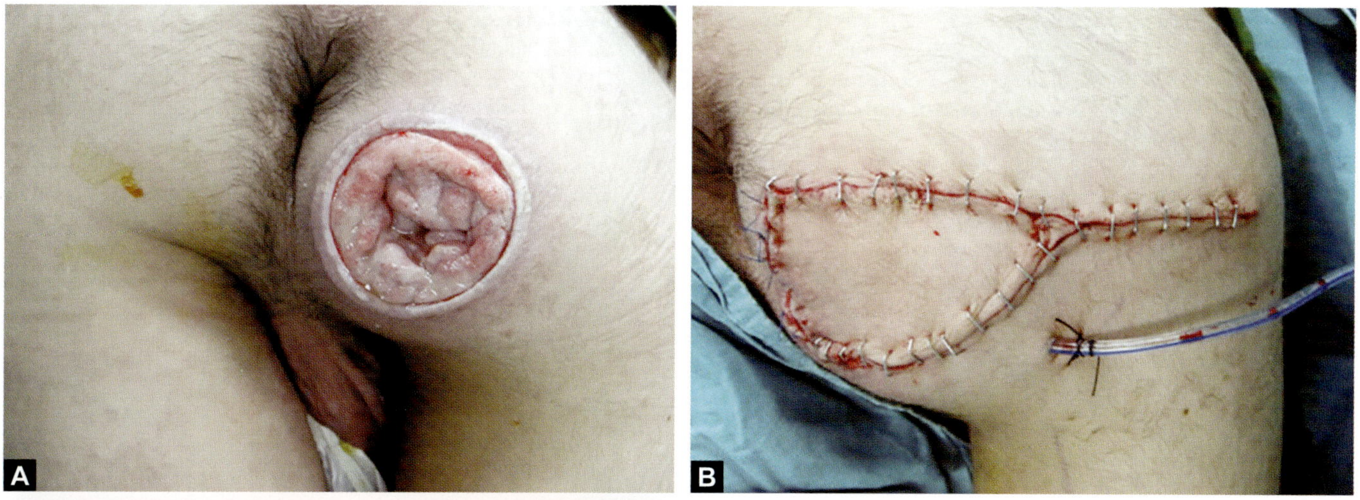

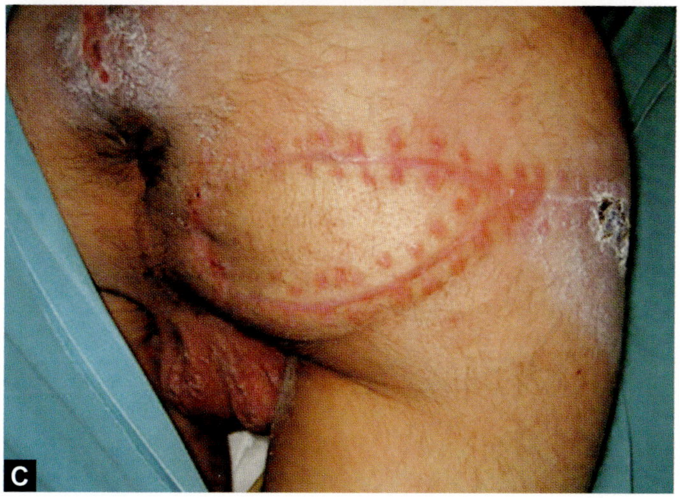

Figs. 14.5A to C: (A) Appearance of an ischial pressure sore before debridement. (B) Early view of the V–Y advancement perforator flap after the operation. (C) Late postoperative view of the same flap.

POSTOPERATIVE CARE

It is imperative to optimize postoperative care for the success of the procedure and to prevent postoperative recurrence. The most important aspect of pressure sore postoperative care is the relief of pressure, shearing, and tension on the newly inset flap. Transfers and positioning require minimal pressure on the flap and minimal tension on the suture line. Urinary catheterization is used to prevent the patient from turning side to side for either micturition or intermittent catheterization. During this time, it is important to continue nutritional support as needed. The initial surgical dressing combined with a nonpermeable dressing can be left in place for 3–5 days postoperatively to help prevent fecal and urinary contamination if necessary. The decision to remove surgical drains should be determined on a patient-to-patient basis and generally removed between fifth and seventh postoperative days.

REFERENCES

1. Taylor GI. The angiosomes of the body and their supply to perforator flaps. Clin Plast Surg. 2003;30(3):331-42.
2. Wei FC, Jain V, Suominen S, et al. Confusion among perforator flaps: what is a true perforator flap? Plast Reconstr Surg. 2001;107(3):874-6.
3. Koshima I, Moriguchi T, Soeda S, et al. The gluteal perforator-based flap for repair of sacral pressure sores. Plast Reconstr Surg. 1993;91(4):678-83.
4. Verpaele AM, Blondeel PN, Van Landuyt K, et al. The superior gluteal artery perforator flap: additional tool in the treatment of sacral pressure sores. Br J Plast Surg. 1999;52 (5):385-91.
5. Higgins JP, Orlando GS, Blondeel PN. Ischial pressure sore reconstruction using an inferior gluteal artery perforator (IGAP) flap. Br J Plast Surg. 2002;55(1):83-5.
6. Ishida LH, Munhoz AM, Montag E, et al. Tensor fasciae latae perforator flap: minimizing donor-site morbidity in the treatment of trochanteric pressure sores. Plast Reconstr Surg. 2005;116(5):1346-52.
7. Hallock GG. The propeller flap version of the adductor muscle perforator flap for coverage of ischial or trochanteric pressure sores. Ann Plast Surg. 2006;56(5):540-42.
8. Scheufler O, Farhadi J, Kovach SJ, et al. Anatomical basis and clinical application of the infragluteal perforator flap. Plast Reconstr Surg. 2006;118(6):1389-400.
9. Coskunfirat OK, Ozgentas HE. Gluteal perforator flaps for coverage of pressure sores at various locations. Plast Reconstr Surg. 2004;113(7):2012-17.
10. Meltem C, Esra C, Hasan F, et al. The gluteal perforator-based flap in repair of pressure sores. Br J Plast Surg. 2004;57(4):342-7.
11. Seyhan T, Ertas NM, Bahar T, et al. Simplified and versatile use of gluteal perforator flaps for pressure sores. Ann Plast Surg. 2008;60(6):673-8.
12. Hallock GG. A primer of schematics to facilitate the design of the preferred muscle perforator flaps. Plast Reconstr Surg. 2009;123(3):1107-15.
13. Ahmadzadeh R, Bergeron L, Tang M, et al. The superior and inferior gluteal artery perforator flaps. Plast Reconstr Surg. 2007;120(6):1551-6.

15 Using Radiofrequency Energy for Heat-Mediated Tissue Tightening: Minimally Invasive and Noninvasive Modalities

Diane I Duncan, Anna Petropoulos, Brian Kinney, Karen S Harkaway, R Stephen Mullholland

INTRODUCTION

A myriad of new devices for nonexcisional skin tightening has been introduced in recent years. This rapidly expanding market[1,2] has been created by an ever-increasing demand for effective procedures with little to no recovery time. As more medical disciplines offer cosmetic services, both the demand and availability has increased. The decision-making process for medical practices interested in offering these services can be difficult. With so many devices to choose from—all claiming exceptional results—how can a person decide upon one or two? A good method for controlling expenses is offered by Pozner.[3] He advises looking at the conditions you are trying to treat and suggests that in the early phase of a cosmetic practice, one should consider “something for red and brown spots, something for resurfacing, a laser hair reduction device, and something for skin and tissue tightening.”

Energy sources commonly used in devices claiming skin and soft tissue tightening include laser, ultrasound, broadband light, and radiofrequency (RF). Sadick[4] evaluated these modalities and presented the recommendation that RF is the best for tissue tightening. However, controversy among his peers still exists regarding which is “best.” Coagulation versus ablation[5] (Lapidoth, Paris) is a primary issue. While many devices have histologic proof of neocollagenesis following treatment,[6-8] an “increase in dermal collagen” does not translate to visible tissue tightening.

RF BASICS

Should we seek ablation or coagulation when the desired response is a decrease in the expanse of skin plus underlying soft tissue? Most surgeons have noted the “drawing together” of subcutaneous tissue when a Bovie cautery is used. This is the desired response when one wants to initiate tissue tightening. In fact, many of us have used this device to tighten a lax breast capsule or to correct a small region of SMAS laxity. Coagulation more effectively appears to “draw together” the skin/fat complex than ablation, which removes tissue.

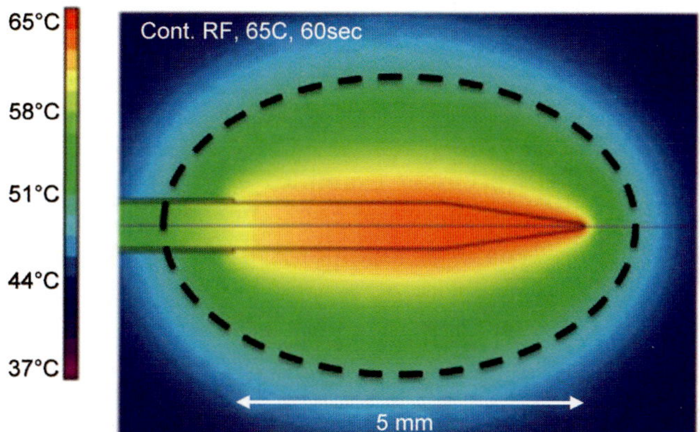

Fig. 15.1: Isotherm of monopolar radiofrequency device. Isotherms can show the distance the energy extends from the device tip, including length and width. Isotherms can also show the maximum temperature at the tip, and the maximum temperature achieved at the edge of the energy field.

One of the factors influencing the effect of the RF device is the isotherm, or “spot size” of the RF tip.[9] Another is the polarity of the device. Ablative devices generally have a small isotherm. The isotherm is the region thermally and therapeutically affected by the device (Fig. 15.1). Therefore, a needle type electrode would usually cause ablation, and an electrode with a larger surface area would generate more of a coagulative response. This principle is expressed by Joule’s law, which notes that energy density directly correlates with the size of the area that the electrical current flows through.

When using a RF device, the treatment provider should then consider the desired effect before choosing the proper device. For example, if the treatment plan is nerve ablation to create a long-lasting relaxation of the corrugators, a small ablative type RF needle or probe would be used. If coagulation or drawing together of tissue is desired, a slightly larger RF tip with lower power would be used. Bipolar energy an easier modality with which to create the "drawing-together" response than monopolar energy is. In order to induce sub-necrotic heating or collagen remodeling, a much larger treatment tip, usually a square centimeter or larger, would be indicated. Due to the large size of the sublative devices, these are generally used externally.

Monopolar or Bipolar?

Monopolar devices, by definition, need a grounding pad (also called the return electrode) in order to close or complete the electrical circuit. Examples of monopolar devices are electrocautery units and nerve ablation devices. In a device using bipolar or multipolar RF, the electrodes are relatively close to each other, and the electrodes create an equal thermal effect. These devices can create a larger zone of thermal injury. Most commonly, monopolar devices are used for cutting or ablation, while bipolar devices are more frequently used for coagulation. Newer multipolar devices can create several levels of subnecrotic heating for noninvasive tissue tightening. Multipolar RF needling devices can insert into the dermis, causing a local coagulative effect.

Principles of RF Tissue Tightening

The focus on an epidermal and dermal target has changed during recent years; now the hypodermis or subcutaneous adipose layer has emerged as a much more responsive target.[10] Thermal effects on tissue have been intensely studied,[11-14] and the temperature at which different types of tissue respond to heat by shrinking has been established.[15] Arguments over the effect of "bulk heating" versus heating a specific target are common. Heating a pinpoint target, as an RF needle or microfocused ultrasound does, will create a small zone of thermal destruction that will cause some inflammation, focal internal scarring, and tissue contraction. A broader spread of energy will result in a more diffuse effect, and more tissue will be affected. Therefore, when a large amount of tissue needs treatment, the use of a bipolar or multichannel monopolar device makes the most sense.

Tissue Tightening Guidelines

Many noninvasive devices claim to combine tissue tightening effects with fat loss. In order to be able to control the degree of tightening and the amount of fat loss, one has to understand the mechanism of action of each.

Tightening of the fibroseptal network is the principle behind heat-mediated tissue tightening. This is more effectively achieved with minimally invasive devices, such as the Invasix BodyTite or the ThermiGen monopolar device, than with totally noninvasive devices. The tissue must be heated to a minimum of 55°C in order to cause visible collagen contraction. While a definite effect can be achieved with noninvasive external devices such as Viora's reaction device or the Endymed multipolar phase controlled device, a series of noninvasive treatments is needed in order to be able to see a definite clinical effect.

In targeting the fibroseptal network—with either minimally invasive or noninvasive device type—the following guidelines should be considered:

- A multilevel treatment can create much more of an effect than treating at only one level. This principle is well demonstrated by the Ulthera multifocused ultrasound device. Treatment at both 4.5 and 3 mm depths causes much more visible lift due to tissue contraction than the use of a single tissue level alone. The reaction device can treat multiple soft tissue levels at once. By using the "Refit" protocol,[15] three levels of tissue heating occur with a single pass. This increases time efficiency as well as cost effectiveness.
- Optimal impedance can help improve the selective uptake of heat energy by the collagenous stromal vascular fraction of the fatty layer. Few physicians really pay attention to impedance. This is an important predictor of long-term effect. Fat is a good insulator since it repels heat. The tissue absorption of electrical energy can be enhanced by making that tissue wetter. The infusion of tumescent fluid in the treatment region can enhance the contractile capability of the FSN by lowering electrical impedance.
- Choosing the correct target is a third key in the achievement of an optimal outcome. Just treating the submental neck does not create a beautiful jawline. A defined mandibular angle, and a straight, lateral jawline with a clearly defined submandibular shadow are equally important aspects. The ability to look at the whole "frame" rather than the center of the picture will improve preoperative planning.

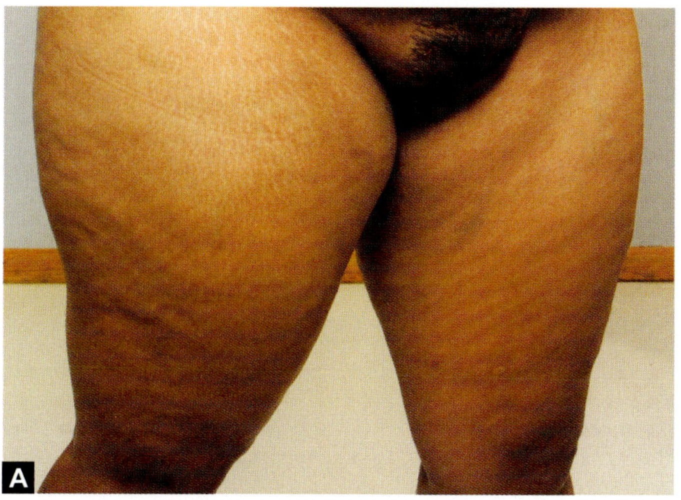

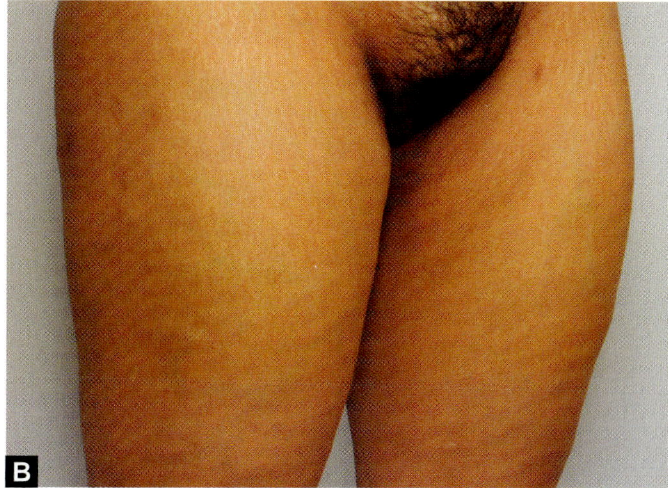

Figs. 15.2A and B: (A) This 28-year-old Native American lost 80 lb, but still complained of large thighs. Circumferential RFAL was performed with the Invasix BodyTite device. (B) Result at 1 year. No skin was excised. RFAL, radiofrequency-assisted liposuction.

- Deciding how much tissue tightening versus how much fat reduction is needed is also an important step in planning. What percent of the deformity is due to fat, and what part is due to tissue laxity? If there is pendulous hanging tissue, a great deal of time and effort will be needed to achieve a nonexcisional success. If the arms are mostly fatty, with very little soft tissue laxity, the majority of time and effort can be devoted to liposuction or noninvasive fat reduction, with less time spent on tissue heating for the purpose of apparent skin tightening.
- Settings/energy use is usually the final decision to be made before treatment can commence. Safety of the patient is paramount; more conservative settings and a slower treatment pace are always wise at the beginning of this learning curve. There is a definite enhancement of outcome when the combination of liposuction and RF heating is used. Even with very safe settings, this combination can result in quite dramatic outcomes (Figs. 15.2A and B)

Following the manufacturer's recommended settings is the safest choice. Because burns can occur even when using the external sublative devices, following the rules is essential to patient safety.

Associated Fat Reduction

When laser-based tissue tightening devices were introduced, most practitioners heated the fat only, without performing associated liposuction.[16] However, simultaneous liposuction was rapidly embraced as the original treatment pattern did not always generate an optimal response.

Many of the newer devices are designed to cause fat reduction without the need for aspiration. While devices that cause a disruption of the stability of the electrical current within and just outside of the cell membrane can cause frank cell lysis, it is more common to see the induction of apoptosis (Tiede A, personal communication May 17, 2013). Electroporation as a mechanism of causing cell death has been cited but not well mastered until recently.[17]

Photodynamic therapy or PDT has been used for almost a decade for fat reduction.[18] Reports of modest but definite fat loss persist. The mechanism appears to be electroporation. Biopsy of the superficial treatment regions shows cell wall lysis in 15% of the cells in a high powered field,[19] and recent electron microscopy images show an emptying of the adipocytes with retention of the external cell wall.[20]

This principle has been applied to RF devices. The Tite FX device (Invasix, Yokneam, Israel) operates upon a modification of that principle. A vacuum device is combined with an RF heating system that warms the skin and soft tissue. When an external temperature of 42°C is achieved, a "2nd RF" impulse is sent in an oscillating manner to the treatment region. This strong RF pulse destabilizes the electrical charge of the adipocyte membranes, causing apoptosis or programmed cell death.[21] Images taken with high resolution ultrasound show a 41–63% reduction in fat thickness with four to eight treatments in reproducible

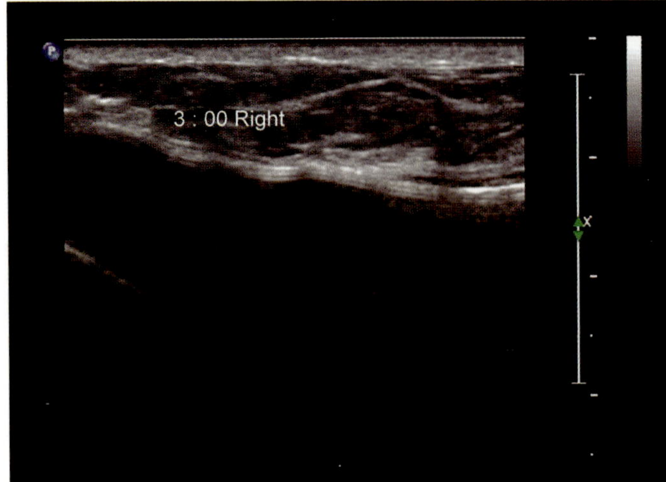

Fig. 15.3: Cross-section of abdomen following treatment with Tite FX. High-resolution ultrasound measurements are used to measure the sequential reduction in subcutaneous fat thickness. The change in fat architecture is also seen as a flattening of the vertically oriented fat lobules.

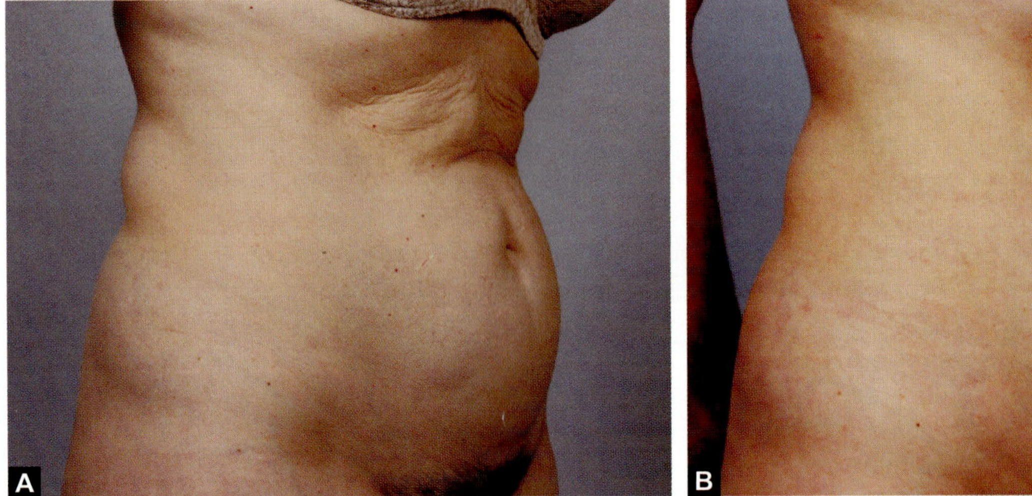
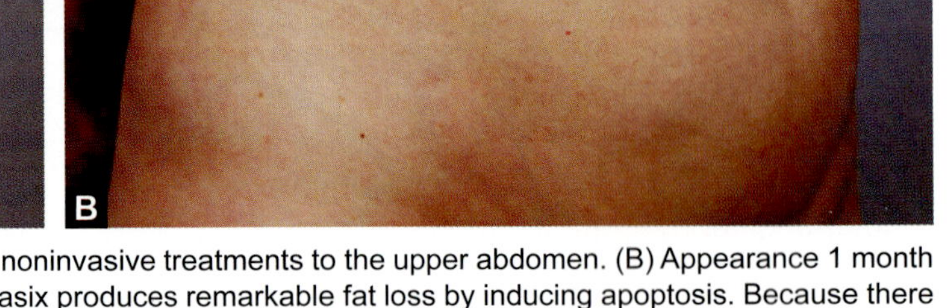

Figs. 15.4A and B: (A) This 63-year-old underwent Tite FX RF noninvasive treatments to the upper abdomen. (B) Appearance 1 month after 8 sequential weekly treatments. The Tite FX device by Invasix produces remarkable fat loss by inducing apoptosis. Because there is very little inflammation and no down time with this device, there is only modest tissue tightening and wrinkle reduction.

defined treatment locations.[22] There is a consequent change in the subcutaneous cross-sectional architecture as well (Fig. 15.3).

If fat loss only without surgery is a priority, a device like this would be recommended. However, the apoptotic process is noninflammatory by definition. Therefore, only mild tightening of the soft tissue is noted with this device (Figs. 15.4A and B). If tissue tightening is more of a priority than fat loss, a device similar to the Viora reaction is recommended (Figs. 15.5A and B). This device is geared toward soft tissue tightening. When used in a defined location with multiple passes, some fat loss is noted as well. Figures 15.4 and 15.5 show results of each treatment with a slightly different effect noted with each device.

TECHNIQUE

Technique varies from one device to another, but also from one practitioner to another. Plastic surgeons used to perform invasive procedures will be more comfortable with minimally invasive devices than with noninvasive devices. Dermatologists and aesthetic medicine practitioners may have a different comfort zone. As Pozner[3] advises, it is important to stay within the realm of your training and experience when choosing and using one of these RF devices.

In order to best offer technique guidance, case examples performed by a variety of practitioners will be presented. These are somewhat limited by the number and

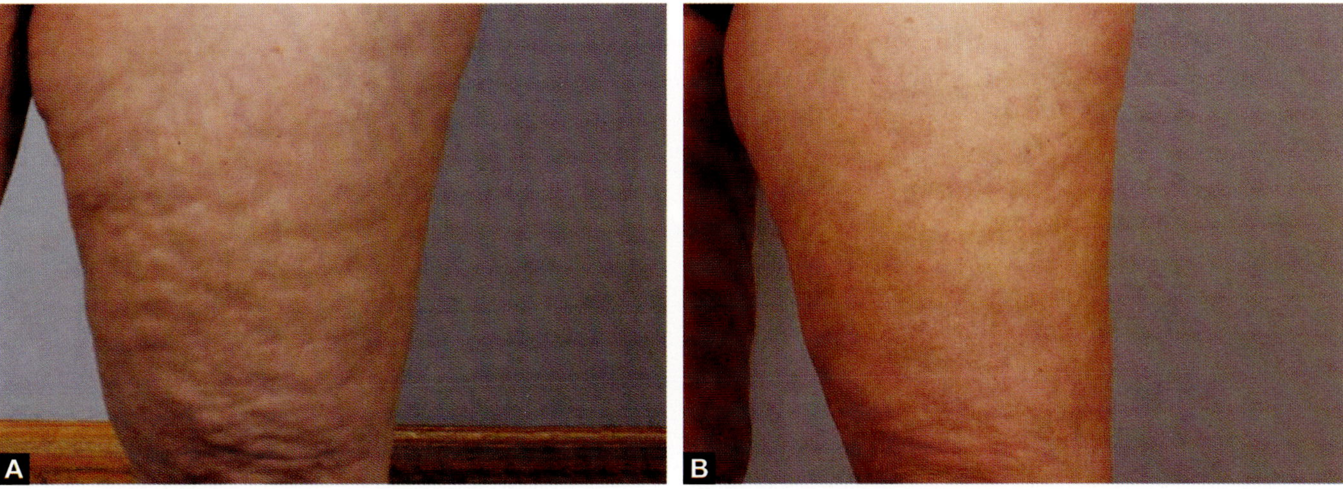

Figs. 15.5A and B: This 53-year-old's left thigh was treated with Tite FX by Invasix for fat reduction and reaction by Viora for tissue tightening. The result at 4 months after eight combination treatments shows a significant improvement in her grade III cellulite.

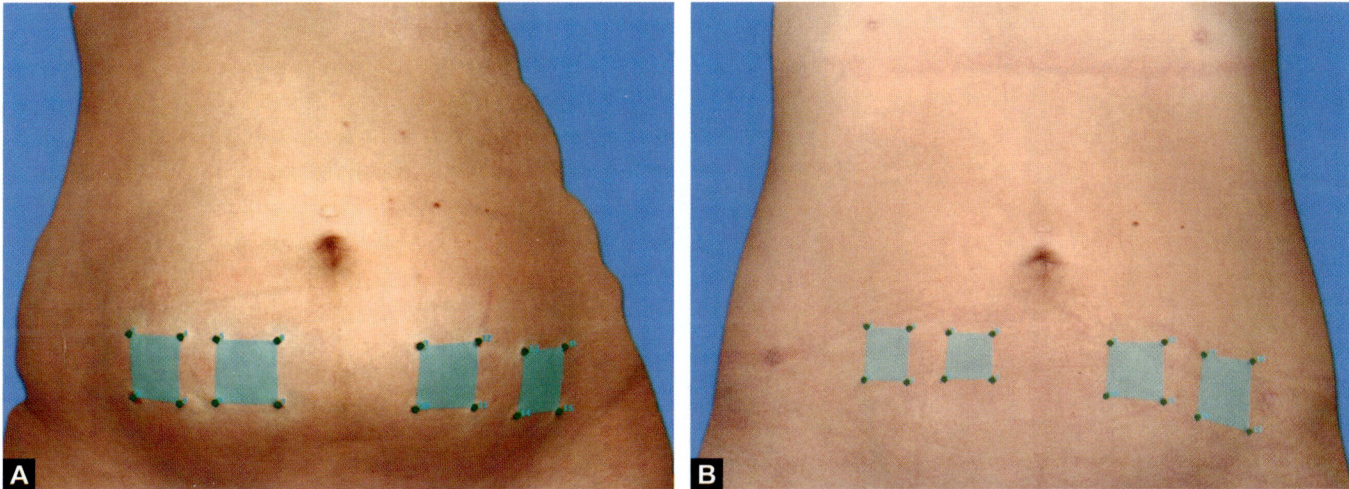

Figs. 15.6A and B: This 21-year-old was part of a prospective randomized study performed with the BodyTite. Small tattoos were placed in a 3 cm^2 pattern before treatment. The right side was treated with tumescent fluid infusion followed by SAL combined with RF heating. The left side was treated with SAL alone. At 1 year, Canfield Vectra measurements showed a 34.5% mean skin surface area reduction on the right, as compared to an 8.4% measured skin surface area reduction on the left.

type of devices owned or in use by the contributors. Indications, settings, and technique tips are included. Before and after photos will demonstrate a variety of outcomes based on device type and treatment style.

Minimally Invasive RF-assisted Tissue Tightening

This is a practice that has advanced greatly during the past years. Even early results showed promise in the quest for tissue tightening and lift without dermolipectomy. A study done in 2010[23] showed that RF heating performed in conjunction with liposuction could create a 26% skin surface area reduction at 6 weeks post-treatment as measured with the Canfield Vectra system. Interestingly, there was a continuing tightening trend until about the 1 year mark. The mean surface area reduction in 24 treatment squares identified with small tattoos was 34.5% at 1 year. While SAL-alone treated regions contracted about 10% at 6 weeks, at a year there was a slight loss of tightening, down to about 8% (Figs. 15.6A and B).

However, more tightening is not always better. A thinner patient with prominent striae had a 60% measured surface area reduction. This caused buckling and visible

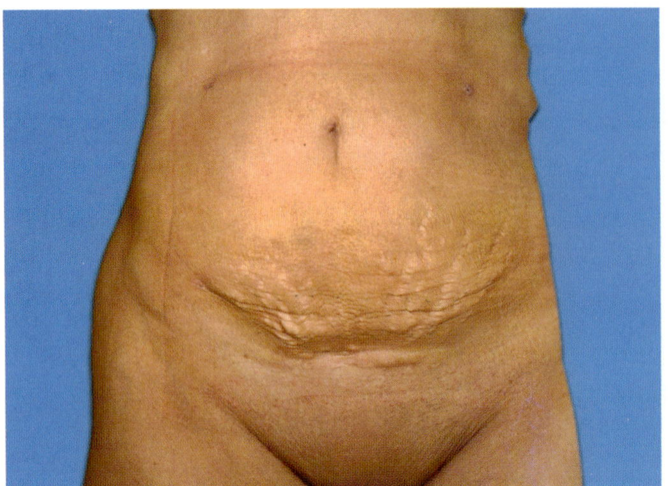

Fig. 15.7: This 51-year-old was treated with SAL only on the left, and with SAL plus RFAL on the right. A measured 60% skin surface area reduction was noted using Canfield Vectra measurements in the right medial tattooed square. While there is a skin contour irregularity on both sides, the right side has more severe buckling due to a combination of preoperatively present striae and overcontraction of the hypodermis below the skin. RFAL, radiofrequency-assisted liposuction.

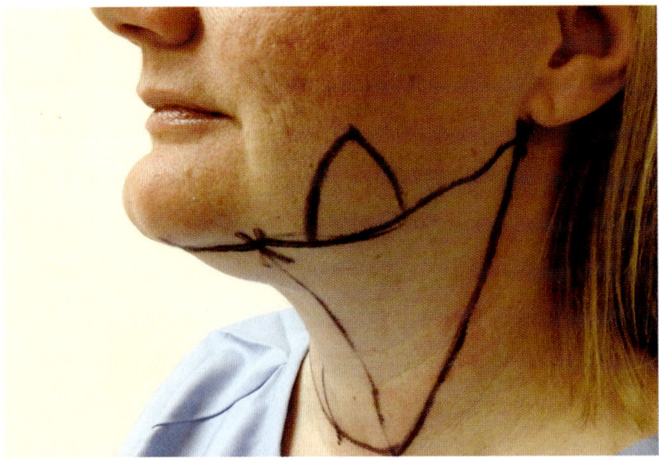

Fig. 15.9: Treatment zones demarcated for ThermiGen RF-assisted neck lift.
Courtesy: Dr Karen Harkaway, Delran, NJ.

surface contour irregularity (Fig. 15.7). A good goal is about 25% or less visible tissue tightening intraoperatively. As the contraction process continues to occur postoperatively, undercorrection of the deformity during the procedure is advisable.

RF-assisted Tissue Tightening

The only currently available minimally invasive device is the ThermiGen monopolar RF platform (Fig. 15.8). It is currently FDA approved for nerve ablation; its use in soft tissue tightening is off-label. This device features an internal tissue thermometer as well as external skin temperature monitoring with the high-resolution FLIR "gun."

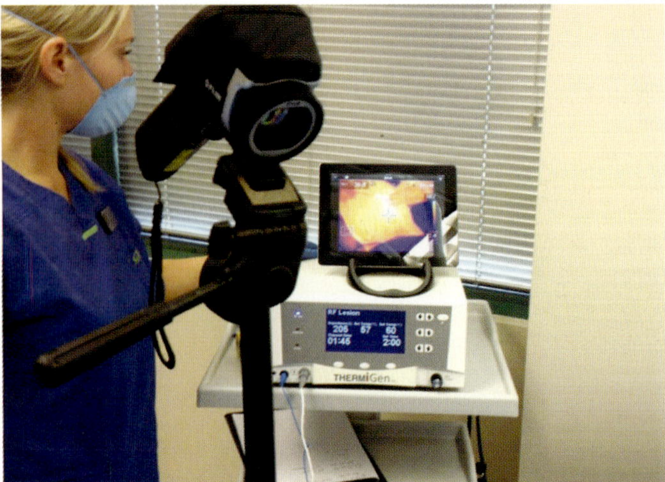

Fig. 15.8: The ThermiGen device with accompanying FLIR camera. This device features an internal tissue thermometer as well as external skin temperature monitoring with the high-resolution FLIR "gun."

Standard ThermiGen neck lifting includes infusion of tumescent anesthesia infusion following sterile prep and drape. Treatment "zones" are marked (Fig. 15.9). Usually three zones (right lateral, left lateral, and submental) are delineated. If jowls are a concern, these are added in separately. Since the treatment probe only measures 10 cm, care must be taken to make each zone slightly <10 cm^2.

Punctate access ports are created with a 16-gauge needle after local anesthesia is introduced at the posterior earlobe base bilaterally and the submental crease. Depending on the size of the neck, between 100 and 200 mL of standard tumescent solution are evenly infused.

Attention is first directed toward the right lateral neck zone. The 10-cm probe is introduced, and the device is set to "RF lesion." Good settings to begin with are 55°C internally, with a 38°C external maximum skin temperature. The probe is slowly moved in and out, spreading in a ray-type manner. Care is taken not to draw back to the same point repeatedly, as the region closest to the probe entry site will become overheated. There are no clinical endpoints to treatment other than temperature. If an area gets too hot externally, it is wise to move on to the next treatment zone.

The 2-minute segments are repeated until all treatment zones have been treated once. A single repeat of each treatment zone is possible, unless the region remains quite

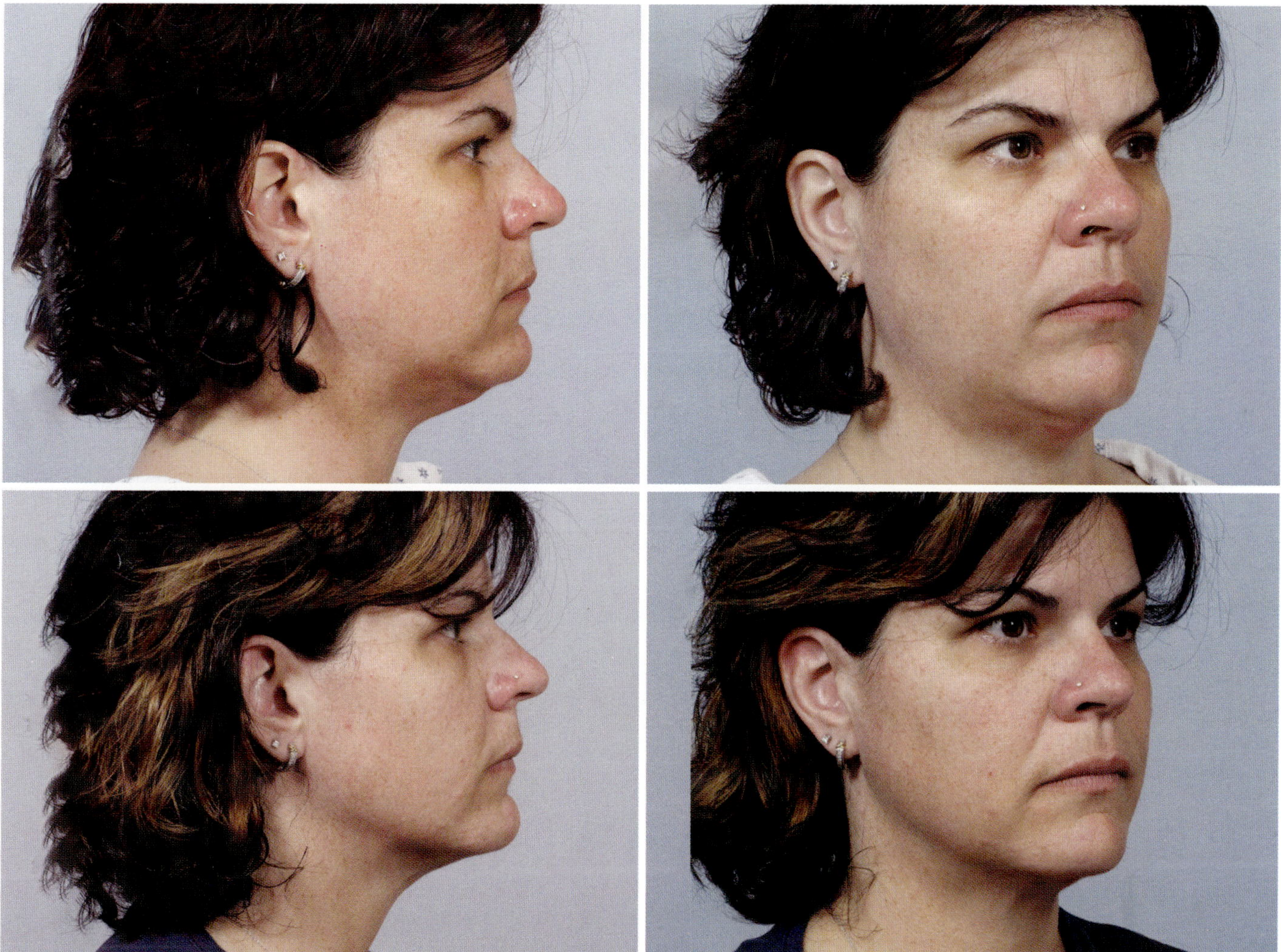

Fig. 15.10: (Left) Preoperative 40-year-old female with residual lipodystrophy and neck skin laxity following 80 lb weight loss. (Right) Two months following RF-assisted neck lift with liposuction. Three 16-gauge needle access ports were created. No skin excision was performed.

hot. If an area of erythema or a spike in skin temperature is noted, immediate application of iced saline on a gauze pad can prevent a burn. Care in closely following tissue and skin temperature is very important.

Liposuction can be performed in conjunction with RF tissue heating. In very thick or fatty necks, half of the liposuction can be performed prior to heating in order to reduce bulk and therefore increase heating efficiency and save time. Care should be taken to avoid aggressive liposuction prior to heating, as this really increases the risk of burns. Usually no sutures are needed to close the access ports. Bandaids can be placed over these. Aftercare includes the wearing of a "jaw bra" for support for several days to a week. The patients are advised to minimize activity for a few days.

Case 1: Invasix FaceTite

A 40-year-old woman had lost 80 lb and had some residual fat and soft tissue laxity in her neck and submental chin (Fig. 15.10). She had a poorly defined jawline. This patient's goals were less pendulosity, a more "firm" appearance, correction of the "gobbler," and a better defined jawline.

Procedure: Device used was Invasix FaceTite. Anesthesia was local with 1% lidocaine plus 131 mL standard tumescent infusion. Settings were 20 W, 37° maximum skin temperature. Energy used was 19.6 kJ. Entry points with 16-gauge needle were at earlobes and submental crease. Local anesthesia was placed at access points, a 16-gauge needle poke was used for access. Small tumescent and

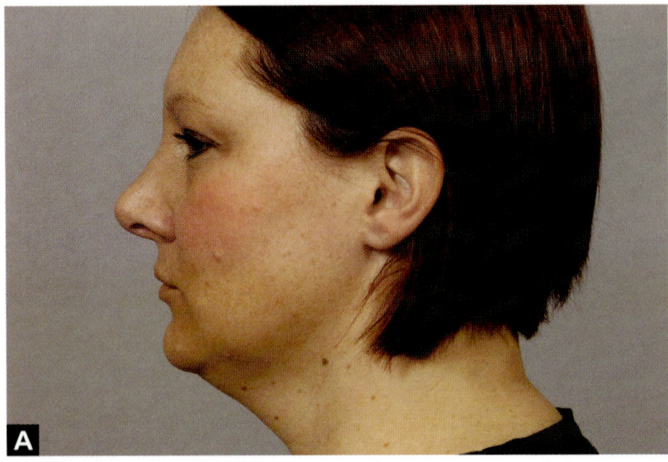
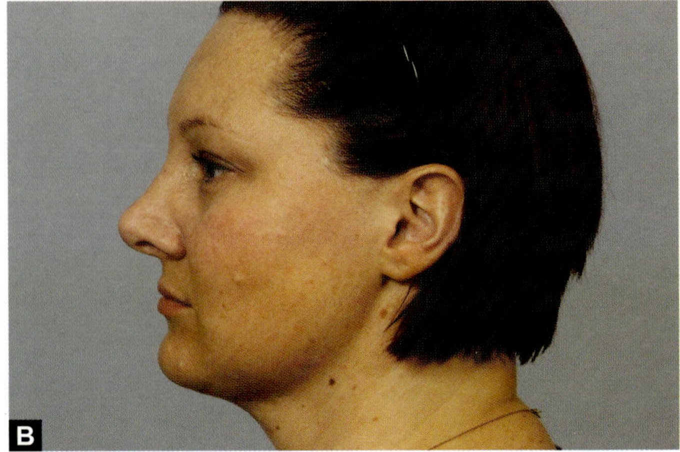

Figs. 15.11A and B: (A) Preoperative 36-year-old with hereditary "chubby neck." (B) Two months following Thermigen neck lift with lipoaspiration 50 mL.

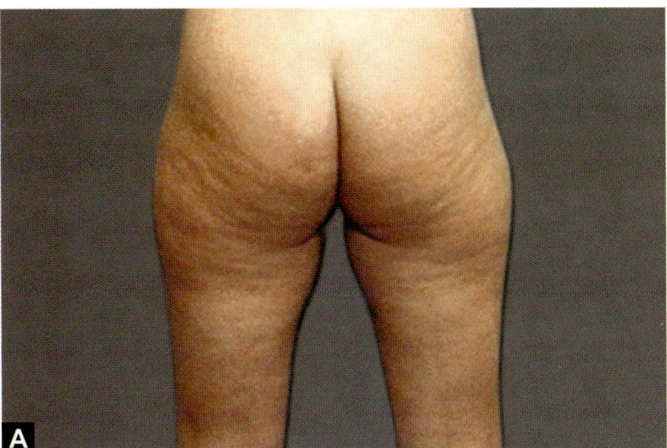
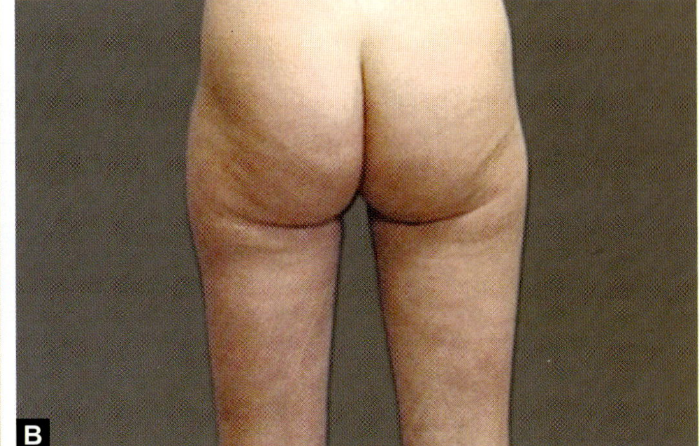

Figs. 15.12A and B: (A) Preoperative 28-year-old with "drumstick" deformity of inner and outer thighs with cellulite. (B) Two months following RF-assisted liposuction.

liposuction cannulas were used. Liposuction was performed first, conservatively, in order to expose more of the fibroseptal network to RF heat. The FaceTite device was used to heat tissue using slow strokes in a radial manner, with a 90°C overlap from the adjacent region when possible. The very conservative 37°C maximum skin temperature prevented any burns. Duration was 1.5 hours.

Case 2: Thermigen RF Device

This 36-year-old had hereditary "chubby neck" (Figs. 15.11A and B).

Procedure: Device used was Thermigen RF symphony with 10 cm probe. Anesthesia was local plus tumescent fluid, 203 mL. Settings were at 60°C maximum internal temperature and 39°C maximum skin temperature. RF device on continuous mode; two sessions per segment. Three entry points using a 16-gauge needle under each earlobe and submental crease. Following injection of lidocaine at access points the tumescent infusion was injected. Conservative liposuction was performed. The path of the marginal mandibular nerve was diagrammed out using the nerve stimulator preoperatively. RF heating was done in three segments: right lateral, central submental, and left lateral. Heating was done in 2 minute time periods as programmed by the device. Once the entire neck had been treated, a second pass was used in a similar manner to heat the treatment region a second time. A FLIR camera was used to monitor the external skin temperature. Duration was 1.5 hours.

Case 3: Invasix BodyTite Device

This 28-year-old had "drumstick" deformity of inner and outer thighs with cellulite (Figs. 15.12A and B).

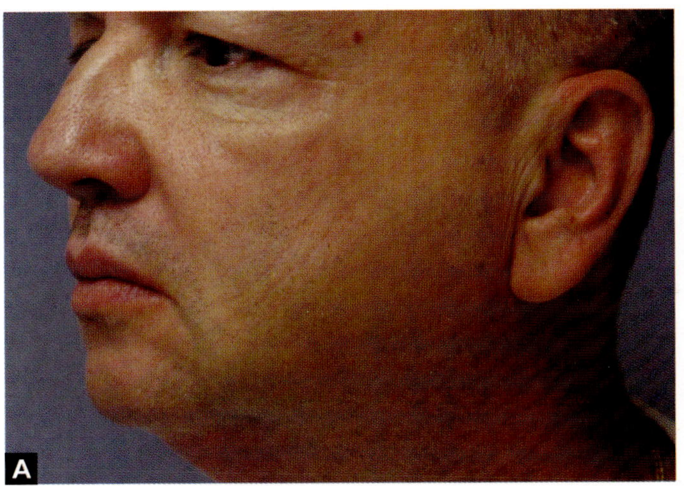
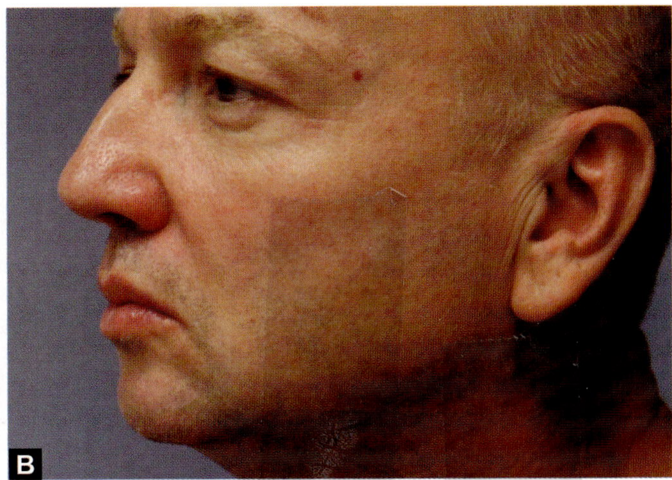

Figs. 15.13A and B: (A) 54-year-old man with laxity plus lipodystrophy of the neck and lower jawline prior to treatment. (B) Seven-week post-treatment with Thermigen RF heating under local anesthesia. No liposuction was performed.
Courtesy: Dr Brian Kinney, Beverly Hills, CA.

Procedure: Device used was Invasix BodyTite. Anesthesia was general with tumescent fluid 400 mL per region. Settings were 45 W, 37°C maximum skin temperature. Eight entry points with 16-gauge needle holes in lateral and medial thigh. Following creation of punctate access points, tumescent fluid was infused into the medial, lateral, and infragluteal thigh. A 3 mm cannula was used to perform about 50% of anticipated SAL in these regions. 10×10 cm^2 were diagrammed in each treatment region. The BodyTite device was used to heat the subcutaneous tissue at 3 depths. Settings were 45 W with a maximum external skin temperature of 37°C. Treatment endpoints of each square were the achievement of warmth and erythema as well as reaching of the skin temp maximum. A visible change in skin texture with a slight drawing together of the skin can be noted. Following RF heating of all squares, completion of the liposuction was performed. Duration was 4 hours and there were no complications.

Case 4: Thermigen RF Neck Lift, Male Patient

This 54-year-old male had laxity plus lipodystrophy of the neck and lower jawline prior to treatment (Fig. 15.13A). Post-treatment with Thermigen RF heating under local anesthesia. No liposuction was performed (Fig. 15.13B).

Case 5: Thermigen Neck Lift, Male Patient

This 58-year-old man had severe skin laxity in the neck and lower jawline (Figs. 15.14A to D). Technique in this case was expanded to include two access ports within each lateral oral commissure. The marginal mandibular nerve can be preoperatively mapped out using the external nerve stimulator. Treatment of the marionette regions and jowls dramatically enhanced overall outcome.

Case 6: Thermigen Neck Lift, Female Patient (Figs. 15.15A and B)

This 49-year-old female had skin laxity in the submental and cervicomental neck (Figs. 15.15A and B). She had and extended neck lift with Thermigen under local tumescent anesthesia.

Case 7: Thermigen Neck Lift, Male Patient (Figs. 15.16A and B)

This 52-year-old male had localized skin laxity in the neck region. Treatment was with RF heating under tumescent anesthesia. Male patients generally decline excisional neck lifts, but are more enthusiastic about the minimally invasive approach.

NONINVASIVE RF DEVICES

Can these devices come close to producing results that the minimally invasive devices can? The answer is yes, but more than a single treatment will be needed. When the goal is tightening of the skin and soft tissue, the results achieved with traditional skin excision techniques remain the benchmark that newer techniques will be compared to. Unmet expectations are more common when these

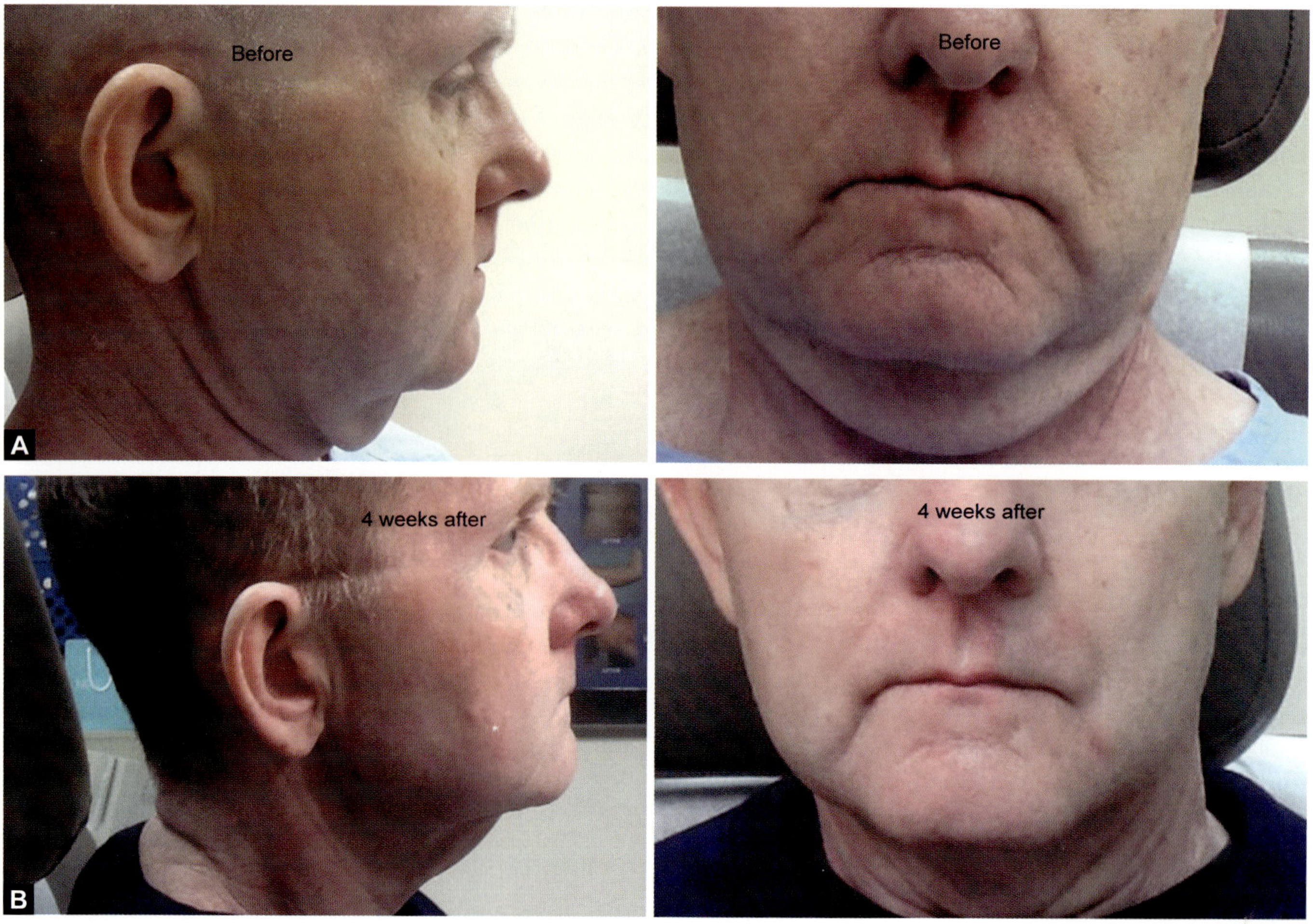

Figs. 15.14A and B: (A) A 58-year-old man with severe skin laxity in the neck and lower jawline. Technique in this case was expanded to include two access ports within each lateral oral commissure. The marginal mandibular nerve can be preoperatively mapped out using the external nerve stimulator. (B) Four-week post-treatment of the marionette regions and jowls. The technique in this case was expanded to include two access ports within each lateral oral commissure. Note dramatically enhance overall outcome.
Courtesy: Dr Karen Harkaway, Delran, NJ.

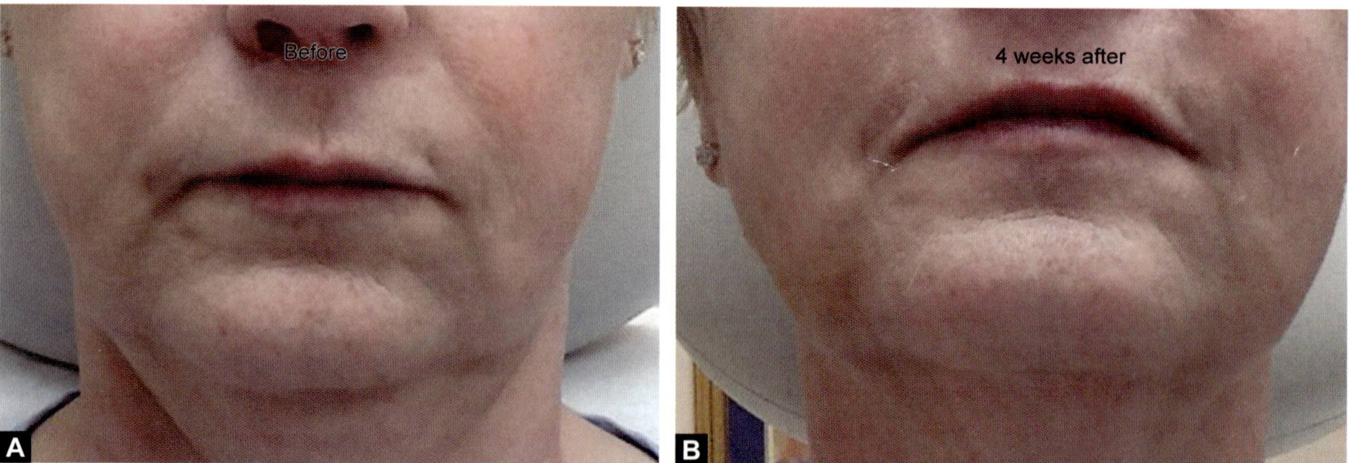

Figs. 15.15A and B: (A) Pretreatment. 49-year-old woman with skin laxity in the submental and cervicomental neck. (B) Three weeks following extended neck lift with Thermigen under local tumescent anesthesia.
Courtesy: Dr Karen Harkaway, Delran, NJ.

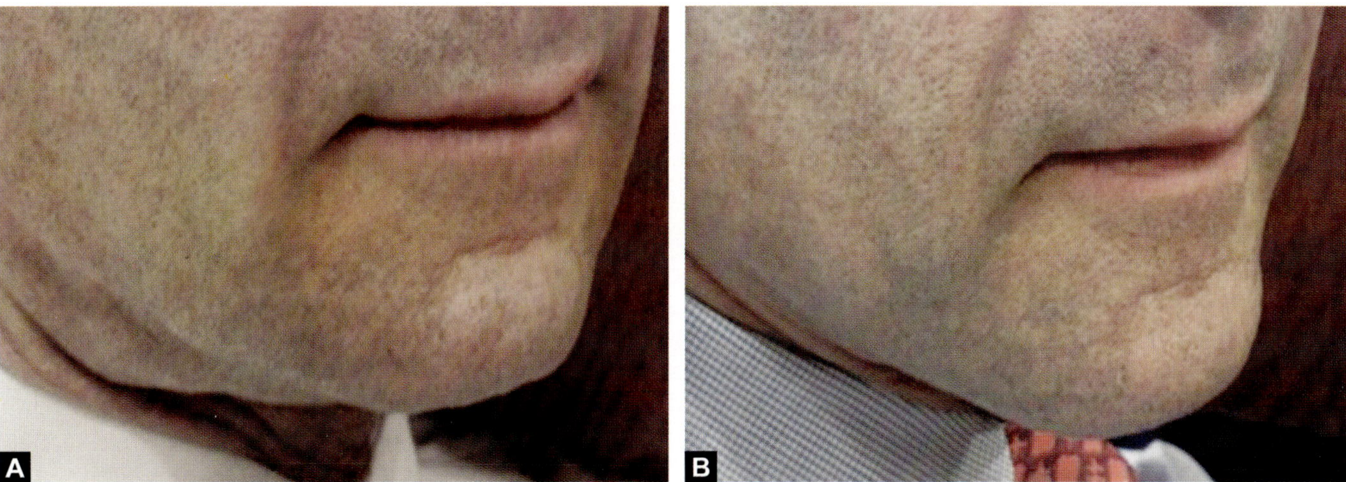

Figs. 15.16A and B: (A) A 52-year-old man with localized skin laxity in the neck region. (B) One month following treatment with RF heating under tumescent anesthesia. Male patients generally decline excisional neck lifts, but are more enthusiastic about the minimally invasive approach.
Courtesy: Dr Anna Petropoulus, Danvers, MA.

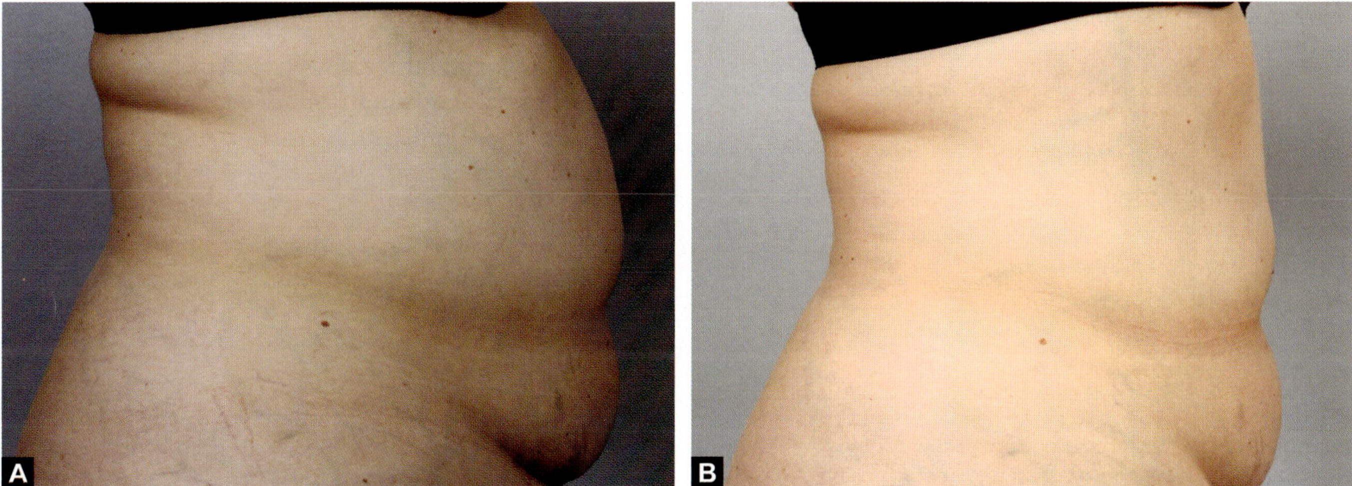

Figs. 15.17A and B: (A) Pretreatment 48-year-old had abdominal lipodystrophy. (B) One month later, after four weekly treatments. No weight loss occurred.
Courtesy: Dr Diane Duncan.

devices are used than with surgical techniques, as the subcutaneous temperatures needed to cause dramatic tissue contraction are much more difficult to reach transcutaneously.

Case 8: Tite FX RF Fat Reduction, Abdominal (Figs. 15.17A and B)

This is a 48-year-old with abdominal lipodystrophy.

Procedure: Device used was TiteFX by Invasix. No anesthesia. Settings were skin temp maximum 42, second RF at 4. The patient was treated on the operating room table. One treatment zone just above the umbilicus and another treatment zone below the umbilicus were delineated. Using the handheld vacuum/RF device, tissue was "stamped" and held in the device while RF heating commenced. Several treatment rows were needed in order to reach the optimum skin temperature. When the device read 42°C, a "2nd RF" oscillating vibration was sent through the tissue. This wave of energy depolarized the adipocyte cell membranes, causing programmed cell death. Four treatments 1 week apart were given. The strength of the "2nd RF" was maximal at a setting of 4. Duration was 45 minutes and there were no complications.

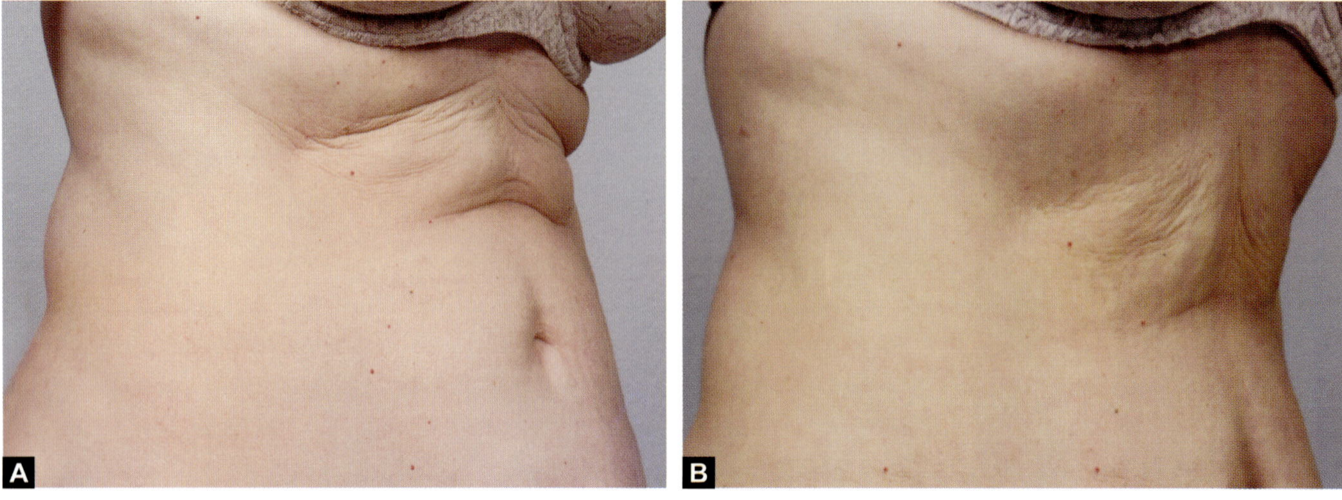

Figs. 15.18A and B: (A) Pretreatment 63-year-old with epigastium wrinkling. (B) After eight treatments of the epigastrium with Tite FX 1 week apart, significant fat reduction is noted. Mild tissue tightening is noted, but some wrinkles still remain.
Courtesy: Dr Diane Duncan.

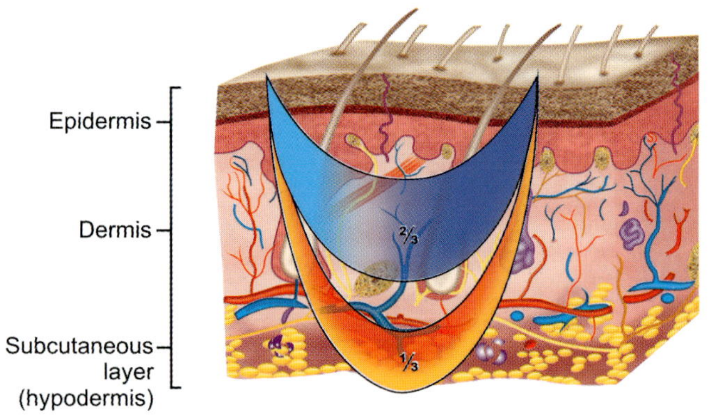

Fig. 15.19: The Reaction device by Viora can simultaneously treat three tissue levels with its bipolar device. Addition of vacuum intensifies the treatment and drives the energy deeper. This diagram shows the approximate location of energy distribution within the dermis and hypodermis.

Because the mechanism of fat loss is apoptosis (by definition without inflammation) less concomitant skin tightening is seen than is noted with devices that induce inflammation. However, some definite tissue lift can be seen, even in older patients.

Case 9: Tite FX Treatment of the Epigastrium (Figs. 15.18A and B)

A 63-year-old patient had four Tite FX treatments in the upper abdomen. Less skin wrinkling is noted after treatment, as well as subcutaneous fat reduction.

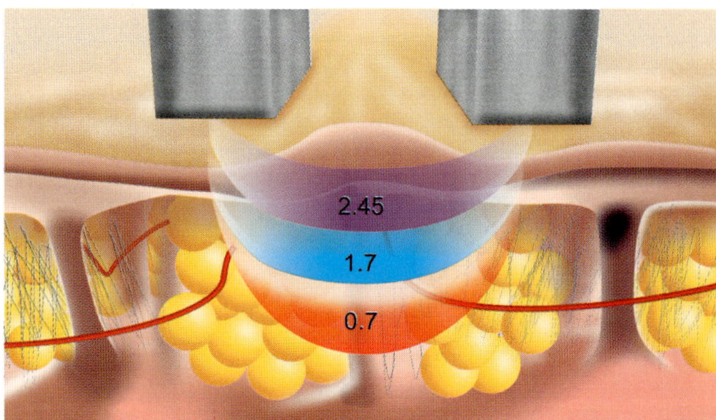

Fig. 15.20: Energy distribution target of the Viora Reaction device.

REACTION DEVICE BY VIORA

This totally noninvasive device is FDA approved for the temporary reduction of cellulite. The RF energy output is bipolar, but can be multilevel. Figure 15.19 shows the relative energy distribution within the dermis and within the hypodermis as well. The device can be set to a single level. For example, on the deepest setting, mode 1, the device can be used to cause apoptotic fat reduction within the superficial subcutaneous layer. Mode 2 treats the superficial hypodermis and lower dermis, while mode 3 targets the papillary dermis. All three modes/levels can be utilized at once in the mode 4 setting (Fig. 15.20).

Use of the mode 4 setting is the most time efficient and effective way to generate skin tightening and some contraction of the superficial fat layer. The technique of use includes the following:

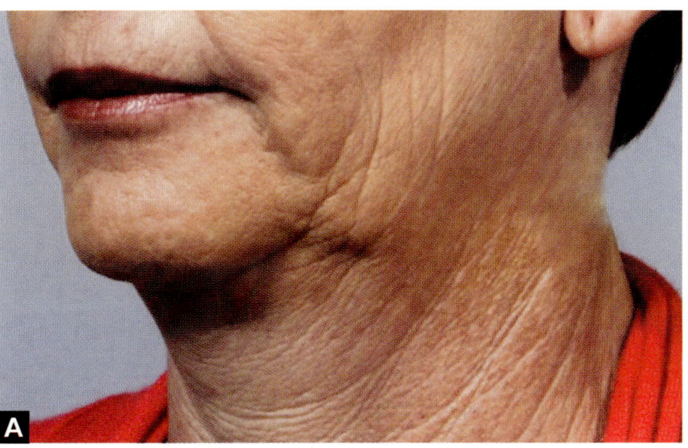

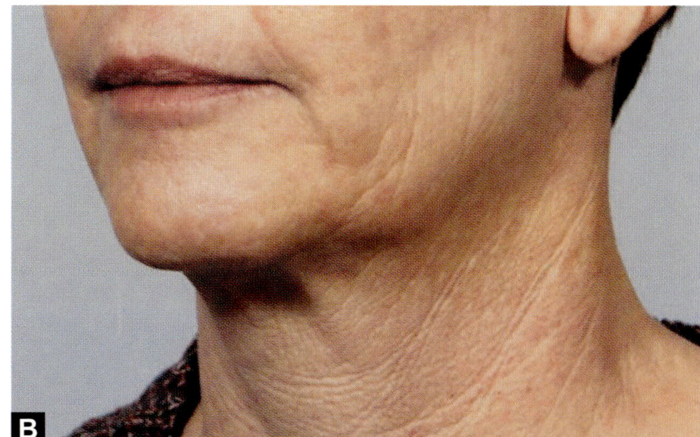

Figs. 15.21A and B: (A) Pretreatment 53-year-old. (B) Two months following three Reaction Refit treatment plus one erbium profractional treatment.
Courtesy: Dr Diane Duncan.

- Set device to mode 4 in order to use all RF frequencies of CORE.
- Set vacuum level, 0–3. The effect of the vacuum is to deepen the RF energy level target, as well as to isolate a treatment region.
- Set RF energy strength as tolerated by the patient.

Megaherz settings of the Viora reaction device:

- *Deep*: One-third at 0.7 MHz—heating below dermis assists in maintaining the temperature and mild effect on subcutaneous layer.
- *More superficial*: Two thirds at 1.7 and 2.45 MHz—targets the dermis directly.

Effect of Vacuum

The dermis and superficial fat are drawn up into the handpiece with the vacuum assist, so the RF energy is delivered at a deeper level. More visible tissue tightening can be achieved when the target is the subcutaneous layer instead of the dermis. Contraction of the fibroseptal network can cause the overlying skin to accommodate. There are limits: skin contraction of >40% can cause rippling and skin contour irregularities.

The Refit mode is illustrated above. Some overlap is recommended in order to maximally expose all tissue in the treatment region to an effective amount of RF heating.

Case 10: Viora Reaction Device plus Profractional Erbium Laser (Figs. 15.21A and B)

This 53-year-old patient had three Reaction Refit treatment plus one profractional erbium treatment.

Procedure: Device used was Reaction by Viora. No anesthesia. Settings were Refit mode 4, vacuum 2, RF power 2–3, and noninvasive. The Refit protocol utilizes the FC (facial handpiece) for face and neck procedures. For this patient, the treatment zone was the jawline and neck extending to the sternal notch. Several treatment zones are delineated, similar to the Thermigen treatment pattern. The four levels of RF energy emitted make this a particularly effective procedure. The vacuum isolates and more efficiently delivers RF energy than devices that just sit on top of the skin. Due to the severe sun damage that this patient had, the Sciton erbium laser Profractional device was also used in order to further correct skin laxity and to reduce hyperpigmentation. Settings were depth of 125 μm and 22% overlap. Two passes were performed in the lower face and neck.

REACTION DEVICE AND RF ENERGY APPLICATORS (FIG. 15.22)

The Reaction device and RF energy applicators: The B-contour device is used on body parts, while the F-contour is used on smaller areas such as the face and neck. Both of these devices combine vacuum with RF energy. The skin tightening device has no vacuum and is used on the skin surface. It targets the dermis directly.

Case 11: Reaction Body Treatment (Fig. 15.23)

This 52-year-old female had epigastric lipodystrophy and skin laxity. After four Reaction treatments to the epigastrium, there is improvement in both skin laxity and fat thickness.

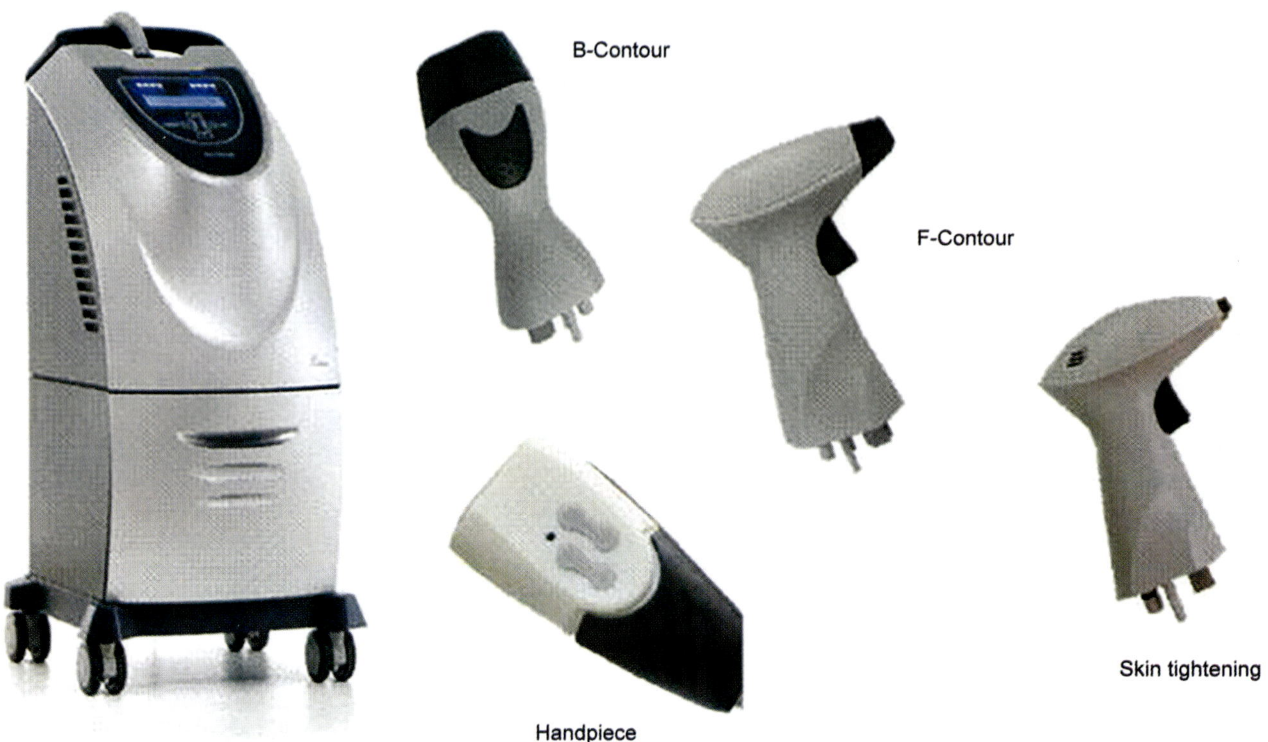

Fig. 15.22: The Reaction device and RF energy applicators. The B-contour device is used on body parts, while the F-contour is used on smaller areas such as the face and neck. Both of these devices combine vacuum with RF energy. The skin tightening device has no vacuum and is used on the skin surface. It targets the dermis directly.

ENDYMED RF DEVICE (FIG. 15.24)

This noninvasive RF device is multipolar, offering a more diffuse energy pattern needing no skin cooling.

Technique

Endymed [multipolar phase controlled radiofrequency (RF) energy]: Depending on the location being treated, the appropriate handpiece is chosen (Fig. 15.25). The medium handpiece was chosen for the jaw line and the large handpiece for the legs. 5 × 10 cm^2 areas to be treated were marked with a white marking pencil, corresponding to inframandibular areas left and right, supramandibular left and right, and the submental area. A treatment gel was applied to the area being treated, which is essential to provide adequate moisture and connectivity between the treatment handpiece and the patient's skin. The handpiece was positioned over the first 5 × 10 cm^2 area to be treated and began moving in a constant circular motion until an audible sound was heard denoting completion of a 30 second pass. After a several passes the patient's skin temperature was measured with an infra-red temperature measuring device. The goal is to have the temperature range of 39.5°C–42°C. If the skin temperature was <40°C the power was increased by 5 W, if the skin temperature was >41°C the power was decreased by 5 W. The treatment was continued for at least 10–12 passes per area.

The delivery of sufficient heat deep into the skin, to the dermal and subdermal layers, creates an immediate effect on the collagen structure and also stimulates neocollagenesis. The heat penetration achieved by EndyMed's proprietary 3DEEP RF technology reaches into the deep dermis and subdermal layers to provide this effective collagen tightening and remodeling. The 3DEEP technology developed by EndyMed controls the power and depth of RF energy delivered to the skin, which is what makes it very effective.

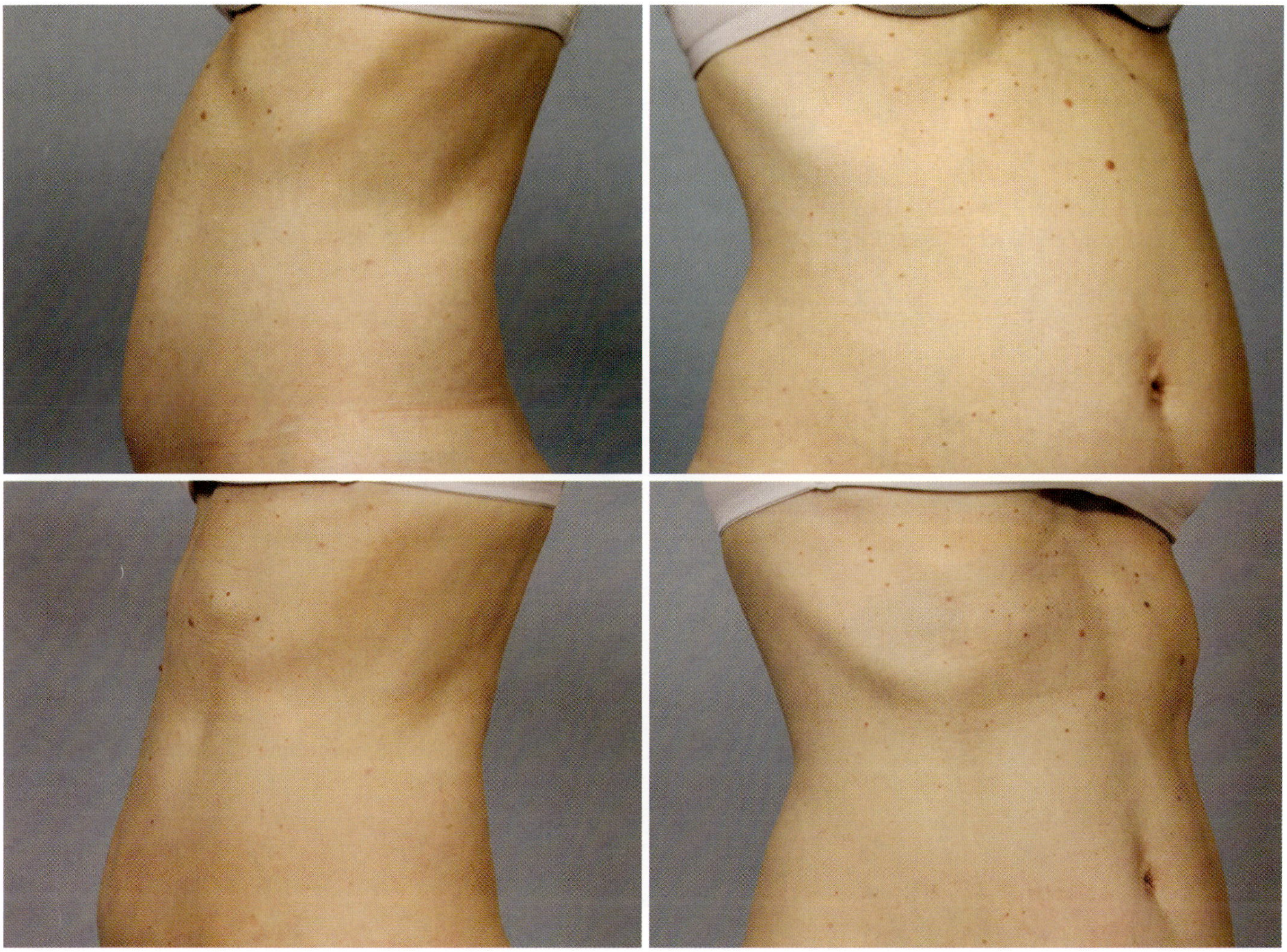

Fig. 15.23: (Top) 52-year-old woman with epigastric lipodystrophy and skin laxity. (Bottom) Six weeks after four Reaction treatments to the epigastrium. Improvement is seen in both skin laxity and fat thickness.
Courtesy: Dr Diane Duncan.

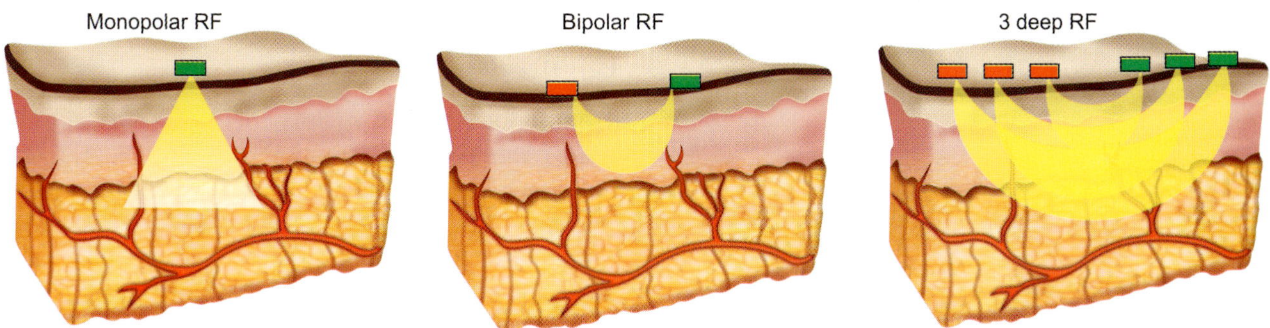

Fig. 15.24: Difference between monopolar and bipolar devices, as well as the energy dispersion pattern generated by Endymed multi-polar RF device.
Courtesy: Endymed.

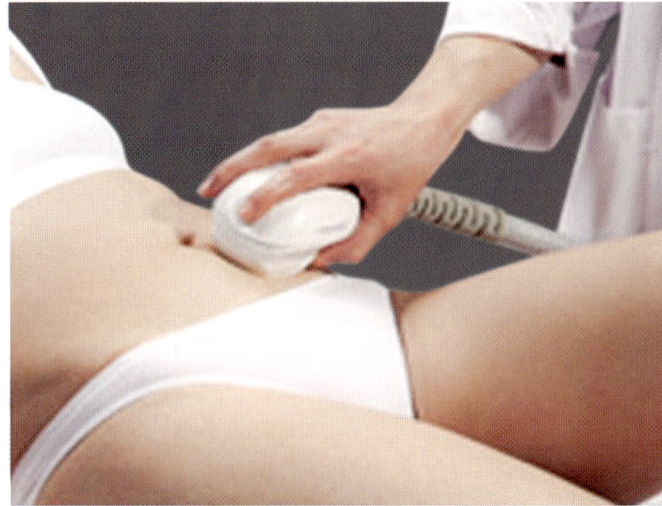

Fig. 15.25: A variety of Endymed handpieces are available to optimize both body and facial treatments.

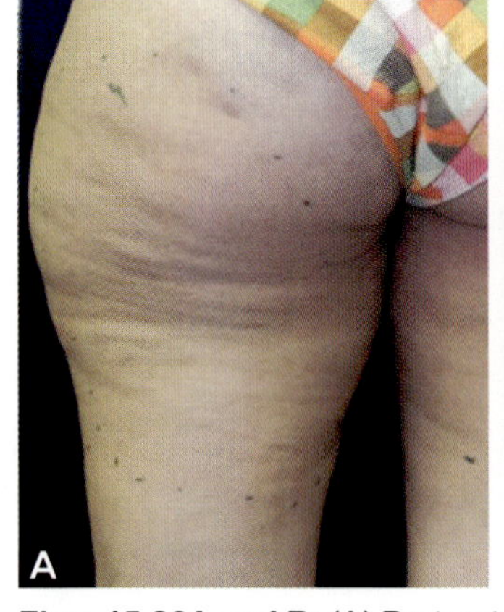

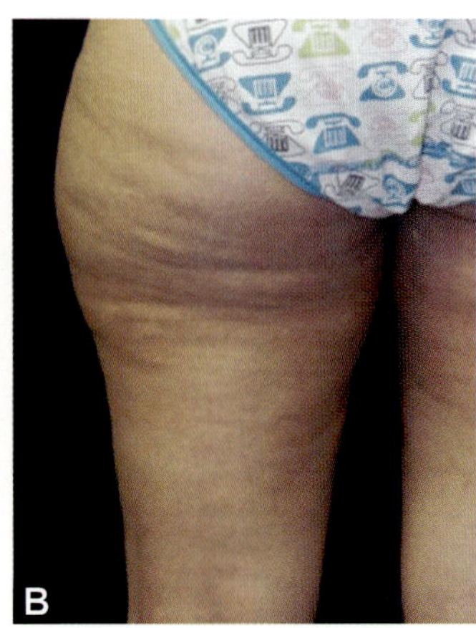

Figs. 15.26A and B: (A) Pretreatment 32-year-old woman. (B) Six weeks following treatment of the posterior and lateral thigh region with the Endymed device shows skin surface improvement plus mild to moderate fat loss.
Courtesy: Dr Anna Petropoulos, Danvers, MA.

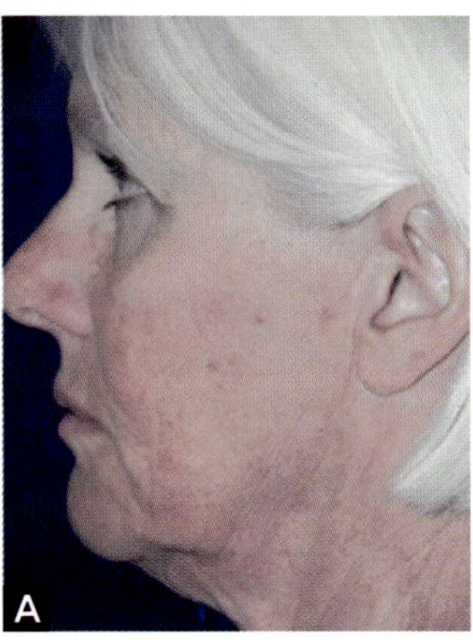

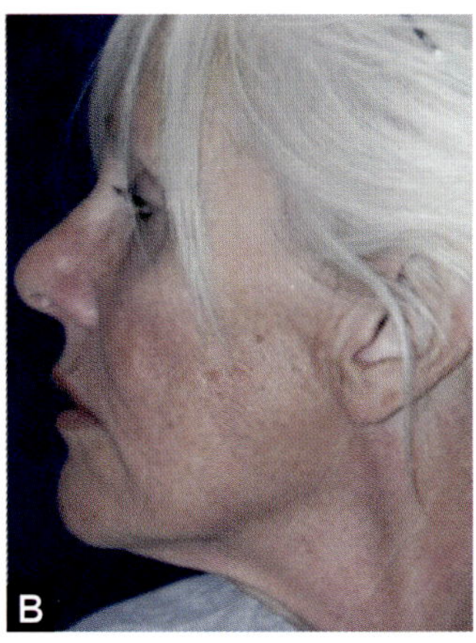

Figs. 15.27A and B: (A) Pretreatment 55-year-old woman with skin laxity. (B) Six weeks after treatment of the lower face and neck region with the Endymed device. Improvement of skin laxity is definite following several treatments.
Courtesy: Dr Anna Petropoulos, Danvers, MA.

Case 12: Endymed for Cellulite (Figs. 15.26A and B)

This 32-year-old woman was treated in the posterior and lateral thigh region with the Endymed device.

Case 13: Endymed Neck Tightening (Figs. 15.27A and B)

This 55-year-old woman was treated in the lower face and neck region with the Endymed device. Improvement of skin laxity is definite following several treatments.

Thermage: Patented Unipolar RF Technology

Thermage has come a long way from the original monopolar RF device first introduced. Figures 15.30A and B outline the way the updated device operates.

The results Thermage can deliver are best seen on the surface: smoother and sleeker skin. But the new Comfort Pulse Technology (CPT) works on a whole new level. The CPT energy algorithm simulates TENS (Transcutaneous Electrical Nerve Stimulation), a proven method for pain relief by affecting sensory nerves and interfering with sensory-discriminative pathways, interspersing cooling bursts with RF heat energy, blocking neural discomfort signals and dramatically increasing patient comfort (Figs. 15.28A to D). Its smart technology works on patient's bodies while working with their mind.

Technique

A return pad is placed on the patient's scapula. The appropriate treatment tip—computer chip (Fig. 15.29) is chosen and attached to the handpiece for the appropriate treatment area, following protocols published by the company (Solta) in its operators' manual. A generous amount of conducting fluid is applied to the skin to ensure conductivity and comfort. The treatment tip is kept perpendicular to the skin ensuring full tip-to-skin contact. Prior to touching down on the skin the button on the handpiece is pressed to deliver the pulse for the duration of the audible harmonic sound that stopped as the delivery of energy is completed. Treatment levels are selected based on the patient's

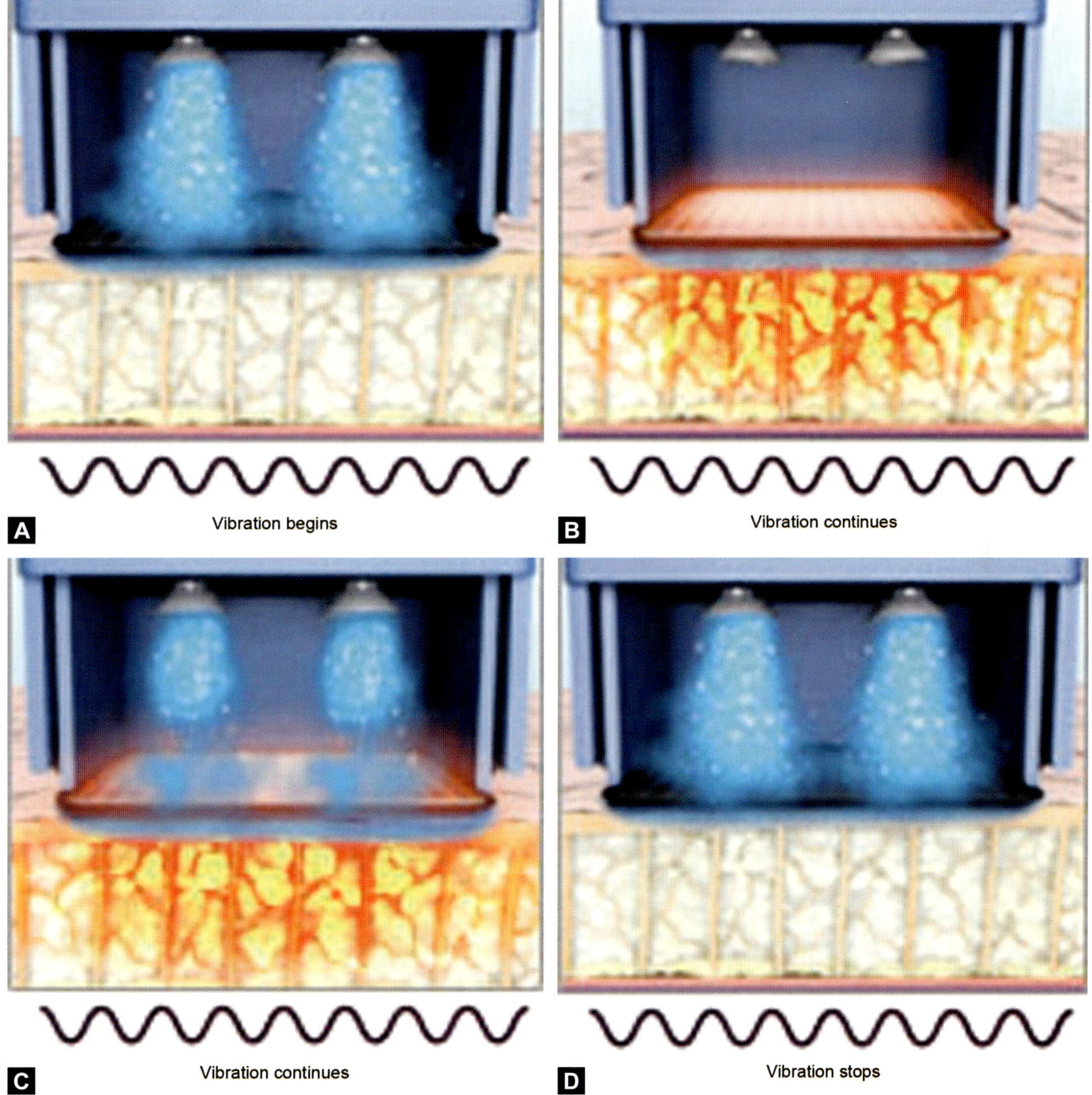

Figs. 15.28A to D: (A) Treatment begins with a cooling effect on the skin for comfort and safety of surface layers. (B) A specially designed treatment tip is placed against the skin in targeted areas. (C) Radiofrequency energy penetrates deep into the skin's tissue, heating the treatment areas, and remodeling the collagen. (D) Final delivery of cryogen to cool the epidermis.

feedback on heat sensation since this has been proven a valid and preferred method for optimal energy selection. On a scale of 0–4, where four is unbearable heat, the level we aim for is a 2 which should feel hot, just starting to hurt but easily tolerable, and over before it is truly perceived. Multiple passes are required for each area treated, performing one row of pulses at a time and restarting at the beginning of each row to perform subsequent or multiple passes, thus allowing for the temperature at any given spot time to cool down, as opposed to "stacking" of pulses on top of the same spot that would cause excessive temperature buildup and even fat melting on occasion. This is thus avoided in most cases, except in an obese neck where we strive to achieve fat melting. The tip is continually cooled

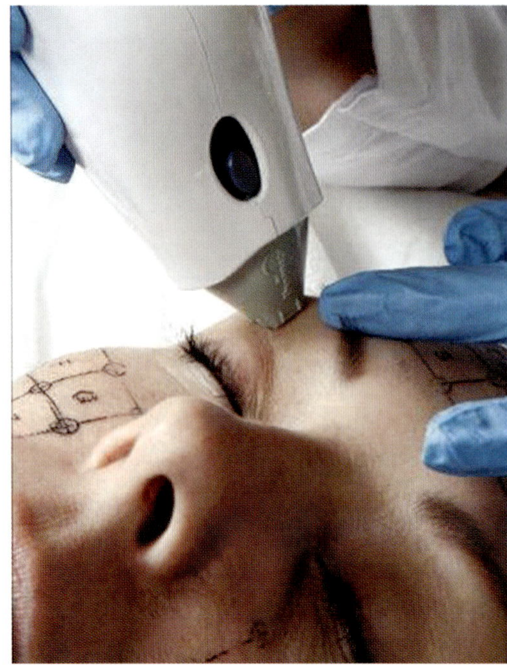

Fig. 15.29: The appropriate treatment tip—computer chip is chosen and attached to the handpiece for the appropriate treatment area, following protocols published by the company (Solta) in its operators' manual.

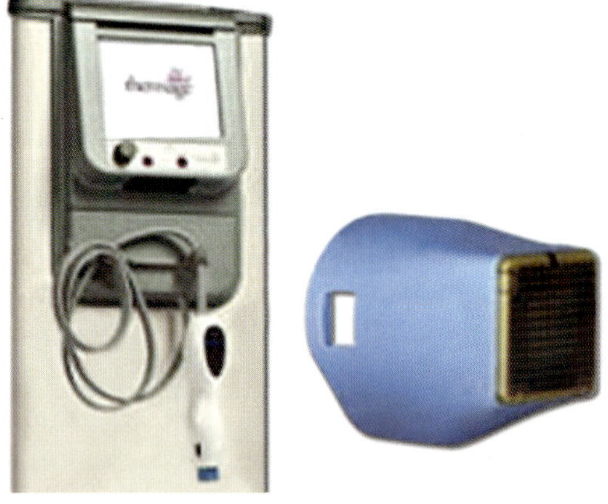

Figs. 15.30A and B: Thermage eyelid treatment.

by automatic expulsion of a built-in coolant during the delivery of energy, thus protecting the skin's surface from heat, but allowing the heat to penetrate to the deep dermal layer with an inverse heat gradient.

When treating the eyelids, anesthetic eye drops were administered onto the globes first in order for the clear plastic scleral protective eye shields to be placed. The treatment tip-computer chip for the eyelids has a total of 450 pulses so we typically divided that by four and delivered approximately 112 pulses to each of the four eyelids (left and right upper and lower), but the number of pulses administered to each area can be adjusted and customized according to its degree of aging (Figs. 15.30A and B).

When treating facial regions, accuracy is enhanced by using a facial grid. This is applied prior to treatment. In varying regions, the use of a vector type pattern can enhance the outcome (Figs. 15.31A and B).

The use of the Thermage RF device on body parts, especially the periumbilical abdomen, has a high patient satisfaction rating (Fig. 15.32). Thermage is a non-invasive RF therapy that addressed skin laxity on many body areas with the appropriate treatment tips selected for each area,

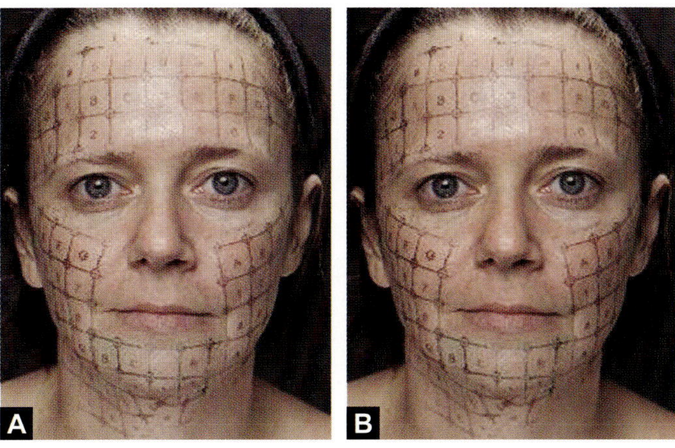

Figs. 15.31A and B: Use of the device on body parts includes a vector treatment pattern for best results.

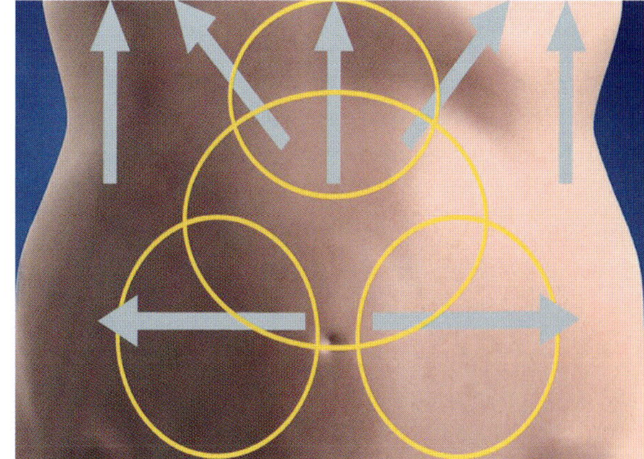

Fig. 15.32: The use of Thermage on body parts.

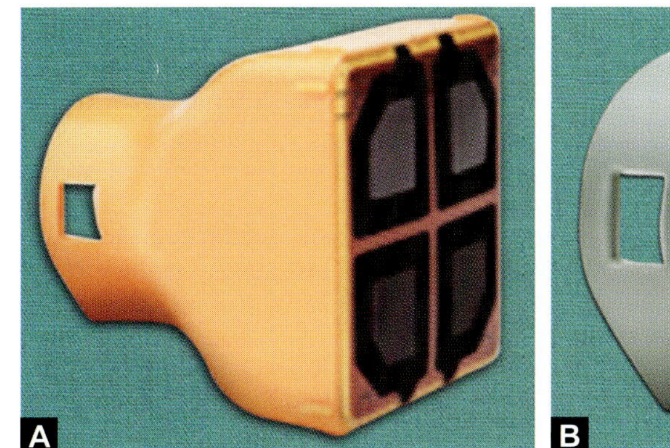

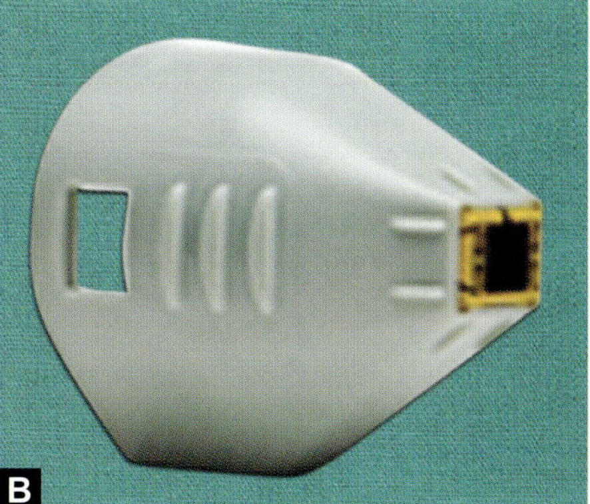

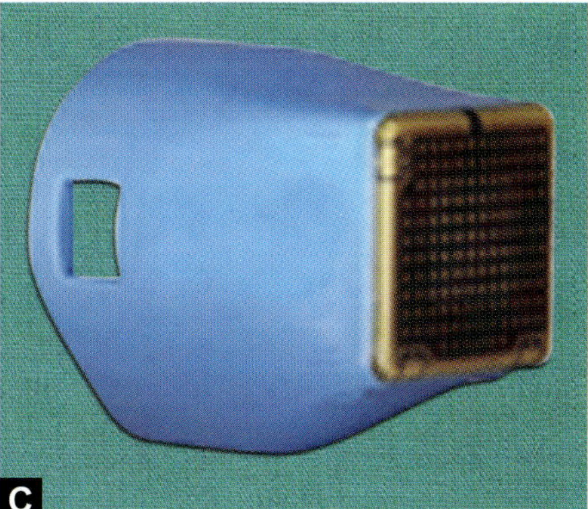

Figs. 15.33A to C: Many treatment tips combined with a computer chip are available for treating a variety of face, neck, and body regions.

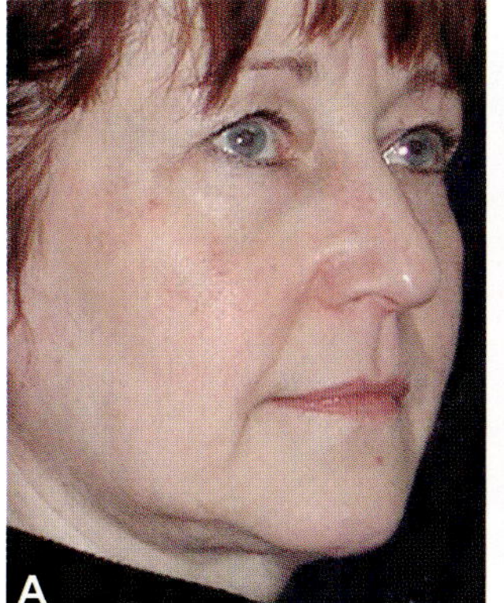

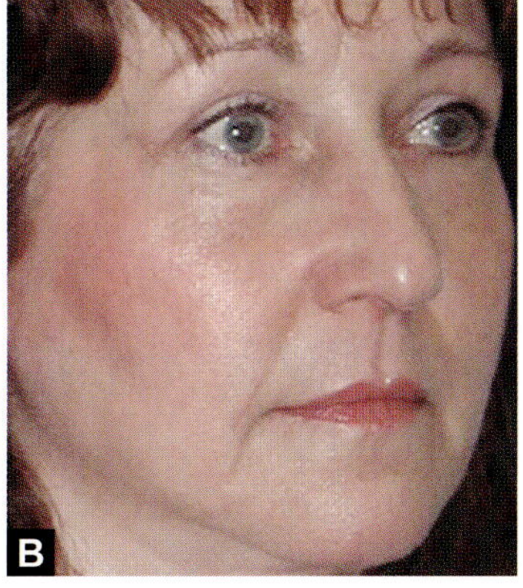

Figs. 15.34A and B: (A) Pretreatment 48-year-old woman. (B) After treatment of the neck and lower jawline with Thermage. *Courtesy*: Dr Anna Petropoulos, Danvers, MA.

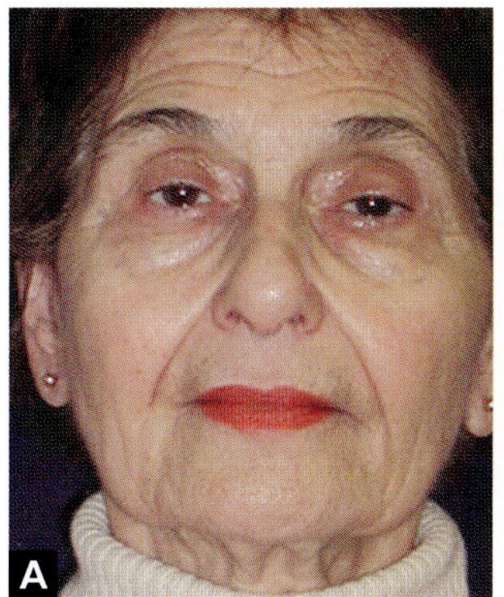

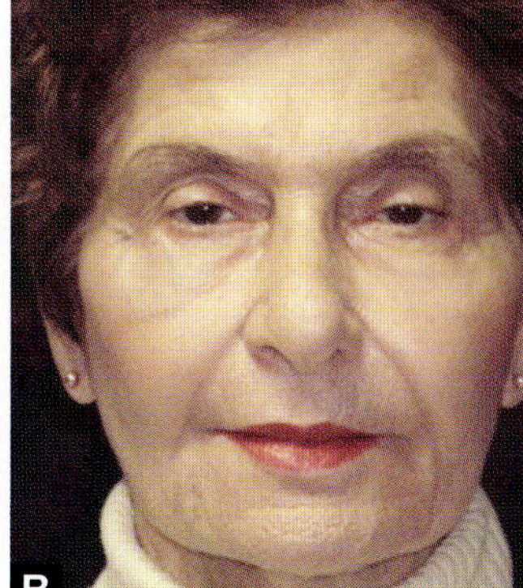

Figs. 15.35A and B: (A) Pretreatment 52-year-old woman. One month following treatment of the neck and lower jawline with Thermage (B).

respectively (Figs. 15.33A to C). Thermage treatments are customized to your needs, and do not require any recovery time. Results of a treatment in the neck region are shown in Figures. 15.34 and 15.35.

CONCLUSION

The use of RF energy for cautery purposes has been available for many years. Interestingly, new uses for the established electromagnetic energy source have recently expanded. The use of RF energy for coagulative tissue contraction is still new, but holds great promise for non-excisional antiaging applications.

REFERENCES

1. Mulholland RS. Radiofrequency energy for non-invasive and minimally invasive skin tightening. Clin Plast Surg. 2011;38(3):437-48.
2. Collawn S. Skin tightening with fractional lasers, radiofrequency, smartlipo. Ann Plast Surg. 2010;65(5):526-9.
3. Pozner J. Laser basics, results and risks. International Master Course on Aging Skin, Paris, January 9, 2008.
4. Sadick N. Energy types and best applications. International Master Course on Aging Skin, Paris, February 3, 2013.
5. Lapidoth M. Comment on presentation "Minimally invasive neck contouring," International Master Course on Aging Skin, Paris, February 3, 2013.
6. Hantash BM, Ubeid AA, Chang H, et al. Bipolar fractional radiofrequency treatment induces neoelastogenesis and neocollagenesis. Lasers Surg Med. 2009;41(1):1-9.
7. Alexiades-Armenakas M, Newman J, Willey A, et al. Prospective multicenter clinical trial of a minimally invasive temperature-controlled bipolar fractional radiofrequency system for rhytid and laxity treatment. Dermatol Surg. 2013;39(2):263-73.
8. Grunebaum LD, Murdock J, Hoosien GE, et al. Laser treatment of skin texture and fine line etching. Facial Plast Surg Clin North Am. 2011;19(2):293-301.
9. Mlosek RK, Woźniak W, Malinowska S, et al. The effectiveness of anticellulite treatment using tripolar radiofrequency monitored by classic and high-frequency ultrasound. J Eur Acad Dermatol Venereol. 2012;26(6):696-703.
10. Mulholland RS, Paul MD, Chalfoun C. Noninvasive body contouring with radiofrequency, ultrasound, cryolipolysis, and low-level laser therapy. Clin Plast Surg. 2011;38(3):503-20.
11. Vangsness CT Jr, Mitchell W III, Nimni M, et al. Collagen shortening: an experimental approach with heat. Clin Orthop Relat Res. 1997;(337):267-71.
12. Lin SJ, Hsiao CY, Sun Y, et al. Monitoring the thermally induced structural transitions of collagen by use of second-harmonic generation microscopy. Opt Lett. 2005;30(6):622-4.
13. Mertyna P, Hines-Peralta A, Liu ZJ, et al. Radiofrequency ablation: variability in heat sensitivity in tumors and tissues. J Vasc Interv Radiol. 2007;18(5):647-54.
14. Hayashi K, Thabit G III, Massa KL, et al. The effect of thermal heating on the length and histologic properties of the glenohumeral joint capsule. Am J Sports Med. 1997;25(1):107-12.
15. Paul M, Blugerman G, Kreindel M, et al. Three-dimensional radiofrequency tissue tightening: a proposed mechanism and applications for body contouring. Aesthetic Plast Surg. 2011;35(1):87-95.
16. Sadick N. Tissue tightening technologies: fact or fiction. Aesthet Surg J. 2008;28(2):180-88.
17. Mulholland RS. Mechanism of electroporation induced by radiofrequency energy: a new look. International Master Course on Aging Skin, Hong Kong, October 3, 2012.
18. Kohl E, Karrer S. Photodynamic therapy for photorejuvenation and non-oncologic indications: overview and update. G Ital Dermatol Venereol. 2011;146(6):473-85.
19. Duncan D. Photodynamic light: histological fat loss. International Master Course on Aging Skin, Bangkok July 13, 2009.
20. Nestor M. Low level laser therapy as viable treatment for reduction of upper extremity adipose tissue. American Society for Laser Medicine and Surgery Annual Meeting, Boston April 12, 2013.
21. Divaris M, Boisnic S, Branchet M, et al. A clinical and histological study of radiofrequency-assisted liposuction (RFAL) mediated skin tightening and cellulite improvement. J Cosmet Dermatol Sci Appl. 2011;1(2):36-42.
22. Duncan D. Tite FX for apoptotic fat reduction: a prospective 20 patient trial. International Master Course on Aging Skin, Hong Kong, October 3, 2012.
23. Duncan D. Abdominal skin contraction with RFAL plus SAL vs. SAL alone: a prospective randomized study. International Master Course on Aging Skin, Paris, January 12, 2011.

Section 6

Extremities

Chapter Outline

- Carpal Tunnel Syndrome
- Improved Double Fusiform Resection Technique for Postbariatric Brachioplasty
- Body Dysmorphic Disorder

16 Carpal Tunnel Syndrome

Cristina Isac, Aurelia Isac, Florin Isac

DEFINITION AND ANATOMY

Ten structures pass through the carpal tunnel: the median nerve, flexor pollicis longus tendon, and the eight flexor tendons to the ten fingers. The carpal tunnel is a narrow structure that is covered by the transverse carpal ligament (TCL), a ligamentous structure that is a continuation of the antebrachial fascia.

Etiology of carpal tunnel syndrome:

1. Congenital:
   a. Persistent median artery
   b. Anatomic variant of lumbrical or superficialis muscle bellies that are unusual long, extending into the carpal tunnel, and compressing the median nerve
   c. Anomalous muscles—reversed palmaris,[1] palmaris profundus[2]
2. Trauma:
   a. Fractures or dislocations of the carpal bones
   b. Repetitive microtrauma from vibrating pick-hammers
   c. Extensive hand injuries or burns leading to severe swelling
3. Tumors:
   a. Lipoma, fibroma
   b. Ganglion
   c. Aneurysm of the median artery
4. Inflammatory:
   a. Rheumatoid arthritis
   b. Gout
   c. Tuberculosis
5. Metabolic:
   a. Amyloidosis
   b. Endocrine imbalanc[3]
   c. Pregnancy
   d. Peripheral neuropathy[3]

SYMPTOMS

Numbness is the most common complaint and it usually involves the thumb, index, and middle finger. It is described by the patients as a sensation of burn and initially it is intermittent to becoming continuous in the advanced stages.

Pain manifests first during the night when the patient is typically awaken by the pain and it diminishes after several shaking of the hands and movements. The patient wakes in the morning with the pain that gradually in the first stages disappears in a few hours. The pain and numbness are often provoked when working with the wrist flexed or in various positions of the wrist, such as when driving or reading a newspaper. They are often alleviated when the upper limb is kept dependent. The pain can irradiate anywhere up to the shoulder.[3]

Clumsiness manifests itself as the inability to close one's buttons or in managing fine gestures. This is due to the loss of sensation or the weakness of the thenar muscles.

EXAMINATION

Muscle wasting: Wasting and weakness of the median nerve-innervated muscles of the hand may be detected (first and second lumbricals, thenar muscles-abductor pollicis brevis, opponens pollicis, flexor pollicis brevis). Thenar atrophy is noticed usually in long-standing compression (Figs. 16.1A and B). The loss of power in the hand particularly for precision grips involving the thumb is an important cause of weakness and clumsiness.

Sensory disturbance: Abnormalities in sensory modalities may be present on the palmar aspect of the first three digits and radial one half of the fourth digit. The sensory

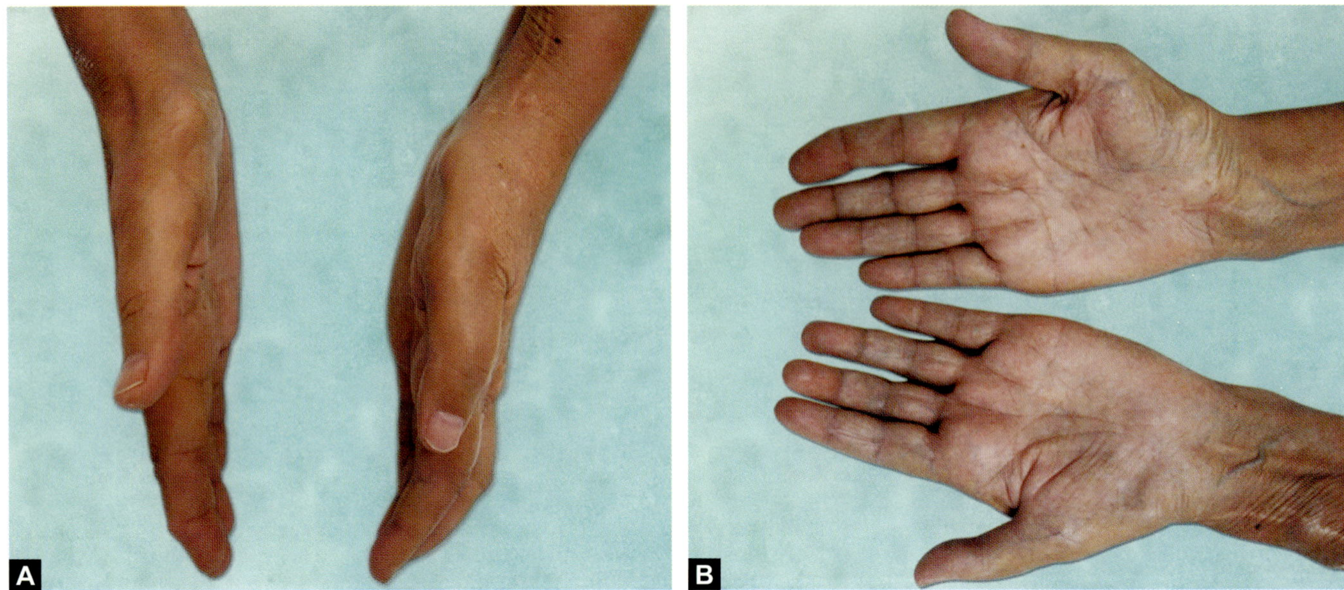

Figs. 16.1A and B: Severe thenar atrophy bilaterally associated with long-standing carpal tunnel syndrome in a chronically dialyzed patient.

disturbance can be checked with Semmes-Weinstein monofilament testing or two-point discrimination test.

Tinel's sign: Gentle tapping over the median nerve in the carpal tunnel region elicits tingling in the nerve's distribution.

Phalen's test: Tingling in the median nerve distribution is induced by full flexion (or full extension for reverse Phalen) of the wrists for up to 60 seconds.

Reversed Phalen's test: Tingling in the median nerve distribution is induced by full extension of the wrists for up to 60 seconds.

Electromyography: Electrophysiologic studies include electromyography (EMG) and nerve conductions studies. They represent the first-line investigations in suggested carpal tunnel syndrome (CTS) and associated with specific symptoms and signs establish CTS diagnosis. They can also exclude other neurologic diagnoses. Electrophysiologic testing can also provide an accurate assessment of how severe the damage to the nerve is (mild, moderate, or severe). In general, patients with mild CTS have sensory abnormalities alone on electrophysiologic testing, and patients with moderate CTS have sensory plus motor abnormalities. Severe CTS has decreased or absent sensory or motor responses distal to the carpal tunnel, meaning axonal loss.[4] According to the severity of CTS, one can establish the prognosis and treatment modalities. Changes in electrophysiologic results over time can be used to assess the success of various treatment modalities.

TYPES OF TREATMENT

Conservative treatment: Wrist splints with the wrist joint in neutral or slight extension worn during night for a minimum of 3 weeks can be used in mild CTS. Steroid injection into the carpal tunnel has been shown to be of long-term benefit and can be tried especially in cases that are contraindicated for surgery, like in pregnancy. Nonsteroidal anti-inflammatory drugs (NSAIDs) and diuretics can be used in patients with fluid retention or with wrist flexor tendinitis.

SURGICAL TREATMENT

Open

The CTS category (as defined by electrophysiologic testing) should be considered for surgery. Surgical release of the transverse ligament provides high success rates and is indicated in patients whose condition does not improve following conservative treatment and in patients with severe CTS.

Open carpal tunnel release: Local anesthesia is used in most cases. The incision is made taking into consideration

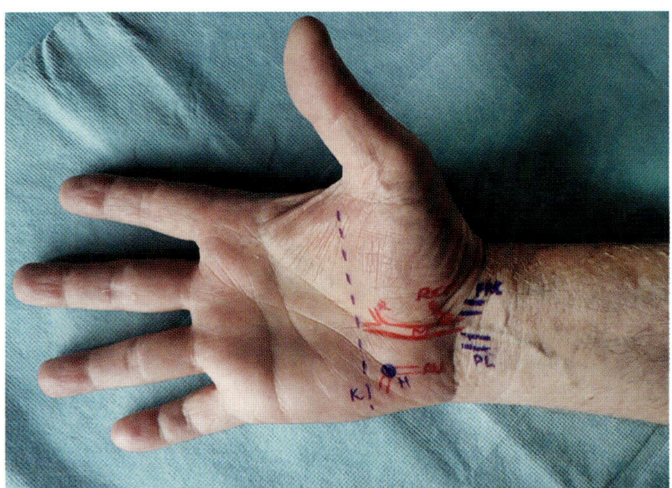

Fig. 16.2: Preoperative markings. RCP, palmar cutaneous branch; K, Kaplan's cardinal line; FRC, flexor carpi radialis tendon; PL, palmaris longus tendon; H, hook of the hamate; T, thenar motor branch of median nerve; AU, ulnar artery; A, superficial arterial arch.

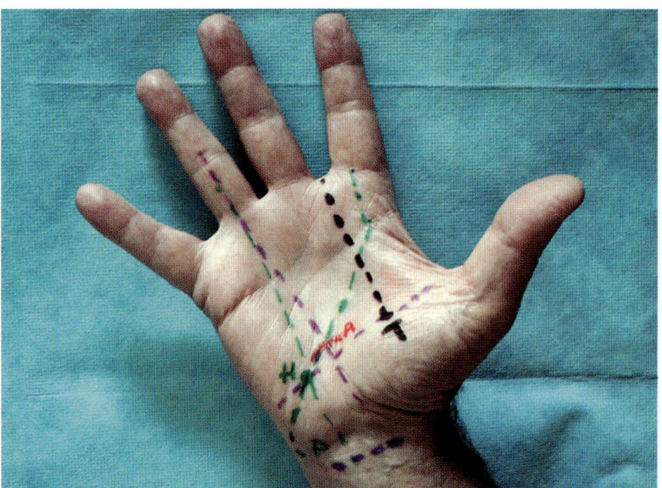

Fig. 16.3: Thenar motor branch and the main anatomic structures that are to be taken into consideration when designing the incision.

several landmarks to avoid injuries to the palmar cutaneous branch (PCB), recurrent motor branch of the median nerve, the superficial arch, and the ulnar nerve and artery:

1. The PCB lies between the median nerve and the flexor carpi radialis tendon at the distal wrist crease; it pierces either the antebrachial fascia or the TCL before becoming subcutaneous (Fig. 16.2).
2. The recurrent motor branch of the median nerve is localized at the point where the flexed long finger intersects the Kaplan's cardinal line (drawn from the apex of the thumb-index web toward the hook of the hamate, parallel with the proximal palmar crease) on the thenar eminence.
3. The deep palmar arch corresponds to Kaplan's cardinal line, the superficial palmar arch lies between the cardinal line and the proximal palmar crease.
4. The ulnar vasculonervous bundle lies radially to the hook of the hamate (Fig. 16.3).

The incision is curvilinear beginning at Kaplan's line and following the thenar crease, then ulnar to the palmaris longus tendon and brought proximally to the distal forearm (Fig. 16.4). Through blunt dissection the antebrachial and palmar fascia are identified, then the transverse carpal.[4] The antebrachial fascia is penetrated proximally and the underlying median nerve is identified (Figs. 16.5A to C). The underside of the TCL is freed from the underlying structures and is sharply divided along its ulnar border, while protecting the underlying elements. The complete division of the TCL should reach its distal end, not reaching, however, the superficial arch. This complete division should be carefully checked.

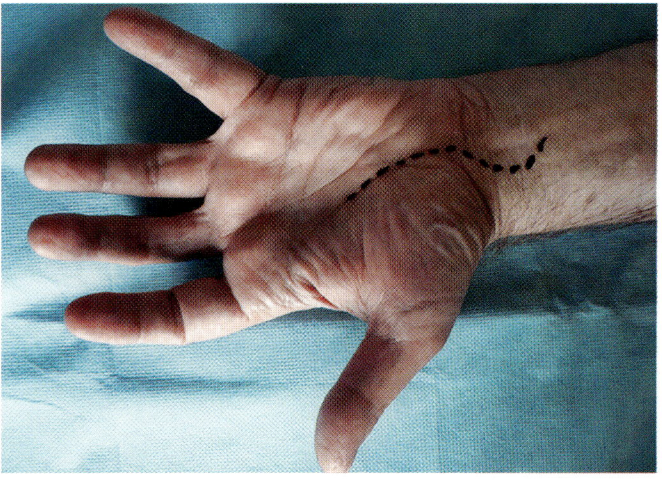

Fig. 16.4: Incision design.

The median nerve with its distal recurrent motor branch is inspected, as well as the flexor tendons and the floor of the canal (for ganglia or osteophytes) (Figs. 16.6A to C).[5] If the synovium of the flexor tendons is thickened, as for example in patients undergoing chronic hemodialysis, where amyloidosis is present in most of the cases (Figs. 16.7A and B), tenosynovectomy is performed (Figs. 16.8A and B). The antebrachial fascia is divided proximally also.[4]

The tourniquet is deflated, meticulous hemostasis achieved, the wound irrigated, and skin is closed with 5-0 nylon sutures. A light splint is applied and kept for 2 days.

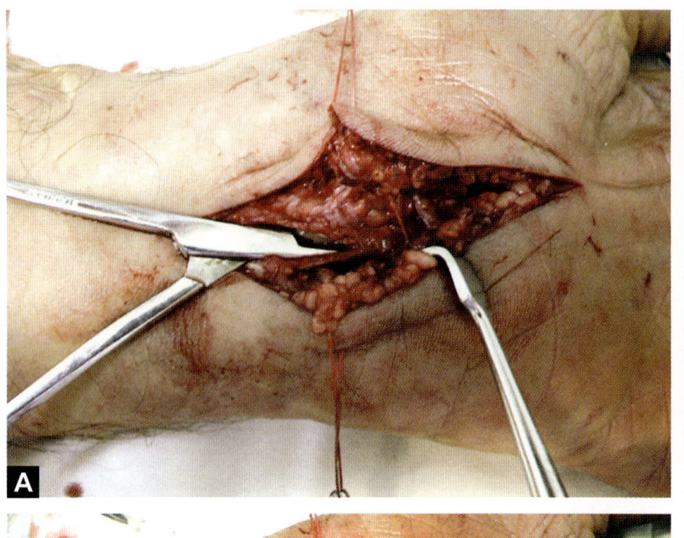

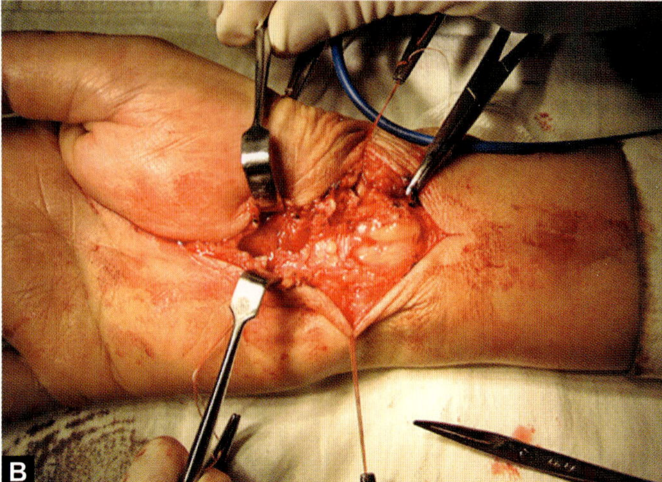

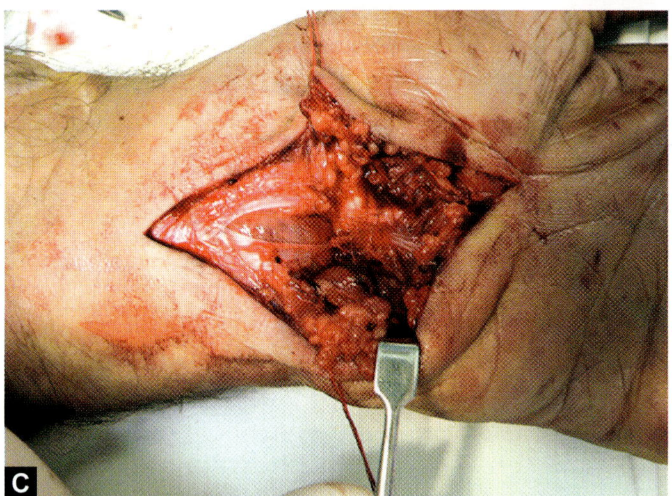

Figs. 16.5A to C: Incising the antebrachial fascia and the transverse carpal ligament. Note that the tight fibrous structures that compress the median nerve.

ENDOSCOPIC CARPAL TUNNEL RELEASE

Avoiding an incision on the palmar surface of the hand, endoscopic techniques claim to decrease postoperative morbidity due to the smaller scar. However, debates are still going on regarding the safety, efficacy, and costs when the endoscopic techniques are compared with the open technique.[5] Regardless of technique, pillar pain has not been reduced and palmar tenderness has not been eliminated.[5] The relative shorter period of rehabilitation gained with endoscopic technique must be weighed against the significant disadvantage of poor or absent visualization, inability to identify anatomic variants involved with the pathology and the attendant risk of iatrogenic injury to the neurovascular structures.[5]

POSTOPERATIVE CARE

The patient is allowed to perform active flexion and extension of the fingers after the splint is removed and he/she may return to activities of daily living progressively after the sutures are removed at 14 days.

COMPLICATIONS

1. If not operated on, CTS may continue to increase median nerve damage, leading to permanent impairment, and disability.
2. Complications during or after surgery may include damage to recurrent motor branch, damage to PCB with numbness in the central palm, incomplete release of TCL and recurrent symptoms, tender scar.

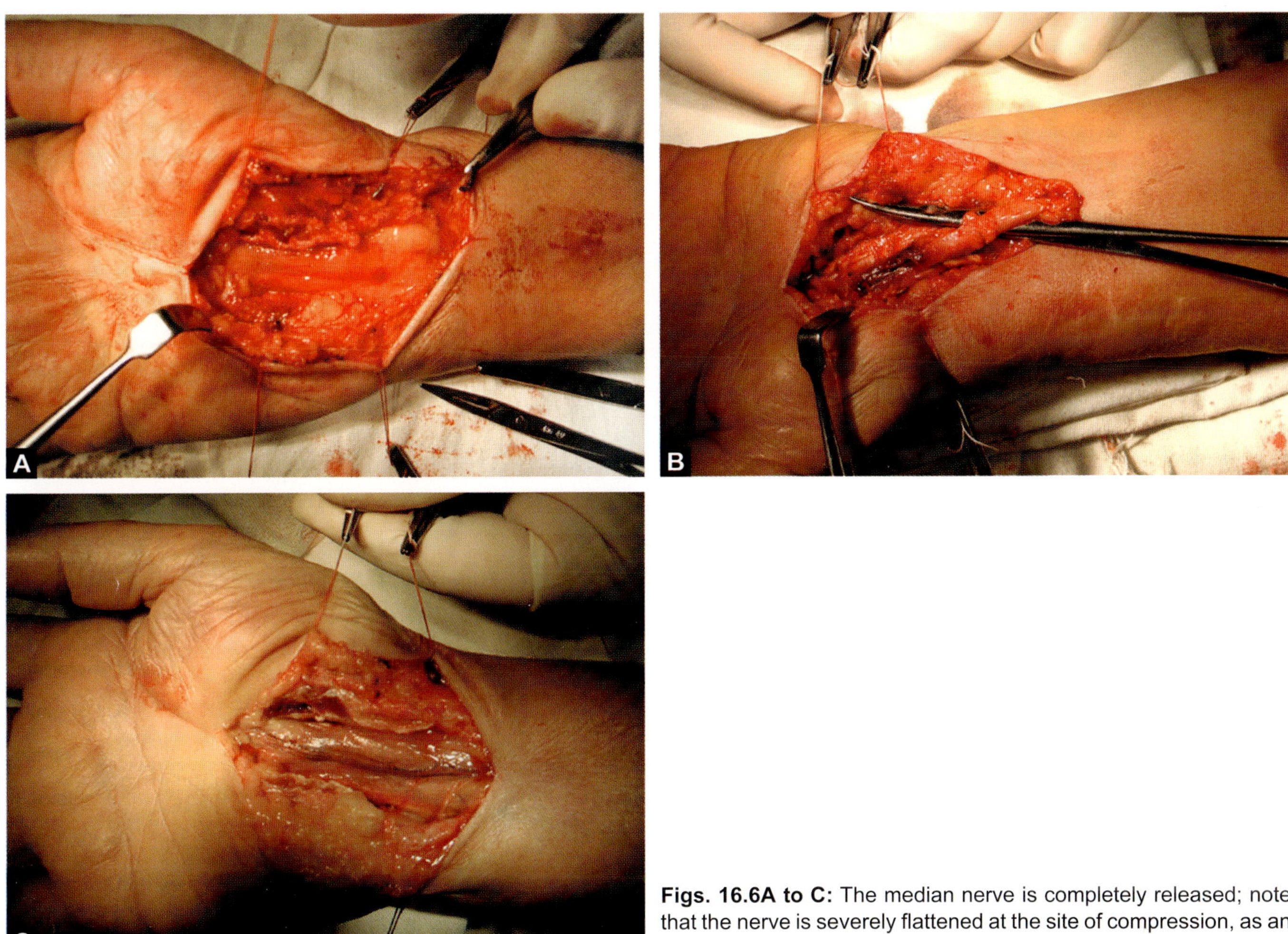

Figs. 16.6A to C: The median nerve is completely released; note that the nerve is severely flattened at the site of compression, as an evidence of long-standing disease.

Figs. 16.7A and B: Deposits of amyloid on the flexor tendons in a chronically dialyzed patient.

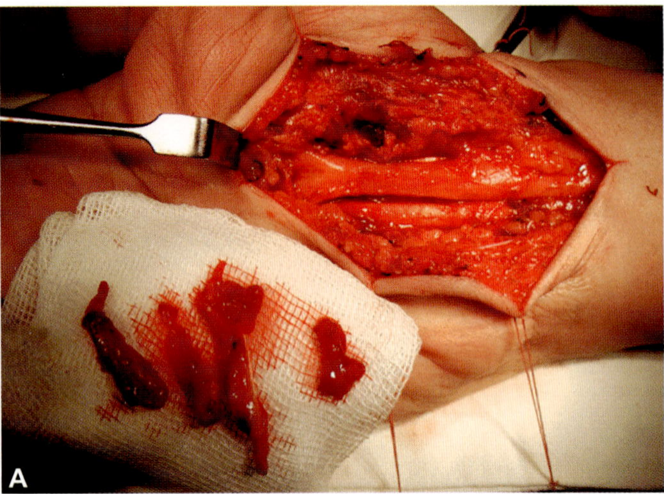

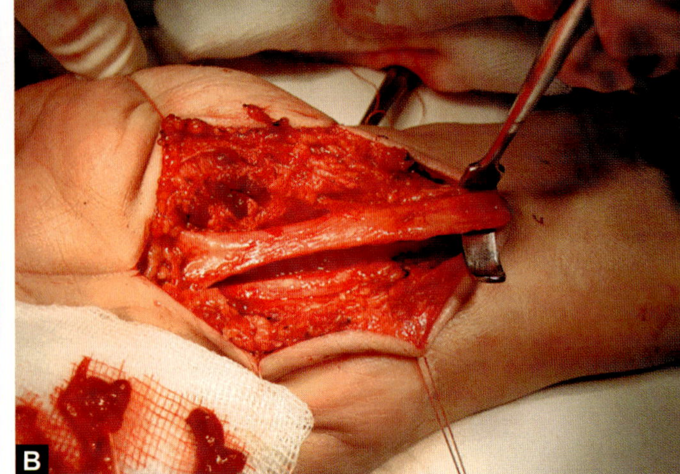

Figs. 16.8A and B: Tenosynovectomy and amyloids removed.

PROGNOSIS

1. Carpal tunnel syndrome (CTS) appears to be progressive over time and can lead to permanent median nerve damage.
2. Patients with CTS secondary to underlying pathology (e.g. diabetes and wrist fracture) tend to have a less favorable prognosis than do those with no apparent underlying cause.
3. Patients with normal electrophysiologic studies consistently have much less favorable operative outcomes (and more complications) than do individuals with abnormalities on these tests. Axonal loss on electrophysiologic testing also indicates a less favorable prognosis.

CONCLUSION

CTS is a serious condition that untreated may lead to permanent functional disability. On the other hand, if recognized and treated as early as possible, it has an excellent outcome through an out-patient surgery with low complication rates.

REFERENCES

1. Carroll M, Montero C. Rare anomalous muscle cause of carpal tunnel syndrome. Orthopaedic Rev. 1980;9:83-5.
2. Floyd T, Burger R. Bilateral palmaris profundus causing bilateral carpal tunnel syndrome. J Hand Surg (Am). 1990; 15(2):364-6.
3. Smith P. Compression. In: Lister's the Hand: Diagnosis and Indications, 4th edition. Edinburgh: Churchill Livingstone; 2002. pp. 271-310.
4. Isac C, Bratu T, Isac A, et al. Sindromul de canal carpian, etio-patologie, clinica si tratament. Timisoara 2010.
5. Szabo R. Entrapement and compression neuropathies. In: Green D, Hotchkiss R, Pederson WC (Eds). Green's Operative Hand Surgery, 4th edition. Philadelphia, PA: Churchill Livingstone; 1998. pp. 1404-47.

17 Improved Double Fusiform Resection Technique for Postbariatric Brachioplasty

Miguel L Modolin

INTRODUCTION

One of the deformities included in the dysmorphism that result from massive weight loss following bariatric surgeries is the arm contour change known as "bat wing" (Figs. 17.1A and B), which is due to a ptotic skin fold along the arm that may extend to the lateral thoracic wall.

This deformity is caused by a partial or total loss of the skin retraction ability after weight loss, whether because of qualitative and quantitative changes in the elastin and collagen contents,[1] or of the laxity due to distension of the superficial fascia.[2]

In these situations, the deformity acquires the shape popularly known as "bingo wings," in reference to the movement performed by the arm when the game is won. This brachial dysmorphism is treated surgically by brachioplasty, whose objective is to provide a more cylindrical arm contour and concomitantly to reduce volume by removing the excess skin fold, thus enabling a wider range of motion, as well as more effective hygiene and the use of more comfortable clothes such as sleeveless shirts.

SURGICAL TECHNIQUE

When the fold is restricted to the arm, its aspect is that of a hammock, and a spindle-shaped skin resection is sufficient to correct it[3] (Figs. 17.2A and B).

With the patient in the sitting position, the anterior line of this spindle-shaped area of skin is medially marked 1–2 cm above and parallel to the brachial sulcus. The posterior line is marked using a bi-digital pinching maneuver, avoiding excessive tension, with the patient's arm at 90° abduction and his elbow at 80° flexion. It is crucial to make careful markings to avoid large resections that could lead to a difficult final wound closure and permanent damage such as transverse grooves or even a tourniquet effect in the distal portion of the upper limb. Both the anterior and posterior lines converge toward the

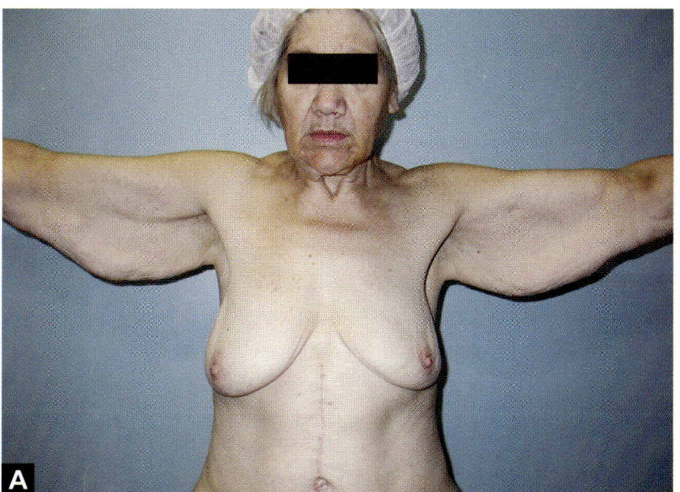

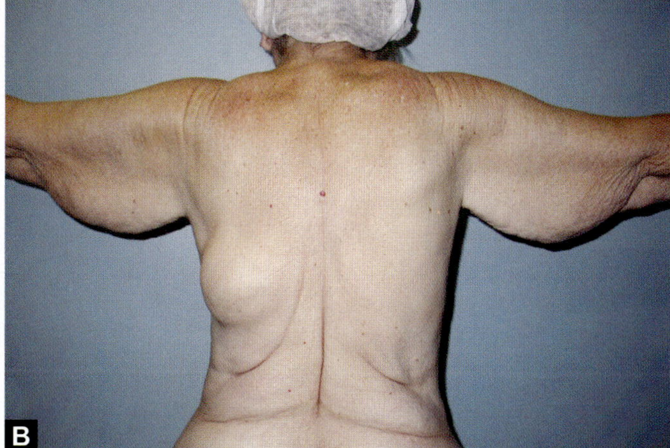

Figs. 17.1A and B: Bat wing brachial dysmorphism.

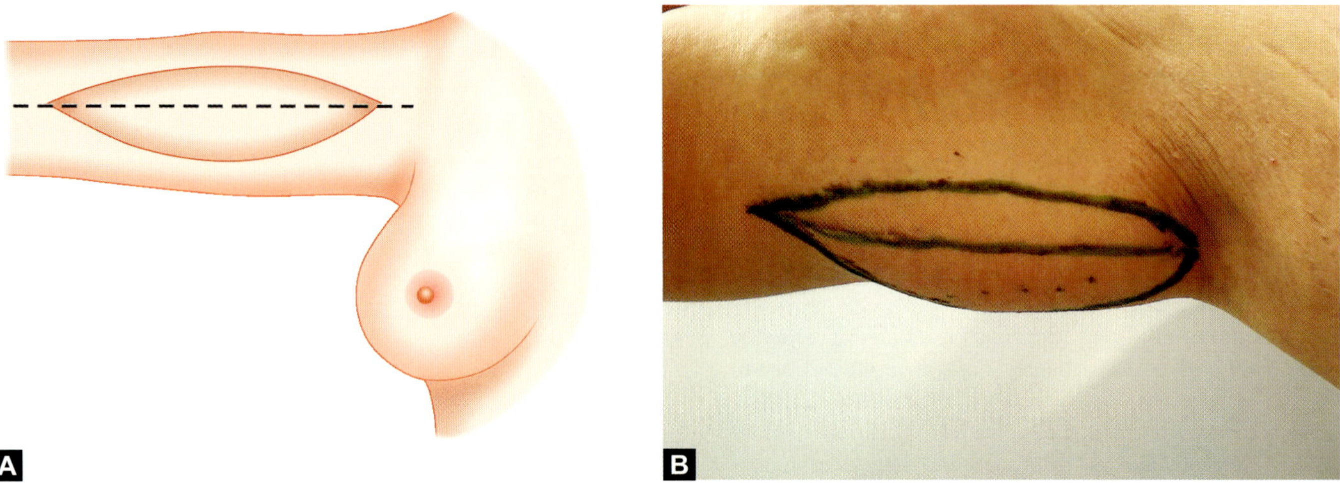

Figs. 17.2A and B: Fusiform technique. (A) Fusiform marking. (B) Preoperative fusiform marking from the epicondyle to the prehairy axillary region.

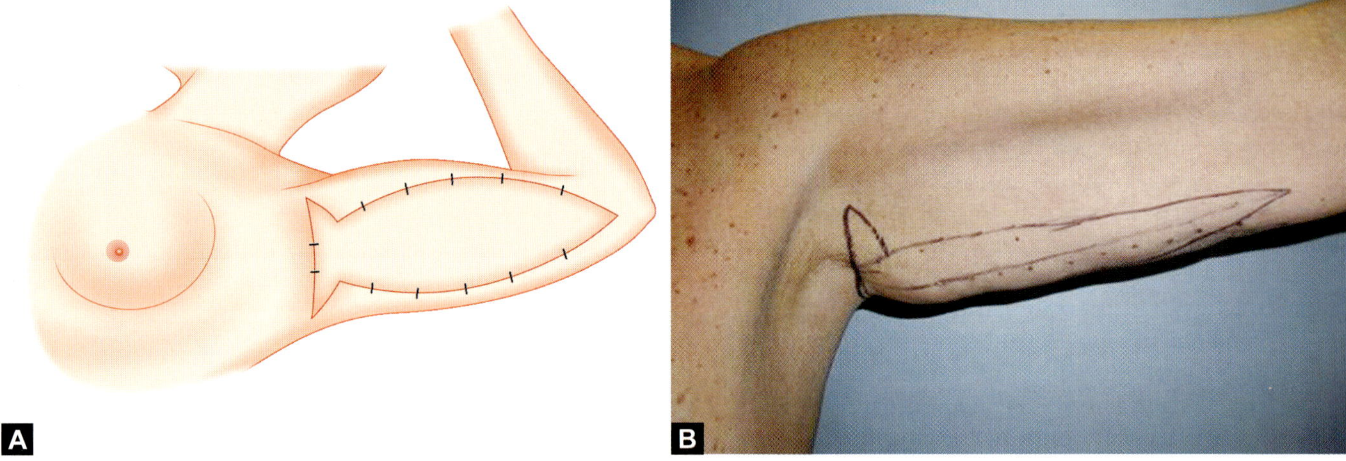

Figs. 17.3A and B: Double fusiform resection technique. (A) The "fish tail" marking. (B) Preoperative marking in a patient.

epicondyle of the humerus and, cephalad, toward the axilla, thus containing the excess skin to be resected. However, as a rule, the fold extends to the axilla, and this excess skin is resected by means of a cross-sectional spindle-shaped area of skin between the anterior and posterior axillary folds, that combines with another longitudinal spindle-shaped area of skin, so that the marking of this double fusiform incision[4] takes the shape of a fish tail (Figs. 17.3A and B).

By using this strategy, the incision does not reach the axilla, which reduces the extent of the longitudinal spindle-shaped area and minimizes the risk of scar retractions. When the deformity extends to the lateral thoracic wall, a brachiothoracoplasty is performed by prolonging the spindle-shaped incision to this region that contains the excess skin (Figs. 17.4A and B). In the axilla, the wound closure line is decomposed using Z-plasty (Figs. 17.5A and B).

The patient is placed in the supine position with his arms abducted upward, thus facilitating the surgical approach (Fig. 17.6). In order to reduce the operative time, the procedure is performed by two teams simultaneously.

Surgery is performed under general anesthesia and, in order to minimize bleeding, 250–350 mL of a solution containing 1 L of saline solution and one epinephrine 1:1,000,000 vial are infiltrated in each arm, depending on the extent of resection. Prophylactic antibiotic therapy with cephazolin is given during the anesthetic induction.

Brachioplasty should be performed above the superficial fascia to prevent damage to the lymphatic vessels and nerves that run in the deeper planes.

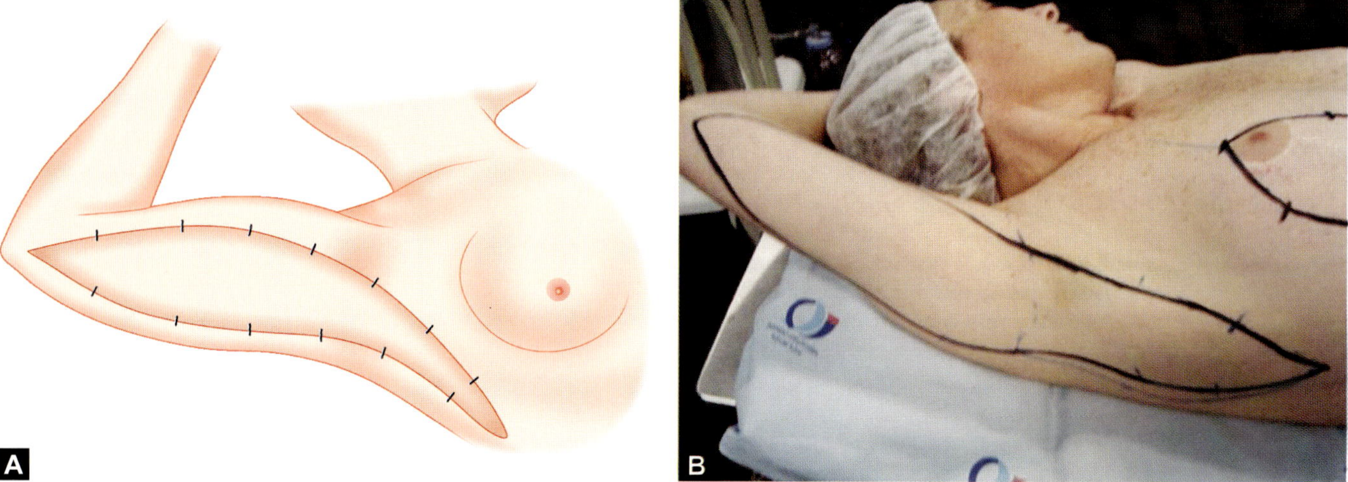

Figs. 17.4A and B: Fusiform marking prolonged from the arm to the thorax, thus defining brachiothoracoplasty. (A and B) Preoperative marking.

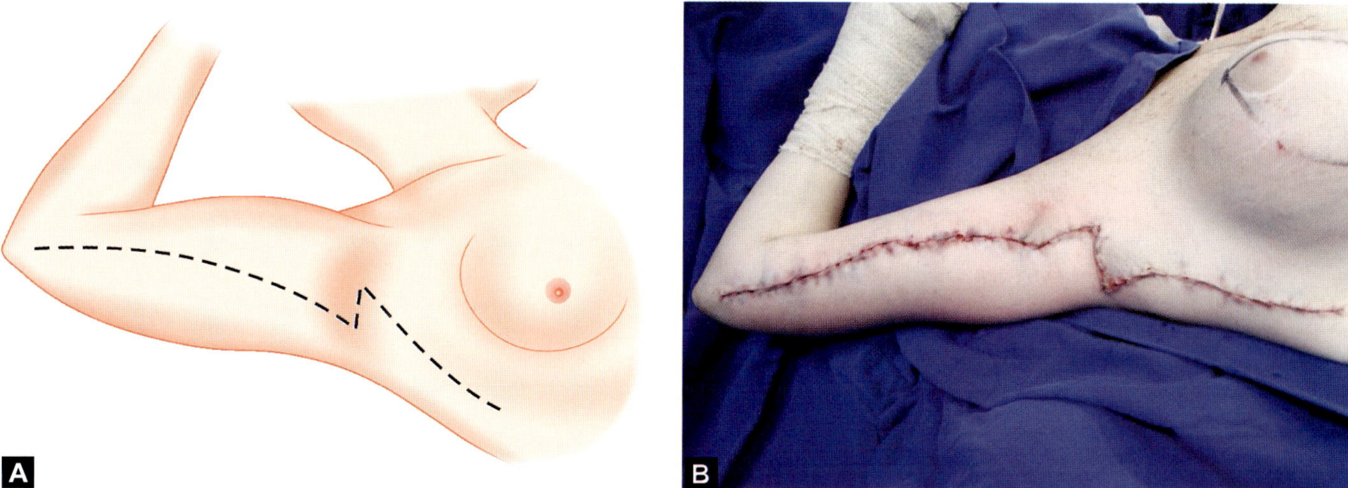

Figs. 17.5A and B: Brachiothoracoplasty with Z-plasty in the axilla. (A and B) Immediate postoperative period.

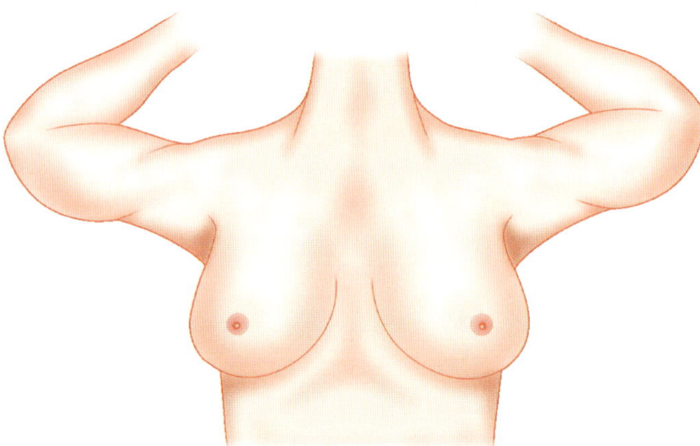

Fig. 17.6: Positioning of the patient's arms during surgery.

Plane closure is initiated after incision, resection, and careful hemostasis. In patients undergoing the axillary approach, the superficial fascia of the arm is fixed to the axillary fascia, thus promoting suspension of the posterior portion of the arm by means of an interrupted suture using 4-0 polyamide. This brings together the tissues that had moved apart and did not retract after weight loss (Fig. 17.6), providing an anatomical looking which is closer to normal.[2] Wound closure in the deep subcutaneous plane, including the superficial fascia, is made with an interrupted suture using 4-0 polyamide (Fig. 17.7). The subdermal suture is made with simple inverted stitches using 3-0 poliglecaprone; a running intradermal suture using 4-0 or 5-0 poliglecaprone is the final suture.

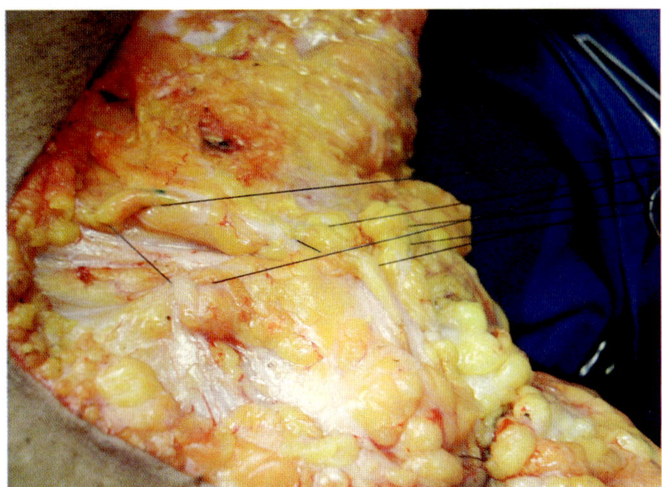

Fig. 17.7: Fixation of the superficial fascia of the arm to the superficial fascia of the axillary region.

When over-resection occurs, closure of the deep subcutaneous plane—which is important for reestablishing the cylindrical shape of the arm, may determine transverse depressions or a tourniquet that are difficult to correct by means other than stitch removal.

Following wound closure, Z-plasty should be performed in the middle of the axilla, in those cases in which the incision extended to the thorax (Figs. 17.5A and B). It could be argued that this maneuver is unnecessary, given that thereis remaining skin. However, precisely because of it, Z-plasty is mandatory to define the axillary dome. It could also be argued that Z-plasty would cause a transposition of a hairless area into a hair area and vice versa. Nonetheless, we should consider that Z-plasty is performed in the middle of the axilla after considerable resection of hairy skin, so that the flaps transposed are practically hairless. Also, female patients are used to hair removal, and in male patients the hairless area will be disguised by the remaining hair. Finally, from a technical point of view, Z-plasty prevents scar contracture.

Wound closure should be performed as fast as possible. In more extensive cases, the use of staples is recommended, to be later replaced by a permanent suture. The purpose is to reduce the edema, which can further make wound closure more difficult and frequently lead to ischemia in the wound area or to a tourniquet effect in the arm.

Dressing is made with sterile micropore adhesive tape woven in a latticework pattern on the surgical wound protected by gauze greased with bactericidal ointment. Drains are not necessary since careful hemostasis is performed and the suture leaves no dead spaces. Compressive wrapping is not routinely used; however, the use of light compression meshes applied from the wrist to the thorax is recommended in larger resections. Meshes that compress only the arm should be avoided because their tourniquet effect may cause distal edema thus affecting the blood flow in the forearm and hand.

Brachioplasty is a relatively safe procedure that provides a good level of patient satisfaction, despite a potentially unfavorable scar.[5,6] Former obese patients who will undergo brachioplasty receive thorough information regarding the scars that are to be expected, and usually accept them in exchange for the excess skin resection. Also, the double fusiform marking results in scars that are located in the posterior portion of the arm and in the axilla. Thus, they can hardly be noticed when the upper limb is adducted. Postbariatric patients undergoing several body contouring surgeries are undeniably familiar with multiple scars of varying extent, so that they are not significantly disappointed with the postbrachioplasty scars.

The double fusiform resection or double-ellipse technique has also been proposed in occasional studies on brachioplasty,[3,7] although with different markings (Figs.17.8 and 17.9). In the technique we propose, the scar lies posterior to the brachial sulcus, in concordance with recent studies.[7]

The use of the double fusiform resection technique, even in the cases in which the incision extends to the thorax, has already been proven[7] to provide remarkable personal satisfaction, with significant improvement of the quality of life. Thus, in terms of contour, the arm resumes an anatomical, cylindrical, and more harmonious shape. Removal of the dermal-cutaneous excess resulting from weight loss reduces the arm volume and, consequently, its weight, thus permitting a wider range of motion. Removal of the large cutaneous fold also provides more confidence thanks to a more effective hygiene. Women's approval is remarkable, as previously described;[4] they start to wear short-sleeve clothes, which was previously embarrassing due to the arm dysmorphism.

COMPLICATIONS

Both the double fusiform resection technique and brachiothoracoplasty are safe and technically simple procedures. However, complications or events may occur. Complications are due to failure to observe an accurate surgical technique, whereas events result from adverse biological factors and, in general, are less severe. These situations, already reported in the double fusiform resection and

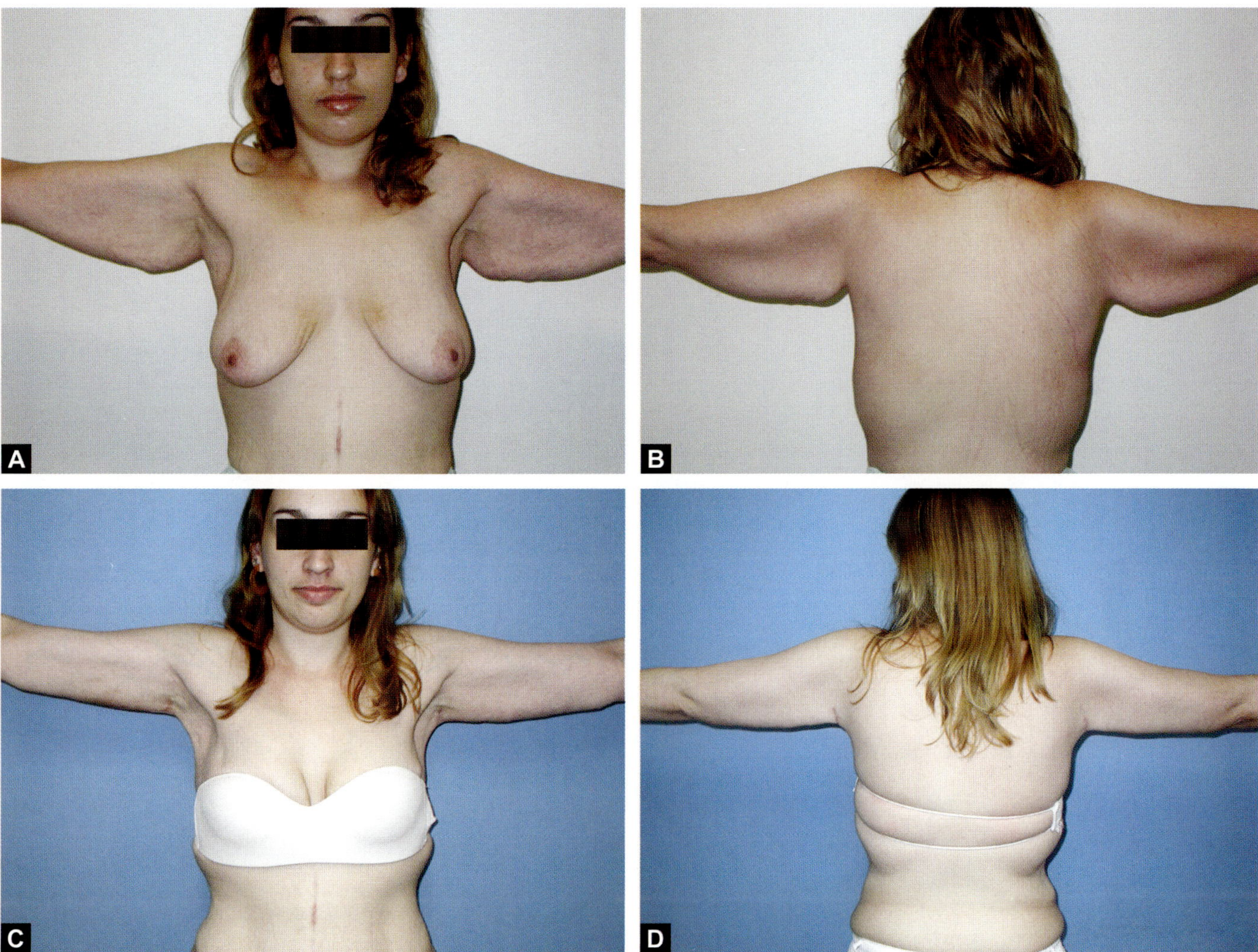

Figs. 17.8A to D: Brachioplasty—double fusiform resection technique. (A and B) Preoperative. (C and D) Postoperative.

brachioplasty techniques,[4] are less severe and frequent in comparison to those mentioned in the references cited:[3,6,8–10]

1. *Edema and seroma*: Both result from surgical damage, and the greater the surgical damage the more severe these events, because they correspond to the inflammatory response to trauma. Edema usually resolves within 1–6 months, and is further improved by upper limb massage, also known as lymphatic drainage, accompanied by flexion exercises of the forearm over the arm. Seroma is a local accumulation of inflammatory exudates; drainage sessions under strict asepsis will solve this condition.
2. *Ecchymosis*: It also results from the surgical damage; soft and delicate manipulation and traction will reduce its incidence. It usually resolves spontaneously in a short period of time. The use of heparinoid creams facilitates the absorption of the blood spilt in the dermal layer of the skin.
3. *Keloid scars*: These are linked to a genetic pattern and are more common in individuals with black or yellow skin color. Once formed, their uncontrolled growth follows a tumoral pattern. In addition to their unpleasant appearance, they may be accompanied by pain and itching. Treatment includes from the use of corticosteroid ointments or scar infiltration with corticosteroids to resection followed by radiation therapy, which seem to be the most effective method.
4. *Hematomas*: They result from failure to observe careful hemostasis techniques. When detected early, they should be drained; recurrence imposes surgical exploration for proper hemostasis. When left inadequately

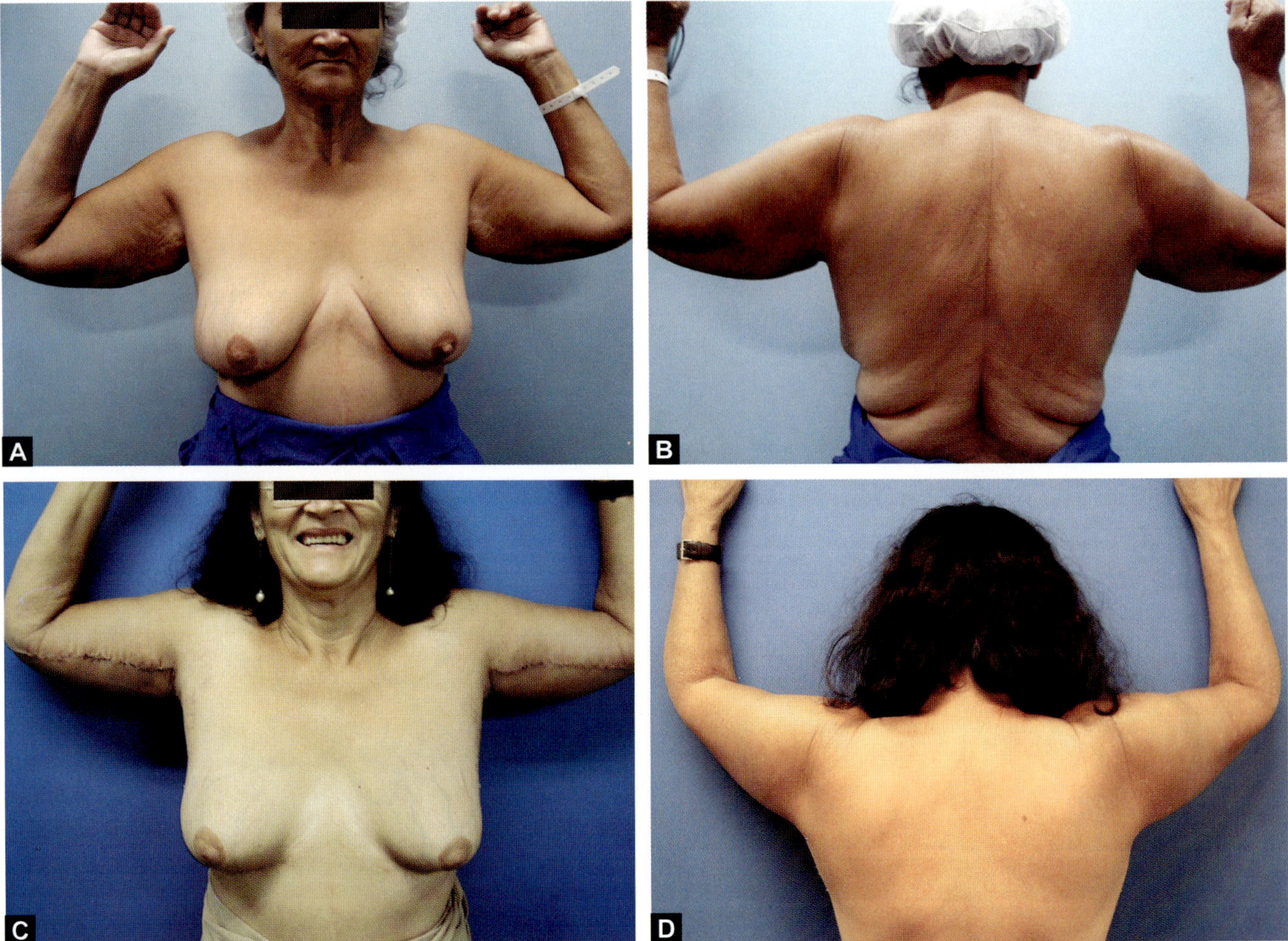

Figs. 17.9A to D: Brachiothoracoplasty: extended fusiform resection technique with Z-plasty. (A and B) Preoperative. (C and D) Postoperative.

treated, hematomas may lead to solid cysts that cause unattractive elevations and sometimes pain, because of compression on subjacent structures.

5. *Dehiscences*: These may be interpreted as complications or events. In the first case, they result from over-resection and tension on the suture; in the second case, since the skin on the medial aspect of the arm is very thin, the final suture may be under tension due to the post-traumatic edema, and the surgical wound breaks open. In both situations, dehiscences are partial and heal by second intention. Larger dehiscences require resuture or even skin grafts.
6. *Lymphorrhea and lymphocele*: Deepening the incision to a plane below the superficial fascia may lead to damage of lymphatic vessels and subsequent lymph leakage through the suture line. This lymphorrhea occurs early in the postoperative period and usually disappears spontaneously within 30 days on average. Sometimes, a cyst, known as lymphocele, may form, and this requires puncture and drainage sessions. However, the best treatment is resection, maintaining suction drainage for 2–3 days.
7. *Infection*: This is an uncommon complication provided that accurate asepsis and antisepsis techniques, including exhaustive and repeated preoperative cleansing of the operative site using antiseptic soaps and plenty of water, are observed. Axillary hair removal should be performed approximately 30 minutes prior to surgery. Hair removal by means of creams or wax is prohibited, because these products can occlude the hair follicle ostium, thus leading to the formation of cysts. Infections are more common in

the axilla and, if they reach these cysts, bacterial colonization within them will occur, and this may infect the surgical site. Infections may determine dehiscence or abscess formation. In the most severe cases, surgical debridement is mandatory. However, infections usually affect small areas and resolve with local cleansing and proper antibiotic therapy.

8. *Necrosis*: This results from excessive tension and subsequent ischemia or infection. Necrosis is partial and requiresresection, butresection of tissues of doubtful vitality should be avoided, to be further reevaluated. In smaller areas, wound healing occurs by second intention, whereas in larger areas, skin grafting is required. In both cases, the outcome is poor and compromises the aesthetic appearance.
9. *Hypertrophic scars*: These result from suture tension. However, we should point out that brachioplasty scars are perpendicular to the tension lines of the arm, thus favoring hypertrophic wound healing. When this complication is suspected, local use of triamcinolone creams and silicone strips on the scar are recommended.
10. *Paresthesia*: If deeper planes of dissection are reached, the anteromedial cutaneous nerve of the forearm may be damaged with subsequent sensitivity impairment. This can also result from the excessive and inadvertent use of an electrocautery. Sensitivity is usually partially re-established within 6–12 weeks. Sometimes, this nerve may also be lodged in the deep plane closure, leading to severe pain. An additional surgical approach is necessary to remove the nodule lodging the nerve.
11. *Asymmetries*: Although fat tissue distribution is not homogeneous in obese individuals, symmetry of opposing segments is always sought in anybody contouring repair. Likewise, although dysmorphism causes some difference between the arms, symmetry is aimed when the double fusiform or brachiothoracoplasty markings are made. When these markings are not carefully made, the result is asymmetry, which, in general, is not commonly noticed by the patients. However, some more demanding patients may occasionally request further correction.

REFERENCES

1. Orpheu SC, Coltro PS, Scopel GP, et al. Collagen and elastic content of abdominal skin after surgical weight loss. Obes Surg. 2010;20(4):480-86.
2. Lockwood T. Brachioplasty with superficial fascial system suspension. Plast Reconstr Surg. 1995;96(4):912-20.
3. Aly A, Pace D, Cram A. Brachioplasty in the patient with massive weight loss. Aesthet Surg J. 2006;26(1):76-84.
4. Modolin M, Cintra W, Faintuch J, et al. Improved double-fuse technique for post-bariatric brachioplasty. Rev Col Bras Cir. 2011;38(4):217-22.
5. Symbas JD, Losken A. An outcome analysis of brachioplasty techniques following massive weight loss. Ann Plast Surg. 2010;64(5):588-91.
6. Baroudi R. Dermolipectomy of the upper arm. Clin Plast Surg. 1975;2:485-94.
7. Samra S, Sawh-Martinez R, Liu YJ, et al. Optimal placement of brachioplasty scar: a survey evaluation. Plastic Surgery 2010, Annual Meeting of the American Society of Plastic Surgeons. Toronto, Ontario, October 4, 2010.
8. Nguyen AT, Rohrich RJ. Liposuction-assisted posterior brachioplasty: technical refinements in upper arm contouring. Plast Reconstr Surg. 2010;126(4):1365-9.
9. Regnault P. Brachioplasty, axilloplasty and pre-axilloplasty. Aesthet Plast Surg. 1983;7(1):31-6.
10. Hurwitz DJ, Holland SW. The L brachioplasty: an innovative approach to correct excess tissue of the upper arm, axilla, and lateral chest. Plast Reconstr Surg. 2006;117(2):403-11.

18 Body Dysmorphic Disorder

Melvin A Shiffman

DEFINITION

Body dysmorphic disorder (BDD) is defined as a preoccupation with an imagined or a very slight defect in physical appearance that causes significant distress to the individual. It was first described by Morselli in 1886[1] who called it "dysmorphobia." The disorder is manifested in people who dislike some aspect of how they look to such an extent that they cannot stop thinking and worrying about it. To other people, these reactions may seem excessive as the supposed problem may not even be noticeable or is related to a very minor blemish such as a mole, or mild acne scarring that anyone else may not even notice. To sufferers of the syndrome the "defects" are very real, very obvious, and very severe.

SYMPTOMS

1. There is preoccupation with the supposed appearance problem.
2. The patient takes actions to "hide" the defect or avoid situations because they feel ugly and do not want to be seen by others.

Some patients with body dysmorphia realize they look worse to themselves than to others and that their view of their appearance is exaggerated and distorted. Others are convinced that their view of their physical defect is accurate. Some have the feeling that other people are taking special notice of the "defect," that people are staring at it and making fun of it or laughing about it behind their backs when in reality, no one may even notice it. Many sufferers feel ashamed and fear being rejected by others.

Most patients with BDD perform one or more repetitive and often time consuming behaviors also known as "rituals" that are usually aimed at examining, "improving," or hiding the perceived flaw in appearance. They usually spend a lot of time checking themselves in the mirror to see whether their "defect" is noticeable or has changed in some way. Others will frequently compare themselves with other people or images in magazines or billboards. Some will spend hours "grooming" themselves by applying make-up, changing clothes, or re-arranging their hair to "correct" or cover up the "problem." Others attempt to camouflage or hide their defect by wearing a hat, a wig, or sunglasses. In extreme cases, people wear a mask or hood over their head. Some try, by acting or standing in a certain way in public, to make the defect seem less noticeable. Others weigh or measure themselves continually or wear big and baggy clothing to hide what they think are "huge" hips or large breasts. Some may wear many layers of clothing to make themselves appear larger or more muscular, and some men (especially those who suffer from "muscle dysmorphia") lift weights or exercise excessively to try to bulk up. They may eat special diets or use drugs such as anabolic steroids to try to build up their muscles.

Patients with body dysmorphia may approach cosmetic surgeons or dermatologists seeking surgery or medical treatments that places the doctor at risk for a continually dissatisfied patient with whatever is done.

CONSEQUENCES OF BDD

Some patients with BDD function well despite their distress. Others are severely impaired by their symptoms, often becoming socially isolated by not going to school or work and extreme cases refusing to leave home for fear of being embarrassed about their appearance. It can be especially difficult for sufferers to go to places such as beaches, hairdressers, shopping, or places where the person may feel anxious about how they look. It is not uncommon for patients with BDD to feel depressed about their problem and the negative impact this has on their life. Some become so desperate that they attempt suicide.

Relationship problems are common and many BDD sufferers have few friends, avoiding dates and other social activities or even getting divorced because of their symptoms.

ASSOCIATED DISORDERS

Many patients with BDD also suffer from depression at some point in their life and there is a high rate of depression in families of patients who develop BDD. The patient develops low esteem, feelings of rejection, heightened sensitivity, and of being unworthy. Other disorders include obsessive compulsive disorder (OCD) such as eating disorders, anxiety disorders, panic attacks, trichotillomania (hair pulling), and abuse of drugs or alcohol.

There is a high rate of suicidal ideation (mean 57.8% of 185 subjects over 4 years) and a mean of 2.6% attempted suicide per year.[2,3]

ETIOLOGY

Several neuroimaging studies have investigated brain gray matter in people with BDD, showing possible abnormalities in the limbic system, orbitofrontal cortex, caudate nuclei and temporal lobes. Buchanan et al.[4] investigated white matter properties in BDD compared with controls using diffusion tensor imaging. This study provided the first evidence of compromised white matter integrity within BDD patients and this suggests that there are inefficient connections between different brain areas, which may explain the cognitive and emotion regulation deficits within BDD patients.

Although previous studies have found functional abnormalities in visual processing, frontostriatal, and limbic systems no study to date has investigated the microstructure of white matter connecting these systems in BDD. Fuesner et al.[5] performed the first diffusion-weighted MR investigation of white matter in BDD. The results suggest a relationship between impairments in insight, a clinically important phenotype, and fiber disorganization in tracts connecting visual with emotion/memory processing systems.

Arienzo et al.[6] did the first brain network analysis in BDD and discovered that the BDD group showed higher whole-brain mean clustering coefficient than controls. Global efficiency negatively correlated with BDD symptom severity. The BDD group demonstrated greater edge between centrality for connections between the anterior temporal lobe and the occipital cortex, and between bilateral occipital poles. This suggests disturbances in whole brain structural topological organization in BDD, in addition to correlations between clinical symptoms and network organization. There is also evidence of abnormal connectivity between regions involved in lower-order visual processing and higher-order visual and emotional processing, as well as interhemispheric visual information transfer. These findings may relate to disturbances in information processing found in previous studies.

SCREENING TOOLS FOR BDD

The Dysmorphic Concerns Questionnaire (DCQ)[7] is designed to screen for people with certain concerns that are often difficult or embarrassing to talk about with their doctor/family/friends and often difficult to find the right help for. Body dysmorphic disorder questionnaire—dermatology version (BDDQ-DV)[8] and body dysmorphic disorder questionnaire—maxillofacial version (BDDQ-MV)[9] are screening questionnaires for body dysmorphic disorder in a cosmetic dermatology and maxillofacial surgery practice. Body dysmorphic symptoms scale (BDSS)[10] is a self-rating instrument consisting of the following 10 items, which estimate the presence of some important psychopathological features of BDD. Body dysmorphic disorder examination—self-report (BDDE-SR)[11] is a self-reporting questionnaire utilized in a variety of articles including plastic and cosmetic surgery.[12–18] The rhinoplasty questionnaire by Veale et al.[19] is a means of diagnosing body dysmorphic disorder in patients requesting rhinoplasty.

Multidimensional body self-relations questionnaire—appearance scales (MBSRQ-AS)[20,21] is a self-report inventory for the assessment of body image. "Body image is conceived as one's attitudinal dispositions toward the physical self." As attitudes, these dispositions include evaluative, cognitive, and behavioral components. Moreover, the physical self encompasses not only one's physical appearance but also the body's competence or fitness and its biological integrity or health/illness." The MBSRQ is intended for use with adults and adolescents (15 years or older). Two forms of the MBSRQ are available. The full, 69-item version consists of 10 subscales: evaluation and orientation vis-à-vis appearance, fitness, and health/illness, plus overweight preoccupation, self-classified weight, and the body areas satisfaction scale (BASS). The MBSRQ-appearance scales (MBSRQ-AS) is a 34-item measure that consists of five subscales appearance evaluation, appearance orientation, overweight preoccupation, self-classified weight, and the BASS. The 12-page MBSRQ manual[21] provides information about its scientific development, its subscales and their interpretation, scoring formulae, gender-specific norms, and reliability data. All subscales possess acceptable internal consistency and stability. References are also given pertinent to the MBSRQ's strong convergent, discriminant, and construct validities.

TREATMENT

Serotonin-reuptake inhibitors (SRIs) are a group of medications that appear to be useful and effective in patients with BDS. The SRIs are a type of antidepressant used successfully in the treatment of both depression and OCD. These include Prozac, Zoloft, Cipramil, and Aropax. Certain medications that have been suggested for treatment of BDD, such as levetiracetam,[22] high-dose glycine,[23] and aripiprazole,[24] are still preliminary and not completely studied although the reports show improvement in BDD.

Cognitive behavioral therapy (CBT) appears to be an effective treatment for BDD.[25] The behavioral component consists of "exposure and response prevention" where the patient exposes their defect in situations that they would usually avoid while response prevention involves helping the patient stop carrying out the compulsive behavior related to the defect. The aim over time is to decrease anxiety involved with that particular avoided situation. The cognitive component addresses the range of intrusive thoughts that accompany the behaviors, or rituals such as mirror checking, in BDS. This focuses on exploring beliefs and values that support and strengthen a person's perceptions about their body. Cognitive restructuring is aimed at developing an understanding of how these strongly held values impact the person's sense of "self" and to progressively build up alternative ways of thinking about the intrusive thought, rather than going through the usual range of behaviors such as mirror checking and reassurance seeking. Restructuring consists of a range of techniques involving making changes to a person's values while not directly questioning the repetitive and intrusive though the person has about their body.

A newly developed modular CBT treatment manual for BDD by Wilhelm et al.[26] appears to be effective and acceptable to patients with BDD.

Inference-based therapy (IBT) "conceptualizes BDD obsessions (e.g. "I feel like my head is deformed") as idiosyncratic inferences arrived at through inductive reasoning processes. Such primary inferences represent the starting point of obsessional doubt and the treatment focuses on addressing the faulty inferences that maintain the doubt.[27] The participants improved significantly over the course of therapy, with large diminutions in BDD and depressive symptoms despite the overall success of cognitive behavioral therapy (CBT) in treating BDD, some people do not seem to benefit as much from this approach. Those with high overvalued ideation (OVI), for instance, have been shown to not respond well with CBT."

DISCUSSION

Understanding body dysmorphic disorder and recognizing the patient with this disorder will prevent many misunderstandings between patient and doctor, especially the dermatologist or cosmetic surgeon. The BDD patient presenting for treatment of minimally abnormal skin findings, if recognized, will prevent unnecessary and potentially unsuccessful treatments.[28-30] Many patients with BDD seek cosmetic surgery and the unwary surgeon will invariably have to deal with a dissatisfied patient. Many eventually fall into the cosmetic surgery victim category of "overoperation." Recognition and deferral of surgery for BDD patients is advised because findings have shown the propensity of these patients to litigate, threaten, and even harm or kill their surgeon.[31]

CONCLUSION

Failure to diagnose body dysmorphic disorder in a preoperative cosmetic surgery patient will almost always leads to the dissatisfied patient. The surgeon will have a patient who is continuously dissatisfied with results no matter what is done to correct the perceived deformity. The treatment for the patient with BDD is medications, usually SRIs, or psychiatric care with CBT. The surgeon has to identify the BDD patients before surgery and tell them that surgery is not the treatment for their problem and refer them to the psychiatrist for treatment.

REFERENCES

1. Thomas I, Patterson WM, Szepietowski JC, et al. Body dysmorphic disorder: more than meets the eye. Acta Dermatovenerol Croat. 2005;13(1):50053.
2. Phillips KA, Menard W. Suicidality in body dysmorphic disorder: a prospective study. Am J Psychiatry. 2006;163 (7):1280-82.
3. Phillips KA, Coles ME, Menard W, et al. Suicidal ideation and suicide attempts in body dysmorphic disorder. J Clin Psychiatry. 2005;66(6):717-25.

4. Buchanan BG, Rossell SL, Maller JJ, et al. Brain connectivity in body dysmorphic disorder compared with controls: a diffusion tensor imaging study. Psychol Med. 2013:1-9.
5. Feusner JD, Arienzo D, Li W, et al. White matter microstructure in body dysmorphic disorder and its clinical correlates. Psychiatry Res. 2013;28;211(2):132-40.
6. Arienzo D, Leow A, Brown JA, et al. Abnormal brain network organization in body dysmorphic disorder. Neuropsychopharmacology. 2013;38(6):1130-39.
7. Oosthuizen P, Lambert T, Castle DJ. Dysmorphic concern prevalence and associations with clinical variables. Aust NZJ Psychiatry. 1998;32:129-32.
8. Dufresne RG, Phillips KA, Vittorio CC, et al. A screening questionnaire for body dysmorphic disorder in a cosmetic dermatology surgery practice. Dermatol Surg. 2001;27: 457-62.
9. Vulink NCC, Rosenberg A, Plooji JM, et al. Body dysmorphic disorder screening in maxillofacial outpatients presenting for orthognathic surgery. Int J Oral Maxillofac Surg. 2008;37:985-91. Maxillofacial version BDDQ-MV.
10. Kaymak Y, Taner E, Simsek I. Body dysmorphic disorder in university students with skin diseases compared with healthy controls. Acta Derm Venereol. 2009;89:281-4.
11. Rosen JC, Reiter J. Development of the body dysmorphic disorder examination. Behav Res Ther. 1996;34(9):755-66.
12. Anderson RC. Body dysmorphic disorder—recognition and treatment. Plast Surg Nurs. 2003;23:125-8.
13. Babuccu O, Latifoğlu O, Atabay K, et al. Sociological aspects of rhinoplasty. Aesthetic Plast Surg. 2003;27:44-9.
14. Hasan JS. Psychological issues in cosmetic surgery: a functional overview. Ann Plast Surg. 2000;44:89-96.
15. Jakubietz M, Jakubietz RJ, Kloss DF, et al. Body dysmorphic disorder, diagnosis and approach. Plast Reconstr Surg. 2007;119:1924-30.
16. Phillips KA, Dufresne RG. Body dysmorphic disorder. A guide for dermatologists and cosmetic surgeons. Am J Clin Dermatol. 2000;l:235-43.
17. Grossbart TA, Sarwer DB. Psychosocial issues and their relevance to the cosmetic surgery patient. Semin Cutan Med Surg. 2003:22:136-47.
18. Dufresne RG, Phillips KA, Vittorio CC. et al. A screening questionnaire for body dysmorphic disorder in a cosmetic dermatologic surgery practice. Dermatol Surg. 2001;27: 457-62.
19. Veale D, Har L, Lambrou C. Cosmetic rhinoplasty in body dysmorphic disorder. Br J Plast Surg. 2003;56(6):546-51.
20. www.body-images.com/assessments/mbsrq.html
21. http://www.body-images.com/assessments/mbsrq.html
22. Phillips KA, Menard W. A prospective pilot study of levetiracetam for body dysmorphic disorder. CNS Spectr. 2009; 14(5):252-60.
23. Cleveland WL, DeLaPaz RL, Fawwaz RA, et al. High-dose glycine treatment of refractory obsessive-compulsive disorder and body dysmorphic disorder in a 5-year period. Neural Plast. 2009;2009:768398.
24. Uzun O, Ozdemir B. Aripiprazole as an augmentation agent in treatment-resistant body dysmorphic disorder. Clin Drug Investig. 2010;30(10):707-10.
25. Honigman R, Castle DJ. Body dysmorphic disorder—a guide for people with BDD. Collaborative Therapy Unit, Mental Health Research Institute; 2003.
26. Wilhelm S, Phillips KA, Fama JM, et al. Modular cognitive-behavioral therapy for body dysmorphic disorder. Behav Ther. 2011;42(4):624-33.
27. Taillon A, O'Connor K, Dupuis G, et al. Inference-based therapy for body dysmorphic disorder. Clin Psychol Psychother. 2013;20(1):67-76.
28. Buescher LS, Buescher KL. Body dysmorphic disorder. Dermatol Clin. 2006;24(2):251-7.
29. Glaser DA, Kaminer MS. Body dysmorphic disorder and the liposuction patient. Dermatol Surg. 2005;31(5):559-60.
30. Mackley CL. Body dysmorphic disorder. Dermatol Surg. 2005;31(5):553-8.
31. Hodgkinson DJ. Identifying the body-dysmorphic patient in aesthetic surgery. Aesthetic Plast Surg. 2005;29(6):503-9.

Index

Note: Page numbers followed by *f* indicate figures.

A

Abdominal lipodystrophy, 201, 201*f*
Accent laser breast lift, 141
Adductor flap, 175
Adductor magnus perforator (AMP) flap, 175, 175*f*
Adipocyte viability, 114*f*
Adipose-derived stem cell (ADSC), 114–115
  derived iPS cells, 10
  homeostasis, 114
  treatments, 113
Aesthetic
  nose goals, 44
  rhinoplasty, 44
  surgery, 116
  treatment, 60*f*
Alar cartilages, 82*f*
American Society of Lasers in Medicine and Surgery (ASLMS), 104, 142
Amyloid, 217*f*–218*f*
Anesthetic eye drops, 208
Antebrachial fascia, 216*f*
Antibiotic therapy, 188
Antiemetic drugs, 118
Anxiety scores, 19
Aquavage canister disposable, 124*f*–125*f*
Areola post-treatment, 138
Areolar marker, 146
Areolar marking, 147*f*
Arm
  lymphedema, 15
  volume reduction, 18
Aspiration, 26
Atypical ectopic niche, 115
Augmentation
  breast ptosis correction, 119*f*
  rhinoplasty, 68, 69*f*
Auricles, 95
Auricular reconstruction, 7
Autologous fat transfer (AFT), 113

B

Bat wing brachial dysmorphism, 219*f*
Biceps femoris muscle, 171
Bikini zone, 100
Bilateral nipple-areolae, 138
Bingo wings, 219
Biologic product, 115
Bipolar device, 103, 191
BodyTite device, 142, 199
Bony defects, 6
Botox injections, 107*f*
Botulinum toxin injection, 102–103
Brachioplasty, 223*f*
Brachiothoracoplasty, 224*f*
Breast
  capsular contracture, 116
  enlargement, 121
  glandular tissue, 140
  inflammation, 129*f*
  ptosis, 133*f*–134*f*, 140
  reduction technique, 113, 144
  tissue engineering, Future, 9*f*
  tissue resection, 148*f*
Breast augmentation, 6*f*–7*f*, 7, 140
  combining silicone implant insertion, 7*f*
  reconstruction, 7
Brow ptosis, 107, 107*f*
Bulbous tip, 83*f*
Bystander mechanism, 115

C

Calcifications, 130
Caliber suction drains, 164
Canfield imaging systems, 116
Canfield vectra
  measurements, 195*f*
  system, 142
Carpal tunnel syndrome (CTS), 218
Cartilage graft, 44–45, 44*f*, 65*f*
  placement, 61*f*
  schematic of the positioning, 48*f*
Cartilaginous
  asymmetry, 87*f*
  grafts, 45*f*
Cell–cell interactions, 114
Cell–matrix, 114
Central breast reduction procedure, 154*f*
Cerebral stroke, 115
Chest incision, 127*f*
Chest lift
  anterior, 154
  lateral, 154
Chin augmentation implant, 66
Chronic ulcers, 115
Cognitive behavioral therapy (CBT), 228
Cognitive restructuring, 228
Coleman technique, 113
Colorado microdissection, 154*f*
  needle, 156
Congenital depressed dorsum, 49*f*
Converse suture, 78
Cooper's ligaments, 144, 149
Coronal brow, 105
Cytokines, 115
Cytori CellBrush injector, 126, 127*f*

D

Deep fascia, 40
  graft, 47*f*, 54
Deepithelialization right breast, 147*f*
Deformed dorsum, 68, 70
Deformity, 69
Dehiscences, 224
Dermal adipose flap, 146, 150
  elevation, 148*f*
  in situ, 149*f*
Doppler
  probe, 171, 176
  signal, 164
  signs, 180
  ultrasound scanner, 164, 179
Drumstick deformity, 198*f*
Dysmorphic Concerns Questionnaire (DCQ), 227

E

Ear, cartilage, 45*f*
Ecchymosis, 223
Edema, 223
  bruising, 129
Electroporation, 193
Elevated flap, 189
Endoscopic
  carpal tunnel release, 216
  dissection, 40*f*
  surgery, 41
Endotechnique, 38
Endotine device, 105
Endymed

handpieces, 206*f*
multipolar phase controlled device, 192
neck tightening, 206
RF device, 204
Epigastrium wrinkling, 202*f*
Epigastric lipodystrophy, 203, 205*f*
Erol report, 60

F

Facial rejuvenation, 5*f*, 108
procedures, 108*f*
Facial volume enhancement, 6
Fascia graft, 46, 53*f*, 66*f*
histological images of, 75*f*
Fascia strip, 65*f*
Fascia-wrapped cartilage grafting, 47*f*
Fat emulsification, vaser in action for, 124*f*
Fat graft, 68, 115
harvesting, sites for, 119*f*
placements, 121*f*
Fat infiltration, 121*f*
Fat reduction, 193
Fat transfer, 131*f*–133*f*
nonindication for, 118*f*
preoperative donor area for, 117*f*
Fat washing, 125*f*
Flap
de-epithelialization, 147*f*
design, 168
harvesting, 168
perfusion, 179
Fragmented cartilage, 66*f*
graft, 60
treatment, 67*f*
Frontalis recruitment, 106*f*
Frontozygomatic suture line, 39
Fusiform technique, 220*f*
FX RF noninvasive treatments, 194*f*

G

Gastric sleeve, 159*f*
Gastroprotectors, 111
GFX device, 104
Glabellar frown lines, 104, 106, 106*f*–108*f*, 109, 197
Glandular ptosis, 149
Glass tube, 115
Gluteal artery, 166
perforator flap, 164–165, 186
Gracilis flap, 172
Gracilis myocutaneous flap, 172
Grade II + ptosis, 141*f*
Growth factors, 115
Gynecomastia, 141, 157

H

Heal radiation damage, 115
Heat mediated tissue tightening, 141
Hematomas, 223
Hematopoietic markers, 114
Hemimammary line, 145*f*, 146
Heparinoid creams, 223
Hereditary chubby neck, 198*f*
HermiGen RF-assisted neck lift, 196*f*
High-energy reservoir, 115
Hump reduction rhinoplasty, 54
Hypertrophic scars, 225
Hypertrophied alar cartilages, 80*f*

I

IGA-P flap design, 168*f*
Iliotibial tract, 171
Incisionless technique, 95
Incisions sites, 120*f*
Inference-based therapy (IBT), 228
Inferior gluteal
artery, 166
perforator flap (IGAP), 186
Inframammary fold, 145*f*, 146
Intestinal stoma, 188
Invasive RF-assisted tissue tightening, 195–196
Invasix BodyTite device, 198
Ischial pressure sore, 189*f*

J

Jowl-chin-neck contouring, 31*f*–32*f*

K

Kaplan's line, 215
Kaplan–Meier curves, 179
Keloid scars, 223

L

Lacrimal sac, 42*f*
Laser resurfacing, 116
Late-stage
ischial pressure sore, 173*f*–174*f*, 177*f*–178*f*
sacral pressure sore, 170*f*
Laxity plus lipodystrophy, 199*f*
Left inner canthus, 42*f*
Lines of concavity, 121
Lines of convexity, 121
Lipectomy, 15
Lipoaspirates, 115
Liposuction
cannula, 16*f*
only breast reductions, 138
technique, 15, 155*f*, 197
Lower blepharochalasis, 28*f*
Luxated nasal tip, 79*f*
Lymphatic bypass techniques, 15
Lymphatic olymphatic techniques, 15
Lymphedema, 15, 19
Lymphocele, 224
Lymphorrhea, 224

M

Male breast, 157
Male chest deformity, 157
Mammary hypertrophy, 152
Mammography, 118*f*
Mandibular condylar fracture, 40
Median nerve, 217
Mesenchymal stem cell-associated markers, 114
Mesodermal stem cells (MSCs), 115
Methylene blue, 170
Midline, 145*f*
Monopolar devices, 191
Motor nerves, 103
Multichannel devices, 103
Multidimensional body self-relations questionnaire–appearance scales (MBSRQ-AS), 227
Multiple sclerosis, 180
Muscle contraction, 103
Muscle flaps, 176, 181
Musculocutaneous flap, 172, 176
Musculocutaneous perforators, 186
Myocardial infarction, 115

N

Nasal dorsum, 46*f*, 63*f*–64*f*, 68
depression, 75*f*
Nasal tip, 77*f*, 84*f*
Neck
chin debulking, 113
laxity, 28*f*
Neck skin
laxity, 197*f*
Necrosis, 225
Nerve ablation, 104
angular, 106
brow, 105
Nipple alveolar complex distance, 120
Nipple–areola complex (NAC), 152
deformities, 157
grafting, 152
line, 153*f*
necrosis, 157
position, 144
Nonexcisional skin tightening, 191
Noninvasive devices, 192
Nonpitting lymphedema, 19

O

Obsessive compulsive disorder (OCD), 227
One-layered temporal fascial patch, 78*f*
Optimal impedance, 192
Oral maxillary cancer, 42*f*
Origins canister autoclavable (glass), 124*f*
Otoplasty techniques, 101
Overvalued ideation (OVI), 228

P

Papaverine, 164
Paresthesia, 225
Parry–Romberg syndrome, 4
Pectus excavatum, 122*f*
Pedicle, de-epithelialization of, 154*f*
Perforator flap, 165, 172, 186
Periareolar incision, 119*f*
Peripheral nerve stimulator, 104
Photodynamic therapy, 193
Physical Medicine and Rehabilitation Services, 164
Pinch test., 144, 144*f*
Piriformis muscle, 187
Pitanguy's maneuver, 145*f*
Pluripotent cells (iPS cells), 10
Postauricular fold, 99
Postfat grafting, 121*f*
Preoperative marking, 145, 145*f*–146*f*
Proangiogenic molecules, 115
Profunda Femoris Artery Perforator (PFAP-AM)
flap, 170–171, 172*f*, 175
Protruding lobule, 96
Pseudogynecomastia, 157
Pure-Graft washing preparation, 113

R

Radiation damage, 116
Radiofrequency
ablation techniques, 103
assisted breast lift, 137*f*–141*f*
assisted tissue tightening, 142, 196
device, 104
energy applicators, 203
lesion, 196
needle, 192
nerve ablation, 108
neuro ablation, 103
probe, 192
tissue tightening, 192
Radiofrequency-assisted liposuction, 193*f*
Radiofrequency nerve, ablation, 103, 109
Radiolesion, 115
Radix augmentation surgery, 68
Reaction device, 202, 202*f*
Recipient bed, 46
Reconstructive Surgery Institute of Jalisco, 74
Regenerative theory, 115
Regnault's classification, 149
Resected tissues, 89*f*
Residual lipodystrophy, 197*f*
Rhinomegaly, 85*f*
Rhinoplasty, 62f, 71*f*

S

Sacral pressure sore, 167*f*, 189*f*
Scarless breast reduction, 141
Scarred skin, 115
Secondary rhinoplasty, 68
treatment in, 70*f*
Self-adhesive dressing tape, 66
SEL technique, 9
Seroma, 223
Serotonin-reuptake inhibitors (SRIs), 228
Severe facial traumatism, 88*f*
Severe skin laxity, 200*f*
SGAP flap, 164–165
design, 166*f*
Shell cartilage, 45*f*
Skin
defects, 98
flap, 8
incisions, 147*f*
laxity, 205*f*
paddle, 171
suture of, 31*f*
Ski slope, 44
Skoog technique, 53*f*
Small puncture holes, 123
Smart Lipo, 142
SoftJet syringes, 121
Spina bifida, 180
Spinal cord tumors, 180
Spindle-shaped skin resection, 219
Sports bra, 148
Stem cell niche therapy, 114
Stromal-enriched
lipograft technique, 4*f*
Stromal-enriched lipograft, 7, 8*f*
Strong crow's feet, 107*f*
Subfascial adipose layer, 156
Suction intensity, 123
Superior gluteal artery perforators, landmarks and markings, 187*f*
Superior gluteal perforator flap (SGAP), 186
Suture of chin incision, 29*f*
Suture-line dehiscence, 179
SVF isolation, 4*f*
Symphony RF device, 102, 104

T

T skin pattern, 140
Teardrop augmentation, 141
Temporal fascia patch, 44, 88, 91*f*
Tenosynovectomy, 215, 218*f*
The reaction device, 204*f*
Thermage
eyelid treatment, 208*f*–209, 209*f*
Thermigen device, 105, 142, 196*f*
Thermigen monopolar device, 192
Thermigen RF ablation device, 108, 198
Thermigen RF neck Lift, 199
Thermigen treatment pattern, 203
Tite FX device, 193
Toomey syringe, 125*f*–126*f*, 126
Topographical skin analysis systems, 116
Translational skin flaps, 100
Transverse forehead lines, 107*f*
Transverse lines, 108
Transverse myelitis, 180
Treatment of gynecomastia, 152
Treatment scheme, 59*f*
Tripollar Apollo device, 141
Tumescent
anesthesia, 123*f*
infiltration, 149
infusion, 26*f*

U

Ultrasound
of breast, 118*f*
guided RF ablation, 103
Upper blepharochalasis, 28*f*
Upper lateral thoracic lift (ULTL), 157
Upside down mastopexy, 140
Urinary catheterization, 190

V

VAC therapy, 166
Vaser system, 30*f*, 33*f*–37*f*, 113*f*
Vaser treatment, 113
Vaser-assisted lipoplasty, 25
VentX cannula, 123, 124*f*
Viora reaction device, 203
VISIA system, 116

X

X-shaped dermal incision, 156*f*

Y

You Tube video, 141

Z

Z-plasty, 100, 222